# ROYAL MARINES
# FITNESS

## PHYSICAL TRAINING MANUAL

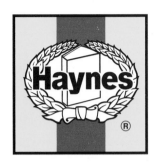

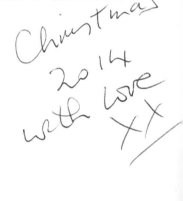

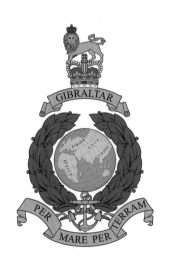

## Sean Lerwill

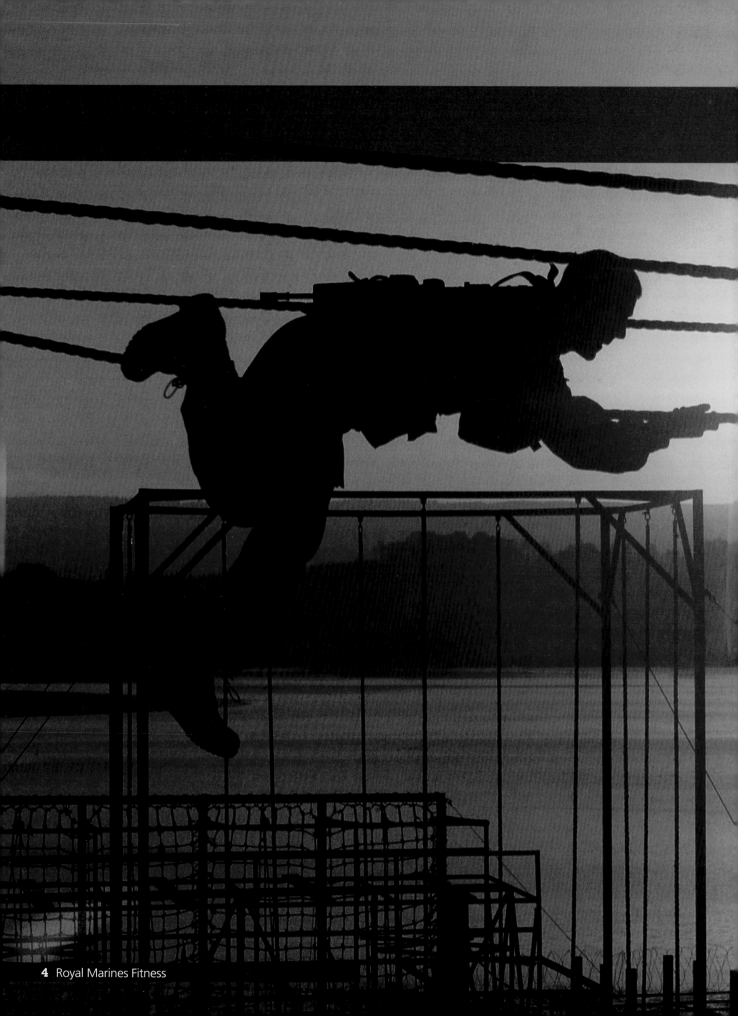

**Dedicated to all Royal Marines past, present and future, but above all to those who have paid the ultimate price. We will never forget.**

First published in December 2009
Reprinted 2010, 2011, 2012 and 2013

A catalogue record for this book is available from the British Library

ISBN 978 1 84425 561 0

Library of Congress catalog card no. 2008926365

Published by Haynes Publishing,
Sparkford, Yeovil, Somerset BA22 7JJ, UK

Tel: 01963 442030  Fax: 01963 440001
Int. tel: +44 1963 442030  Int. fax: +44 1963 440001
E-mail: sales@haynes.co.uk
Website: www.haynes.co.uk

Haynes North America, Inc.,
861 Lawrence Drive, Newbury Park,
California 91320, USA

Printed in the USA by Odcombe Press LP,
1299 Bridgestone Parkway, La Vergne, TN 37086

While every effort is taken to ensure the accuracy of the information given in this book, no liability can be accepted by the author or publishers for any loss, damage or injury caused by errors in, or omissions from, the information given.

It is advisable to check with a medical professional before commencing any exercise programme.

**Author:** Sean Lerwill

**Managing Editor:** Louise McIntyre

**Design:** Richard Parsons

**Photography:** Guy Harrop (www.guyharrop.com)

**Library images:** Images that appear on the following pages are all Crown Copyright: 4, 5, 6, 9, 10, 11, 13, 17, 27, 31, 36, 37, 38, 40, 55, 59, 60, 80
Page 13 Imperial War Museum (image FKD2028)
Pages 44, 45, 100 Andy Blow (www.votwo.co.uk).
Page 36 copyright RNRU (Jenny Lodge)

**Copy Editor:** Ian Heath

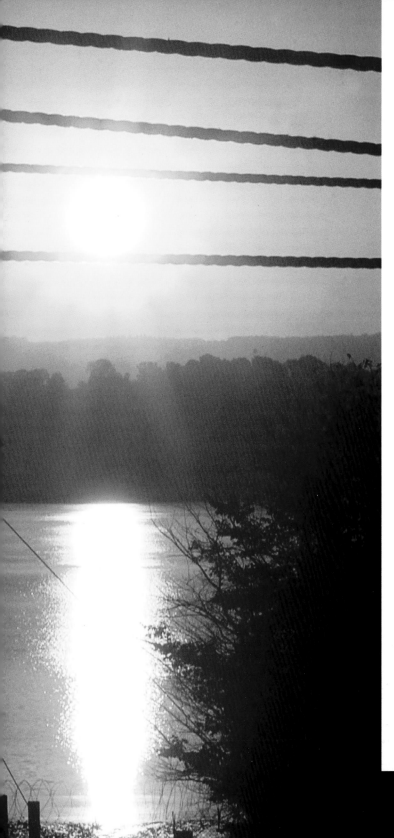

# CONTENTS

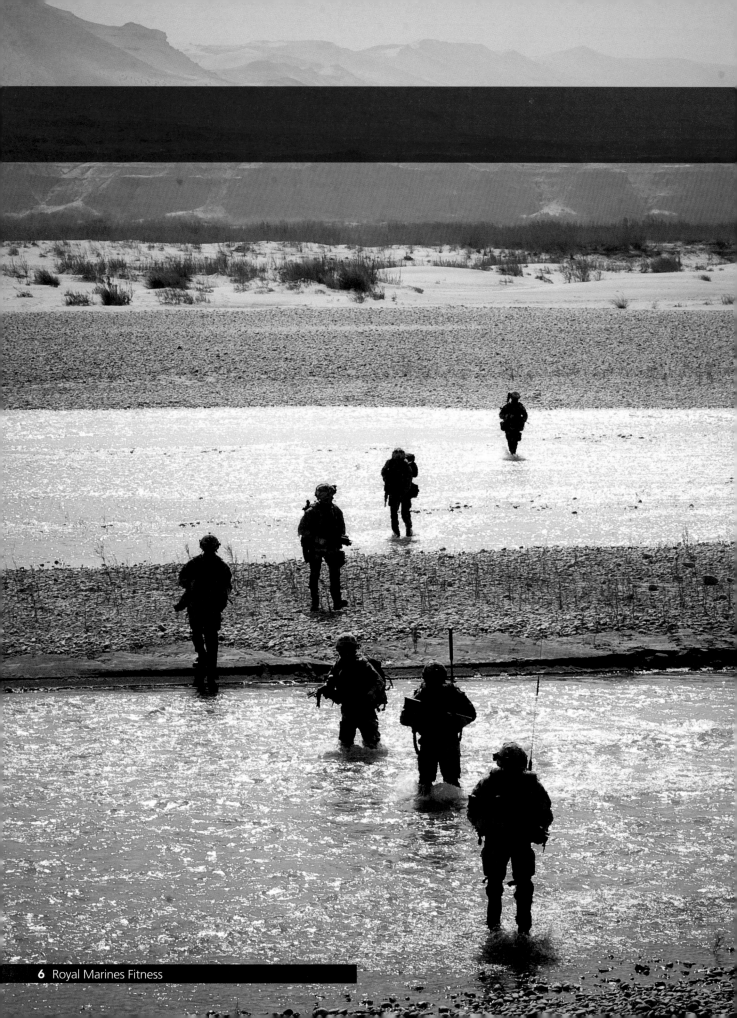

# INTRODUCTION

The Royal Marines have firmly established themselves as the elite infantry fighting force of the United Kingdom. Their Commando status, represented by the coveted green beret worn by all Commando-trained soldiers, is world-renowned. The physical training that all Royal Marines Recruits go through to become Royal Marines Commandos is challenging and demanding, yet structured and achievable, and it is this that you should try to mimic in your own training.

This book gives you a taster of what Recruits go through from the day they walk into the recruitment office to the day when they leave the Commando Training Centre with a green beret. It gives you access to the mindset and lifestyle of a trained Royal Marine beyond his training days, and the importance to him of staying physically and psychologically fit. With its insight into what it takes to be a successful Royal Marine Commando, this book should give you all the tools you need to start your own fitness regime.

By understanding how your body functions in terms of exercise physiology, and how it requires and uses food through nutrition, your physical training can be designed and structured in such a way as to make your fitness goals, whatever they may be, a reality. Although reaching a specific fitness or physical goal can often require considerable time, pain, effort, motivation and dedication, your elation once it is achieved makes it all worthwhile.

The ethos of the Armed Forces, and especially the Royal Marines, is often viewed with awe by the general public looking in from outside. This book tries to explain this culture in such a way as to inspire you to apply some of the Commando values to your own everyday life – to laugh in the face of adversity, to be unselfish wherever possible, and most of all to make physical fitness and physical training a habitual part of your life. If you can learn to use physical training as a tool to enrich your existence, to relieve stress, to socialise and, above all, to make your life more fulfilled, this will stay with you until the day you die, just as it does for every Royal Marines Commando, past, present and future.

### How to use this book

This book does not say 'follow this programme for the rest of your life and you will be as fit as a Royal Marine'. This would not be either practical or realistic. No one can maintain ultimate physical fitness, so fitness training must change, peak and drop off as appropriate. In addition, don't forget that the body adapts, so that the effectiveness of following the same programme day in day out for the rest of your life would soon plateau; it would also become boring and dull. Furthermore, training should be specific to goals and functions – a Royal Marine will train differently for a tour of Afghanistan, for instance, than he would to take part in a Mountain Leader or Physical Training course.

In short, this book will provide you with all the tools and information you need to put together a fitness programme specific to your own short- and long-term goals, and to adapt it as you surpass your own expectations. It does not fall into the trap of trying to provide you with the Royal Marines training programme – because there is no such thing.

Every reader will have different aims they want to achieve; some may be similar, but they will all be subtly different. For example, some readers may wish to get fit for a marathon, others to lose weight, yet others to put on muscle mass, and it needs hardly be said that there are huge differences in the programmes required to achieve each of these aims. It is therefore up to you to select those elements in this book that apply to your own specific requirements and to put together a training programme that incorporates them.

The following are the key fundamentals to keep in mind as you draw up your programme:

- Start gently, with a few light sessions a week.
- Always include rest days – at least one per week, or more likely two or three.
- Be specific – if you want to get better at running, then go running.
- Remember the 'seven components of fitness' – flexibility, endurance, stamina, skill, strength, speed and power – and try to include all of them somewhere in your training.
- Include rest weeks following hard periods of training or overtraining.
- If you exercise a body part one day, rest it the next, even if you aren't having a rest day.
- Don't become lazy – avoid only including 'easy' sessions.
- Don't follow a hard cardiovascular training day with another hard cardiovascular training day – ensure that you alternate between hard and easy days.
- Don't overdo very intense sessions such as intervals and plyometrics – include them at most once a week, or better just twice monthly.
- Always warm up and cool down.

The Royal Marines wish you the best of luck on your quest for health and fitness, whatever your goals may be. Just remember, Royal Marine training takes 32 weeks, and it will take a Recruit this long to get his green beret, providing he does not get injured. During this time he must remain patient, motivated and dedicated; and in the end he will be rewarded by his goal becoming a reality. The same is true for your own training – success will not come overnight, it will take time. But that is what makes it even more desirable. Keep your goal in the forefront of you mind, be patient, stay motivated, and above all be dedicated.

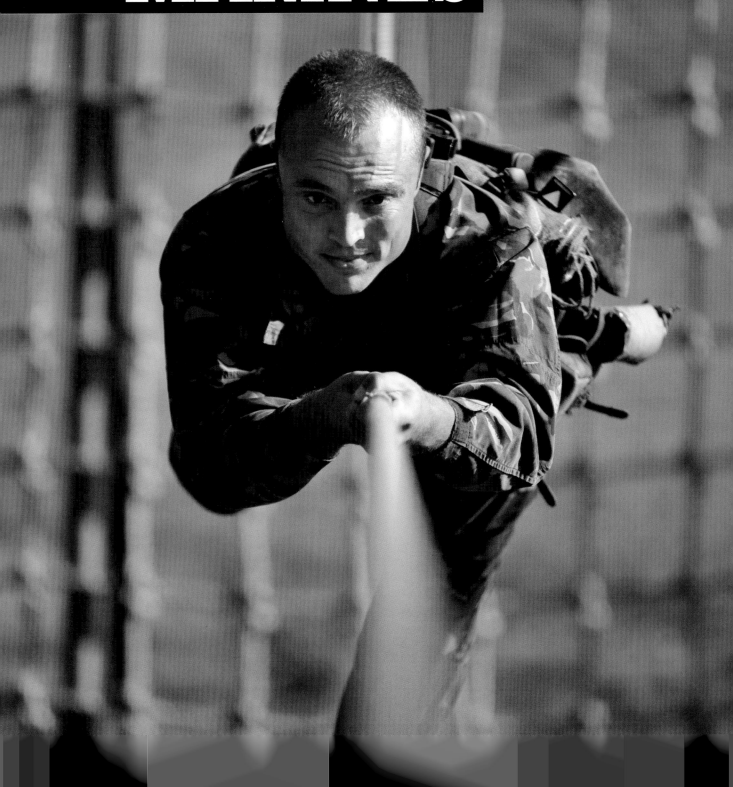

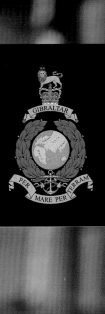

# CHAPTER 1
# THE ROYAL MARINES

The Royal Marines – or the Royal Marines Commandos as they are known today – are Britain's Commando forces. Every single Royal Marine (or 'Bootneck' as they are sometimes referred to) is Commando-trained and wears the coveted green beret symbolising a Commando-trained soldier. Any Commando-trained British soldier who wears a green beret has been trained by Royal Marines at the Commando Training Centre Royal Marines (CTCRM) in Lympstone, Devon.

The Royal Marines are an elite fighting force, highlighted by their specialist capabilities but relatively small size. There are around 6,000 individuals in the Royal Marines, compared to some 102,000 in the British Army and 180,000 in the United States Marine Corps (USMC). Despite their small size the Royal Marines have always been at the forefront of British military, and world military, operations; indeed, the Royal Marines have been involved in nearly every conflict since the Second World War including Palestine, Korea, Malaya, Suez, Cyprus, Radfan, Aden, the Falklands, Northern Ireland, Iraq and Afghanistan.

Due to our limited size the Royal Marines can hand-pick those who join. Consequently we only have the best that Britain and the Commonwealth can offer. Additionally, as we all go through the same training (officers and all other ranks alike) and complete the same Commando tests, we are all capable of feats that many would not dream feasible. This is not just because of the fitness levels we reach while completing Commando training, but also because of the strength of mind we gain and take with us for the rest of our lives.

The Royal Marine Corps was formed on 28 October 1664, a date which is celebrated by the Corps every year. The Royal Marines can be described as the Royal Navy's infantry (yes, the Royal Marines are part of the Navy, not the Army!). Despite a long, active and varied history (many books are available on this subject) the Corps did not take on its Commando status until the Second World War. By 1943 all Royal Marine units had undergone Commando training, though at this point the Army also had a number of Commando Units of its own. Following the war Parliament announced that all Army Commandos were to be disbanded and that only the Royal Marines were to retain this specialisation, as they were 'fully qualified by their long tradition and history to carry out the special role'.

Since the War only a single brigade of Royal Marines has been kept up: this is 3 Commando Brigade, made up of 40 Cdo RM, 42 Cdo RM, 45 Cdo Gp RM, UK Landing Force Command Support Group, Cdo Logistic Regt RM, 539 Assault Squadron RM, 29 Cdo Regt RA, 24 Cdo Regt RE and 1 RIFLES. The Royal Marines take on a number of specialist roles within British military operations, providing amphibious, mountain and cold-weather warfare expertise. However, there is no climate or terrain in which the Royal Marines cannot and have not operated and functioned.

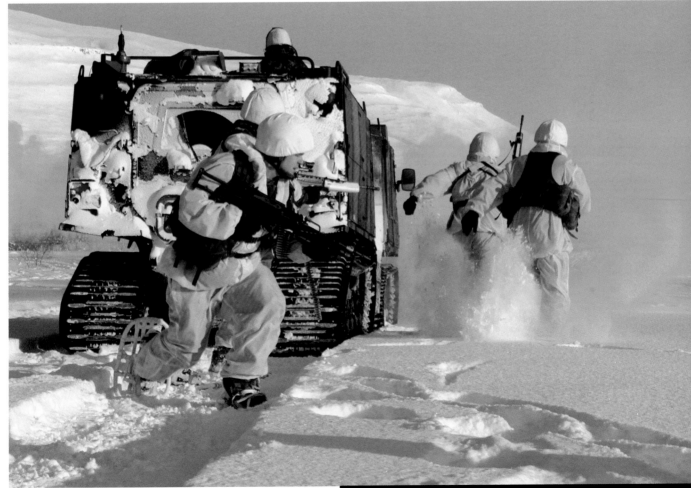

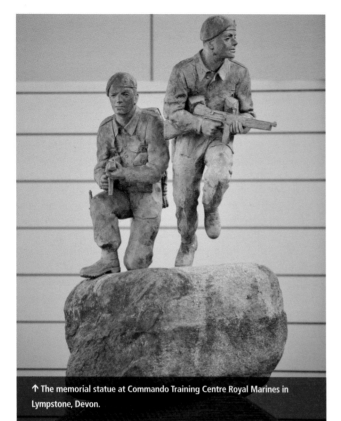

↑ The memorial statue at Commando Training Centre Royal Marines in Lympstone, Devon.

The motto of the Royal Marines is *Per Mare Per Terram* ('By Sea, By Land'). This is believed to have been used for the first time in 1775 but is still as relevant today as it was all those years ago. The Corps holds its amphibious role very dear, with every Royal Marine Recruit having to pass a specific swim test and boating package to ensure that we do not lose this incredibly important specialisation. After all, the Royal Marines *are* part of the Royal Navy.

Three emblems personify the Royal Marines: the Globe and Laurel, the Commando Dagger and the Green Beret. The Globe and Laurel is the cap badge of the Corps, worn on the headdress of every Royal Marine Commando and Royal Marine in training. It is comprised of a number of parts, all having some historical importance to the Corps.

The lion and crown denotes it is a Royal regiment, an honour received in 1802 from King George III.

The globe, symbolising the Royal Marines' successes in every quarter of the world, was granted to the Corps by King George IV, while the laurels that surround it are said that to honour the gallantry the Corps displayed during the investment and capture of Belle Isle in 1761.

The word 'Gibraltar' on the badge refers to the Siege of Gibraltar in 1704, and was awarded by George IV in 1827.

Last, but by no means least, is the fouled anchor, the badge of the Lord High Admiral, which shows that the Corps is part of the Naval Service. This was first incorporated into the Globe and Laurel in 1747.

The Commando dagger has more recently become the symbol most often associated with the Royal Marines, but is also worn by other Commando-trained soldiers. The dagger was first borne at Achnacarry (near Ben Nevis in Scotland), a previous Royal Marines' training centre. This was a slim, stealthy and precise dagger, to be used to swiftly and stealthily dispatch enemies without compromising the user by noise. It is also known as the 'Fairbairn-Sykes Fighting Knife', as it was designed by William Ewart Fairbairn and Eric Anthony Sykes just prior to the Second World War. Wilkinson sword produced the first batch of the knife in 1941. It has since become more of a symbol than a weapon of choice – for example, a solid gold Commando dagger forms part of the Commando memorial in Westminster Abbey. Army Commandos often wear a red dagger on a black patch to symbolise their Commando status, while the emblem worn by all members of 3 Commando Brigade is a black Commando dagger on a green patch (or a desert variant if uniform dictates).

The green beret is now a symbol of Commando-trained ranks from the British forces throughout the world and remains a very prestigious prize, requiring much hard work and dedication to obtain. Initially, during the Second World War, Commando-trained soldiers all wore their own regimental headdress and cap badge, but in 1942 a decision was made to choose a beret that all would wear to denote their Commando status. For a variety of reasons it was decided that green was the most appropriate colour and so the Corps' green beret was born. Since 1960 it has been the daily headdress for all Royal Marines who have completed training. The previous blue beret is now worn only by Recruits and Young Officers undergoing training, and by the Corps band.

Training to become a Royal Marines Commando has always been surrounded in awe and mystery. To this day, it is not a road to start upon lightly. Royal Marines training is still regarded as the longest and hardest initial military training in the world. The Royal Marines have moved their training establishment over the years. Initial training was originally at RM Deal in Kent, with volunteers wishing to become Commandos travelling to Achnacarry in Scotland for Commando training, which eventually became compulsory for all Royal Marines. Nowadays all training has moved to the Commando Training Centre Royal Marines in Lympstone, Devon. It has to be emphasised, however, that although the location has changed the Commando tests performed today are taken directly from those undertaken in Achnacarry, ensuring that every Commando-trained Royal Marine has earned his green beret in just the same way as his predecessors.

Once a Royal Marine has passed out of training and gone on to take his place in arguably the best infantry force in the world, he then has the option of specialising within the Corps. For example, Royal Marines can become drivers, chefs, clerks, weapons instructors, Royal Marines Police, vehicle mechanics, signallers, assault engineers, landing craft operators or mountain leaders to name but a few, or physical training instructors like myself. All of these specialists play their part not only on Operations, but also in peacetime and while training new Recruits.

## The Green Beret

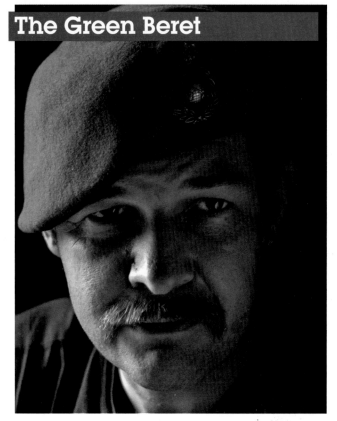

## The Globe and Laurel

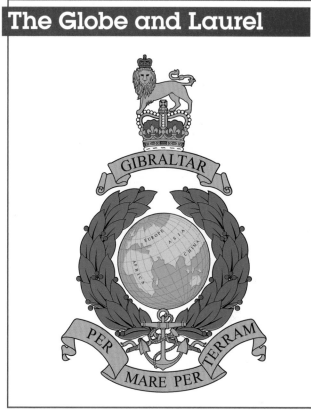

Royal Marines have always been credited for their intelligence and level-headedness in all situations. This is particularly apparent when one looks beyond their normal 'war-fighting' role, and has been seen most recently in Afghanistan. The Royal Marines have also conducted a large number of peaceful operations for the United Nations and have been praised for their ability to switch – sometimes overnight – from a fighting role to a peacekeeping one. They have worked with many relief and humanitarian support teams in countries where natural disasters have occurred or where there is ongoing internal conflict.

It may appear that all a Royal Marine needs is to be incredibly fit, but this is a little way from the truth. We can train almost anyone to our standards who possesses some degree of potential fitness, but for the majority of Recruits it is not just about raising their personal fitness, it is about teaching and conveying our attributes and ethos. Of utmost importance is the strength of mind that every Royal Marine must have, and the personal values that will allow him to understand and contribute to the ethos of the Royal Marines. Without this strength of mind, a Royal Marine Recruit will never complete Royal Marine training, let alone take up his place in the wider Corps.

This book will try to explain the Corps' values and ethos and their relation to physical fitness. It will show you how extremely physically demanding training can be completed by increasing your fitness and by using your mind to push your body, not just further than you might believe possible, but also further than its fitness might allow.

## The Commando Dagger

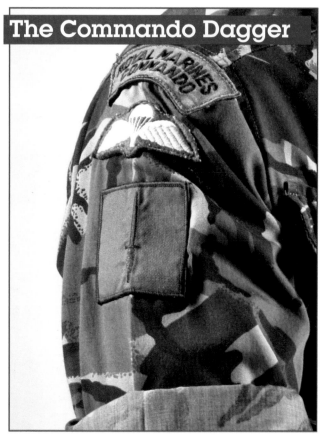

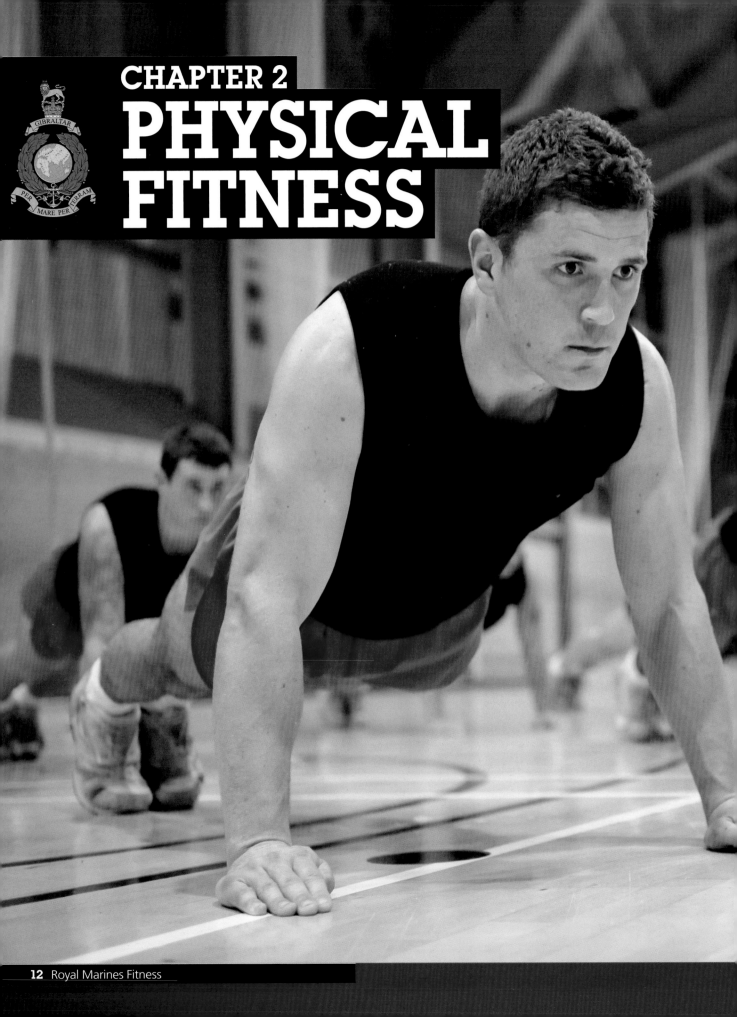

# CHAPTER 2
# PHYSICAL FITNESS

The Falklands Conflict of the early 1980s provides an excellent example as to why physical fitness is so important to the Royal Marines. After disembarking from ships at San Carlos on East Falkland on 21 May 1982, a large number of Royal Marines 'yomped' (walked carrying full kit on the back in a Bergen) with their equipment across the island, covering 56 miles (90km) in three days carrying loads in excess of 80lb (36kg). This was achieved with limited water and rations, as everything had to be carried. In addition the Royal Marines completed their march with little rest, and on completion moved straight into offensive operations to take the high ground surrounding Port Stanley. Without their exceptional physical fitness these men would not have been able to complete this task and therefore take the offensive action needed.

Prior to their 56-mile yomp, the Royal Marines had spent a considerable amount of time aboard ship sailing south to the Falkland Islands. Though they had little space and specific equipment to conduct physical training, they still trained hard, maintaining and improving their fitness. It was this physical fitness that enabled them to operate at extremely high physical intensity immediately after landing, and take part in what is now considered a very prominent piece of British military history. It was 'Commando fitness' that ensured they could operate at this level.

At this point it seems sensible to examine what exactly Commando fitness is. The aims of Commando fitness (relevant to the trained and untrained Royal Marine) are:

■ To prepare the Recruit physically for war. This includes the development of all-round physical fitness, the teaching of purposeful military skills, the development of mental alertness, the development of character and the development of leadership.

■ To maintain the trained Royal Marine's physical fitness for his particular role. This includes maintenance of a high standard of all-round physical fitness, the application of purposeful military skills to training for war, the development of leadership and self-confidence, and the development of willpower and endurance.

Although only two aims exist, they are both extensive and should not be taken lightly. A significant amount of time and effort is required from both the trainer and the trainee to make these aims a reality.

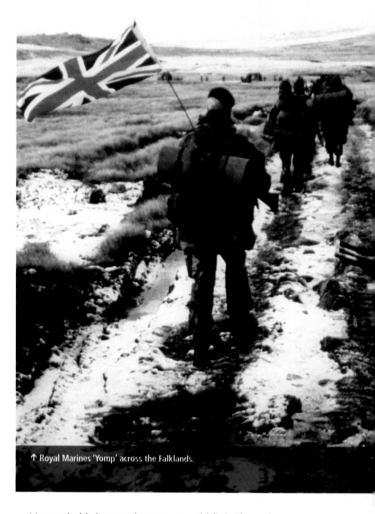

↑ Royal Marines 'Yomp' across the Falklands.

### Physical fitness

Physical fitness can mean a number of different things these days, and cover a myriad of ideas and physical states. To some it is just the ability to live life healthily and complete daily tasks with relative ease; to others it is the ability to compete at a given sport or activity without undue stress or after-effects; and to others again it is an ongoing quest to improve themselves physically as far as they possibly can.

You probably know where you would fit in if people holding these three viewpoints were placed in line, with the first group at the far left, the last group at the far right, and the middle group somewhere near the centre. Most Royal Marines would be somewhere on the right-hand side, many at the far right end. You may well find that once you have read and tried some of the training in this book, you may drift further towards the right-hand side as well.

It is important to note that Royal Marines are not only prepared by training to be physically fit but are also mentally prepared; pushed to and taught to push themselves up to and beyond perceived limits, thus allowing their physical and psychological strength to be increased, so that when the body says no, the mind will still push on.

The idea of physical fitness is not a new concept. Various sorts of physical training were in fact practised in both the East and West the many, many centuries ago. The Ancient Greeks

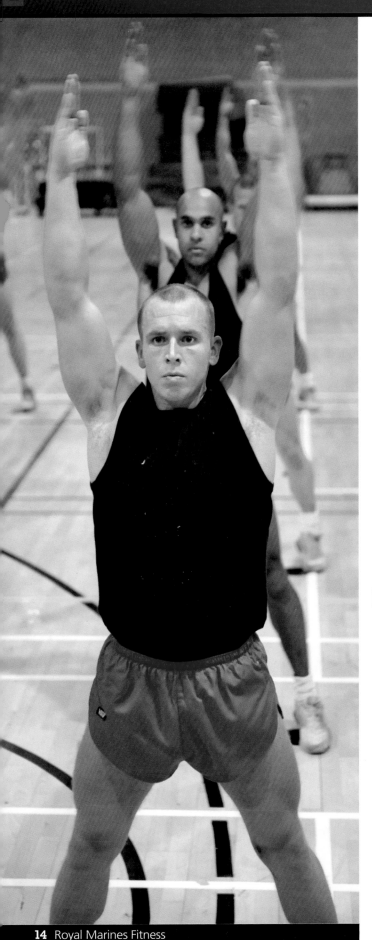

designed and implemented a wide range of physical training, culminating in the Olympic games, which are still with us today, although in a considerably different format. Military physical fitness is also an old concept, as the Ancient Chinese are said to have had specific physical training systems to prepare their soldiers for war.

Initial Royal Marine physical training includes a system called 'Swedish PT', adopted from a system designed by a Swedish scholar and fencer named Pehr Henri Ling and introduced into England in the 1860s. Its longevity can be credited to its basis being focussed on an understanding of the anatomy and physiology of the human body.

The Swedish system was very effective in a number of areas, firstly in its delivery, being instructor-led in a very formal 'command, response' format, *ie* instructor says, class does, all at once. Additionally, Swedish PT required little or no equipment so could be done anywhere in the world without any additional kit. This was, of course, perfect for onboard ship, where space-saving is crucial. Lastly, it did not lead to the development of large muscles, which can often be an unwanted consequence of lifting heavy weights. The system was consequently perfect for the military, so much so that by the end of the 1960s the Royal Navy and the Army had also adopted it.

These days the Army, Navy and RAF all have their own 'PT Schools', designing, testing and delivering appropriate physical training to meet their specific needs. The Royal Marines also has its own separate PT School, located at the Commando Training Centre (CTCRM) in Lympstone, Devon. The Royal Marines PT School, run by specifically handpicked Physical Training Instructors, not only writes and designs physical training for the Corps to ensure that individuals receive the best training to prepare them for today's Operations, but also selects and trains the next generation of Physical Training Instructors to ensure that the training continues to be delivered in the best possible way.

## Components of fitness

When we are asked to think of someone who is physically fit, we all picture someone different, be it an Olympic athlete, a professional footballer, the World's Strongest Man or, while reading this book, a Royal Marines Commando. Yet although they may all be fit in their own specific areas, they may be very unfit in other ways.

To be regarded as having all-round fitness, anyone training must bear in mind the 'seven components of fitness'. Arguably someone can appear, and indeed be, fit without actually having all of the components. However, to avoid injury and be at the top of their game, it is important to at least train each component to some degree. It is true that one component may be more important than another depending on the sport trained for, but ignoring one or two because they do not seem applicable to your sport or training goals could potentially leave you open to injury or a lack of overall fitness. Royal Marines, however, must have a great all-round fitness base, and it is therefore essential that Recruits are introduced to all seven components during training.

# The seven components of fitness

## 1 Flexibility

Flexibility is defined as 'the maximum range of movement around a joint allowed by the muscles, tendons and ligaments'. Wherever possible, every training session should involve a comprehensive warm-up including mobility work and dynamic stretches. If static stretches are included they should be held for 8–10 seconds.

Far more important is the post-exercise stretch: each training session should end with a comprehensive cool-down and static stretch session. This will have a marked improvement on recovery time and help produce strong healthy muscles. These 'maintenance stretches' should be held for around 10 seconds. Better still would be to stretch the muscles for up to 30 seconds; these are known as 'developmental stretches' and are extremely beneficial for improving the flexible range of a joint/muscle. Remember, a healthy muscle is a flexible muscle.

## 2 Endurance

Endurance fitness is said to be the body's ability to resist fatigue whilst performing relatively prolonged exercise of low to moderate intensity. All Royal Marines require a high level of endurance fitness. In fact it is probably the most important component for a Recruit or trained Royal Marine. Having a good level of endurance will ensure a Royal Marine can keep performing for long periods of time, whatever the task, and not feel tired prematurely. The easiest way to train endurance is to go on long, slow- to medium-paced runs. This is a gradual process and either time or distance should be used as a marker and built on. For example, running 20 minutes one session, then 25 minutes the next, then 30 the next etc, or two miles one session, two and a half the next, three miles the next etc.

Another great way to train endurance is using a heart rate monitor. The efficiency of the heart in pumping oxygen can be a limiting factor to your ability to endure and perform during endurance activities. Remember, the heart is a muscle, and just like any other muscle it must be trained for it to strengthen and grow. For anyone wanting to get fit, the heart is the most important muscle to train, so train it well.

Long runs are particularly relevant to Royal Marines' training due to the fitness requirements of a trained Royal Marine. In terms of your own training, long runs may not seem specific to your chosen goal or sport; however, they will help your overall fitness considerably and aid in the production of healthy muscles, cardiovascular fitness, a healthy lifestyle, and weight management. I would therefore recommend that any basic fitness regime involves at least two long endurance sessions (runs/cycles/swims/rows) a week.

## 3 Skill

A skill is said to be the ability of the mind/body to know when and where to use a specific technique to successfully complete a fitness activity or sport. For general fitness developing skills is not important. However, for a gymnast, a footballer or a Royal Marine in certain scenarios it is obviously very important.

You might think that for the general gym-goer developing skills will not be at the top of the fitness priority list. Actually, there are a number of techniques that need to be mastered when training in the gym, from how to run economically to how to perform exercises with specific pieces of kit such as

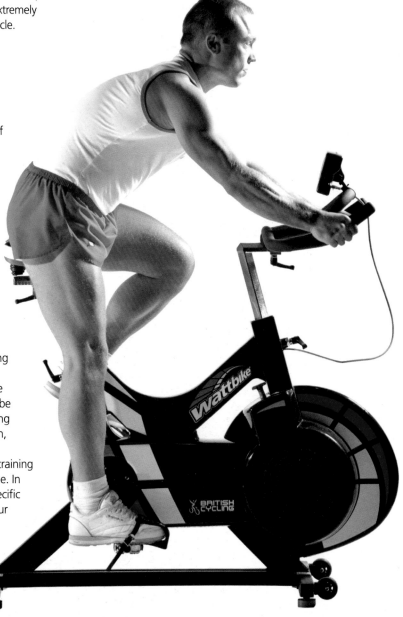

kettlebells. However, mastering these techniques, or even doing these activities, is not imperative in order to get generally fit, but is if you plan to do such exercises.

For Royal Marines and Recruits it is important to master certain techniques skilfully, so that they become second nature and can be used under pressure. The perfect example is weapon drills. If a Marine's rifle stops firing or becomes jammed, he has a specific set of drills to sort it out and get it firing. The skill is knowing which drills to use when. Another physical example is the regain (see Chapter 9), which once mastered must be completed under pressure and when tired – the true mark of a skill.

Everyone reading this book has probably heard the phrase 'practice makes perfect'; you may have even used it if you have children or younger siblings, to encourage them to practise piano, a football turn or their handwriting. If so, then the following will probably surprise you: practice does *not* make perfect! What practice does is make *permanent* – in other words, if something is practised (*ie* repeated) over and over it is committed to muscle memory and becomes the way your body performs the practised task. The problem is that if the *wrong* technique is practised over and over then a bad technique will become permanent. Which is why practice certainly does not make perfect. When thinking about developing skills and training techniques, a far better phrase to use is 'perfect practice makes permanent'.

## 4 Stamina

Stamina is said to be the ability of the body to resist fatigue whilst performing repetitive high-level intensity work. Royal Marines require a good level of stamina to ensure that they can keep performing at the high intensity required throughout either an entire fitness session or an entire battle, ensuring that they do not slow down significantly towards the end.

The best way to train stamina is to perform repetitive sprints/intervals a set number of times. Whether for Royal Marines, a local sports team or a casual gym-goer, training stamina is essential for all-round fitness, and is also an excellent way to lose weight – the level of work required when performing sprints or interval training burns a lot of calories. Furthermore, stamina training raises the metabolism for a period of time after the session, leading to the same end goal.

## 5 Strength

Strength is said to be the maximum force that specific muscles can generate against resistance. Strength training is very important to young men training in a gym, but they often overdo it and ignore the other equally important areas of fitness. For Royal Marines, whether fully trained or Recruits in training, strength training is important, but it is important to achieve it without too

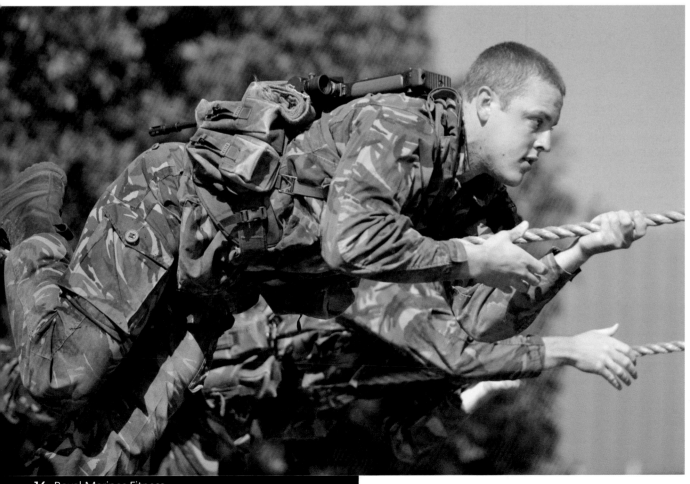

much weight gain. Good overall strength will ensure that we can perform all techniques without risk of injury, making the body quicker when sprinting and able to jump further and higher, and allowing the muscles to pull or push harder and faster; and, of course, it will also aid overall fitness.

Strength training and in particular resistance training also strengthens tendons, ligaments and supporting muscles to help limit injury. This is especially important for sports such as rugby or football, where the muscles are often put under stress in a contact situation. Furthermore, strength training improves core strength. A strong core is paramount in avoiding injuries.

## 6 Speed

Speed is said to be how fast the muscles can move given a set objective. We often think of this as our sprint speed, but it could be our reaction times, and the speed of any specific action. To train speed, you need to do repetitive drills when not overly fatigued. Doing so when fatigued will lead to bad technique, and if the body is too tired can lead to injury. Speed training is performed only over shorter distances, so that it does not become interval training.

## 7 Power

Power is said to be the functional relationship between strength and speed. Power is a key component to athletic performance. This power is the combination of the strength of a muscle and of how quickly it can apply that strength. There are three types of power:

- **Explosive power** – The muscles continue to generate the initial force quickly, with the movement usually being heavily resisted, so training will usually focus on strength development with heavy resistance.
- **Reactive power** – The muscles generate the initial power accompanied either by a change in direction or by a rapid reversal of the range of movement just performed.
- **Fast power** – The muscles generate the force very quickly to oppose the resistance, so training will focus on using less resistance.

Jumping (long, high and triple) and sprinting are the exercises of muscular power. However, endurance running and swimming are also enhanced by increased power. By improving power the efficiency and quickness of muscle movement is maximised, which in turn creates further efficiency and a greater VO2 max for endurance.

Training for power requires some muscular strength beforehand. Increasing the strength levels by controlled resistance and moderate repetition can improve performance in many areas.

As both speed and strength training are being undertaken anyway, power will increase. However, specific 'plyometric' sessions, involving jumps, bounds, hops etc, will see power increase more so, which in turn will see you become more explosive, have better reactions and be generally faster.

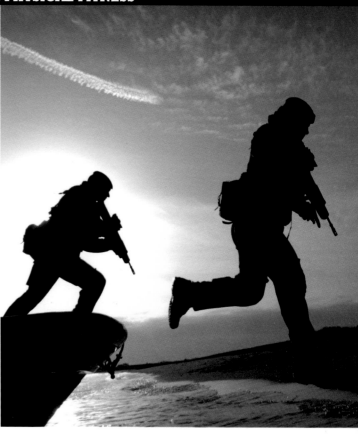

### Fitness for purpose

A common misconception of Royal Marines is that they are all muscle-bound as a result of intensive training; this is certainly not the case. It is important for Royal Marines to have strength, but only so as to react to operational requirements, and the ability to shift one's body weight quickly and efficiently is vital. Muscle-bound individuals do not necessarily have the ability to endure long distances with weight (though some do, and do it very well, often better than very slim endurance runners). However, being big does have its problems in terms of fitting into vehicles, helicopters or even sleeping bags! It is far more important for a Royal Marine to have muscular endurance to perform repetitive activities than to have muscular size and incredible strength. Commandos passing out of training are therefore far from muscle-bound – they are always lean, fit, and well-proportioned.

For success in any sport it is important that individuals have an all-round fitness training programme, and do not concentrate too heavily on one area. Although it is not necessary to train all the seven components of fitness every day, or even to train them equally, it is important that all get some attention to ensure all-round fitness and injury avoidance. For the casual gym-goer, a training programme that includes all the components of fitness in some form or another is an ideal way to train. Obviously if the end goal of the gym-goer is to complete a marathon then power training may not be at the top of his agenda. However, if the end goal is to lose weight, then sessions covering all seven areas will be worthwhile.

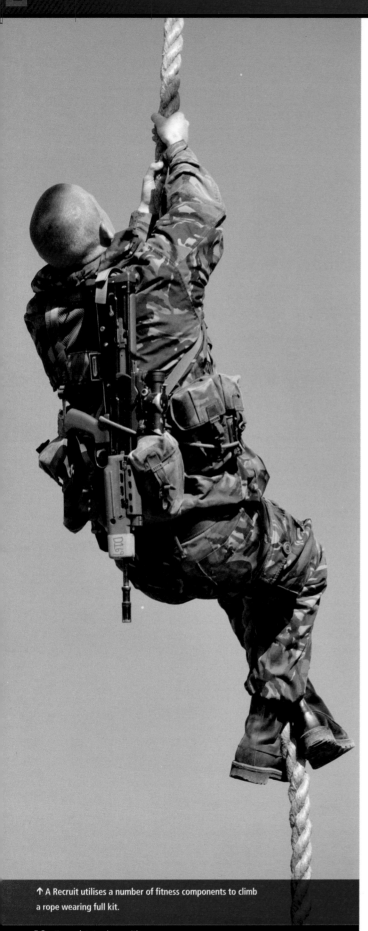

Not all of the components need to be trained in one session – they can be mixed together from one training session to the next. However, one type of training may interfere with another type, so the following order should be kept to if being performed on the same day or in the same session:

- **Warm-up**
- **Skill**
- **Power/speed**
- **Strength**
- **Stamina**
- **Endurance**
- **Flexibility**
- **Cool-down**

The order is quite obvious when you think about it. For instance, it would not be sensible to concentrate on a specific skill if stamina training had been performed just before it.

## The effects of training

Exercise promotes adaptations in the body that improve performance, which for many of us is the reason we train. Overall performance is improved through an all-round training regime, and tolerance to hard exercise is increased. 'Specific adaptations to imposed demands' (SAID) is the way we describe the changes the body makes as it adapts to a training regime. It is therefore important that although you should try to incorporate the seven components of fitness where possible, you must also be aware that the training undertaken should generally reflect the physical tasks to be performed.

In Recruit training we concentrate on 'functional fitness', fitness that relates specifically to the tests and roles a Royal Marine/Recruit will encounter. For example, to improve the cardiovascular system, swimming or cycling at 75–80% of your maximum heart rate will improve your VO2 max, cardiovascular efficiency and thus your running. However, if the end goal is to improve running for a race or marathon, then running should be specifically trained. Swimming or cycle training will increase swimming and cycling performance, but the ability to run economically will diminish, as the body adapts to the functions demanded of it (*ie* swimming and cycling). 'The body becomes its function' is something I have kept in my mind ever since being taught it on my first PT course. It suggests that whatever you ask of your body (*ie* what you train) is what it will become good at.

## Physical fitness in Royal Marine training

Physical fitness is a primary aim of Commando training, and during training Recruits will have to endure intense periods of physical and mental strain. To keep it current, Commando training is constantly being reviewed and developed, not only by the Royal Marines Physical Training branch but also by the Institute of Naval Medicine, which together ensure that the training delivered – and therefore the Royal Marines produced – reflects the output demanded of the Commandos and the environment in which they are operating. In today's world a Recruit may complete

↑ A Recruit utilises a number of fitness components to climb a rope wearing full kit.

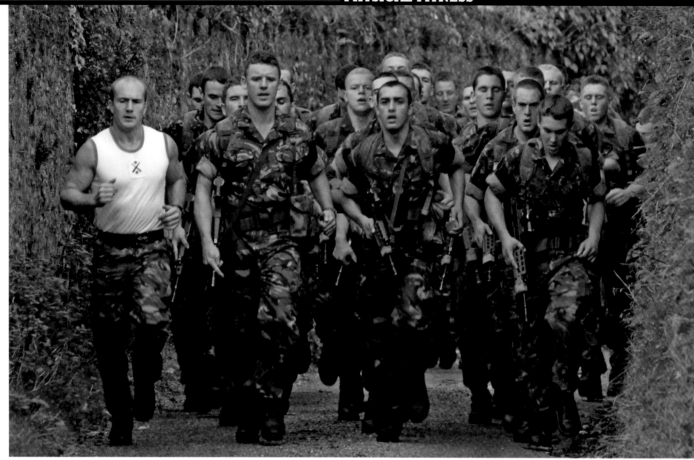

32 weeks of Commando training and then find himself on the front line in Afghanistan a week or so later.

At week 30/31 of their training Recruits complete and hopefully pass their Commando tests, and although they have other landmark tests throughout training this is our main 'race', if we use the model of a professional sportsman. However, unlike a professional sportsman we intentionally pre-fatigue the Recruits and sleep-deprive them prior to completing the four Commando tests, allowing us to test not only their fitness but their mental resolve as well.

The methods used to increase a Recruit's fitness are vastly different from those used in the civilian world. Although this will be enlarged on considerably in later chapters, an excellent example is our use of rope climbing. The climbing of 30ft (9.14m) vertical ropes is rare in civilian training, but it is required of every Royal Marine. Rope climbing increases upper body strength tremendously, leads to confidence at height, and is a technique (and skill) that has to be learnt, and therefore tests the trainee's ability to concentrate when fatigued. Every Recruit will eventually

have to climb a 30ft rope outside, whatever the weather, in combat boots and carrying 31lb of kit.

Often when a Recruit leaves CTCRM and arrives at a Commando Unit as a trained Royal Marine he will be at the peak of 'Commando fitness', having just passed his Commando tests. Among the majority of Royal Marines, a significant loss of fitness will never truly occur thereafter. This is down to the innate personal pride ingrained into every trained Royal Marine Commando from his time at CTCRM. It is as if letting his fitness decline will be letting others down, or that physical weakness will lead to his losing face amongst his peers. This need for fitness seems to be built into the psyche of all of us, and for many Royal Marines continues well into retirement!

### Commando fitness

Throughout history, Royal Marines Units have been called upon at very short notice and had to go directly on Operations without any pre-deployment training. This obviously calls for all Royal

## Physical fitness is a primary aim of Commando training, and during training Recruits will endure periods of physical and mental strain

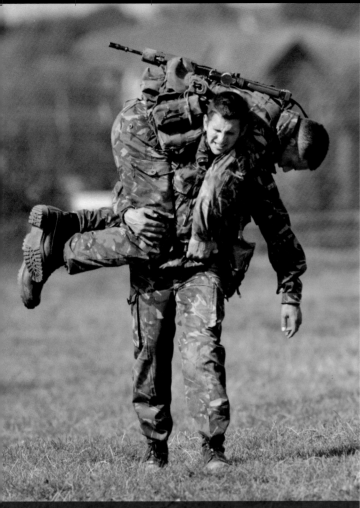

↑ **A Recruit utilises his Commando Fitness to endure the Fireman's Carry.**

In the evenings it will be up to individuals to do their own training, be it weight training, running training or perhaps a chosen sport. Furthermore if an individual is particularly weak at a specific area he will concentrate on that in his own time, to ensure that he will not let himself, his eight-man section or his Troop down. The bottom line is that there is something within each Royal Marine that compels him to do his own training outside of that done as part of his usual working routine. However, this is still not specific to Operations, and therefore a pre-deployment training programme is the best way of ensuring that an entire Commando Unit is physically fit for its specific role.

## Maintaining physical fitness

Whether we are considering a Royal Marine Recruit, a trained Commando, an Olympic athlete, a professional Boxer or a member of your local gym, no one can remain at peak fitness indefinitely. It is not only a huge strain on the body, which can lead to injury, it is also a huge strain on the mind and can be mentally fatiguing. A professional sportsman will have off seasons and on seasons, *ie* times when they are training and times when they are recovering, when they are either resting or just doing 'maintenance' training. Perhaps around three months before the on season they will start to prepare, hopefully enabling them to reach peak performance just at the time of the first event or race. If they tried to keep at this peak level throughout the year they would eventually hit a plateau or a period of fatigue or even injury, and if this coincided with their race it could spell disaster.

The same scientific approach of 'build-up' training is applied to Royal Marines, whether fully trained or Recruits. Although the general level of fitness for all Royal Marines is above that of most civilians – and in fact most other Services – again, it cannot be maintained at the very top level indefinitely. Just as with professional sportsmen, a basic level of fitness will be maintained which can be increased in specific areas or for specific roles when necessary.

## Physical training used in the Royal Marines

A combination of methods are used in conjunction with the time and resources available, and allowing for injury, to achieve the aim of Commando fitness, both in Recruit training and in Commando Units. What follows are not the only methods, since individuals often bring their own ideas into play as well. As with any good all-round civilian fitness regime, variation and determination are the keys to progress.

### ■ Daily exercises (DEs)
A series of callisthenics-style basic exercises, which can be different every day. They can be performed in a short time frame and with minimum space and resources. Examples would be press-ups, squats and sit-ups.

### ■ Circuit training
Similar to DEs in that basic exercises can be used. However, a circuit usually requires a little more planning and imagination.

Marines to be physically fit all year round. Although the gold standard is for the Unit Physical Training Instructor to plan and implement pre-deployment fitness training to an entire Commando Unit prior to its deployment, this is often not practical due to the ever-changing world we live in and the role Royal Marines play in British foreign policy. Therefore it is imperative that Royal Marines have the innate ability to keep fit, stay fit and, more importantly, have the state of mind to believe that they can achieve whatever is required of them. The foundations for all of this are set in Commando training at CTCRM.

When not on Operations or pre-deployment training for Operations, it is still imperative that all Royal Marines stay fit. To achieve this daily fitness training takes place, consisting of an hour's 'Troop Phys' in the morning, involving either about 30 Royal Marines if at Troop level or about 100 Royal Marines if at Company level. If a PTI is available he will organise and instruct the Physical Training; if not, the other Royal Marines will take it in turns to organise and run the training themselves. The daily PT concentrates on runs (intervals, long-distance endurance or shorter stamina routes) and body-weight circuits – basic 'maintenance physical training'.

# Physical training programmes

Any physical training programme must be monitored carefully, and the Commando training programme used for Recruit training, as well as any Unit PTIs' training programmes for Commando Units going on Operations, are no different. To become physically fit an individual must train, or be trained. Following a well-planned and produced Physical training programme is a great start, and, as Royal Marines Recruit training shows, produces great results. However, alone it is not enough; no one can maintain themselves at their physical peak indefinitely. Therefore every training programme needs to include changes and rest periods to ensure that the body is truly physically fit.

Remember, general muscular development is essential. Do not fall into the trap of concentrating on specific muscle groups because they look best on the beach; the body's systems work best when responding to progressive all-round exercise. It is important to always start slowly – master the easier exercises and techniques before attempting the harder ones. This will lead to greater gains and will avoid injury.

Circuits may be specific to a task (*eg* muscular endurance) or an area of the body (*eg* leg overload) or may be dependent on the equipment available.

## ■ Weight training
Used to increase the strength/size of muscles, often in specific areas of the body for a particular task. Can be used to increase muscle tone for the entire body, increasing metabolism and all-round fitness.

## ■ Five basic exercises (5BX)
These are similar to DEs but more prescriptive. Usually the same five basic exercises need to be achieved in a short time, with minimal resources and fuss. Generally they include warm-up, arm, trunk, leg and sprint exercises. (An example would be press-ups, pull-ups, sit-ups, burpees and sprints.) Competition can be introduced by requiring a certain number of each exercise to be completed within a set time.

## ■ Free activities
These are a combination of activities and games with a specific theme and a fun element, similar to 'It's a Knockout', the idea being to get people to perform physical activities while enjoying themselves. Games are usually performed as team events rather than as individuals, with the emphasis of each game being different, *eg* skill, strength, endurance or stamina.

## ■ Recreational training
This is anything from regular sporting activities to adventurous outdoor activities. Examples are football, climbing, mountain biking and skiing.

## ■ Battle Physical Training (BPT)
This is the main fitness training of Recruits during Commando training. It is done with the basic yet essential equipment that individuals will use on Operations: a set of 'combat order' webbing weighing 21lb and an SA80 assault rifle weighing 10lb. It is always conducted in boots and camouflage uniform (called Combat Soldier 95, CS95 for short). BPT involves such activities as the Assault Course, rope climbing and the Fireman's Carry.

## ■ Swimming
All Royal Marines have to achieve a certain level of swimming and pass the Battle Swim Test (BST), which is performed wearing CS95 shirt and trousers, webbing weighing 10lb and a dummy SA80 rifle weighing 10lb. This test is well above the requirement of other forces due to the Royal Marines working on board ships and boats of all sizes. It is consequently imperative that all Royal Marines can pass this test.

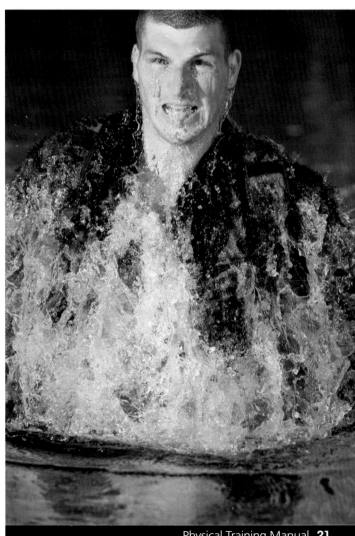

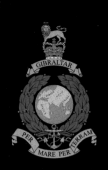

# CHAPTER 3
# FITNESS PSYCHOLOGY

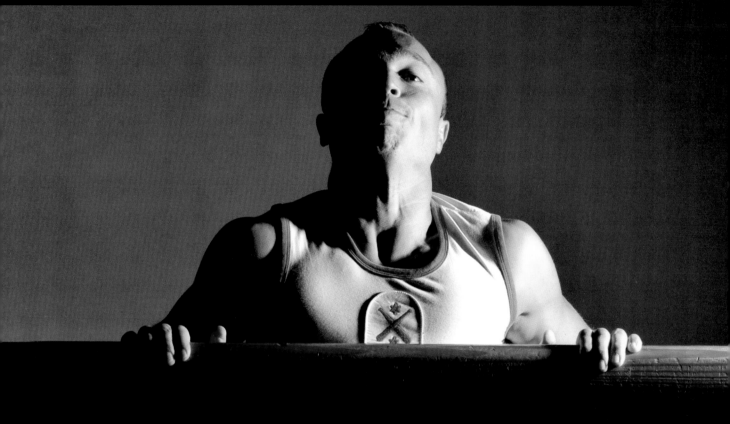

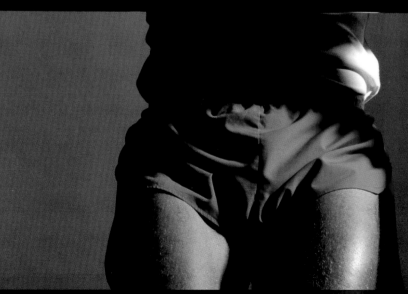

A good training programme and a willing trainee are an excellent start to becoming physically fit. However, they do not guarantee it. Whether we are considering RM Recruits or someone who just wants to get fit at home, a third equally important factor is often the missing ingredient to achieving true physical fitness: the willingness and strength of mind to push through the difficult days, through the pain barrier, to say no to a night of binge drinking, and to concentrate wholeheartedly on the goal, whether it is to be a Commando, to run a 36-minute 10km race, or to have a size eight figure.

The Potential Royal Marines Course and Potential Officers Course both test young men to see if they have the 'potential' to become Royal Marines. We get some very fit men on these courses, and, yes, we are testing their physical potential; but often it is not because they are lacking in physical fitness that candidates fail – it is because they lack mental strength. The majority of young men joining Royal Marines training do not know how to push themselves. When given a 1.5-mile best effort run in week 1 of training, most Recruits get to a certain 'comfortable' speed and stay at that, never pushing the body that little bit more. They are fit because their 'comfortable' speed is generally good enough to pass. However, by week 9, when they repeat that test, most understand that the mind controls the body, and even if the body hurts, it can still give more, it can still go faster. By the time they get to the Commando tests every Recruit knows and understands this, and even if he really dislikes the fact, he will use it to his advantage.

Individuals from certain backgrounds already have the ability to push themselves, and understand that the psychological side of fitness means the mind can control the body and ensure that it is pushed as hard as it can be to reach the goals and the physical fitness needed. Such individuals have usually taken part in a specific type of sport and trained to a relatively high level. Examples of such sports are running (cross-country or track), swimming, boxing, gymnastics, and rowing. It is not true that everyone who takes part in these activities has a psychological advantage in fitness training over everyone else, far from it. Most casual runners never really push themselves to the point of being physically sick, yet competitive runners often will. Similarly, many casual gym-goers will push themselves very hard during organised circuit sessions just to get one up on the man next to them. However, most people do not really know how to push themselves physically, and this is because they do not appreciate the psychological side of fitness.

## Psychological skills

There are a number of ways of 'tricking' the mind to enable a better physical performance to be achieved. These are not difficult to understand or utilise, but every 'trick' does not work for every person. This list is not extensive, but provides a few ideas and examples.

The first is counting in smaller denominations: for example, let's say someone can do 23 press-ups but no more. Every time they do press-ups, they get to 20 and struggle – suddenly it gets really difficult. They manage to squeeze out another three, but then always fail. But counting in fives may allow them to do more. Obviously they know that the fourth set of five is equal to the normal 20, but the mind is occupied with not forgetting how many fives have been done so the brain does not tell the body 'Oh no, 20, this is where it gets hard!' This technique can be used for pull-ups, sit-ups or any other repetitive exercise.

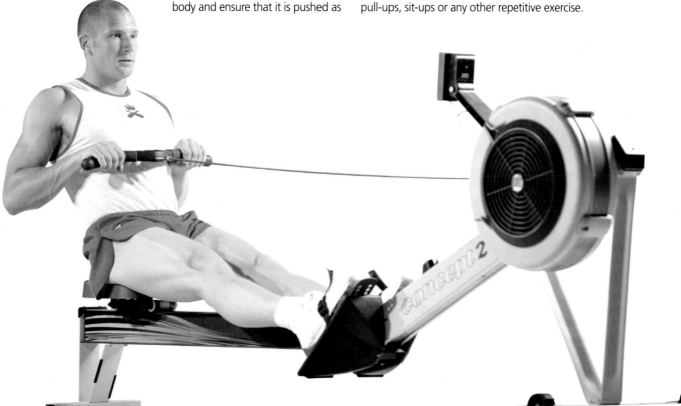

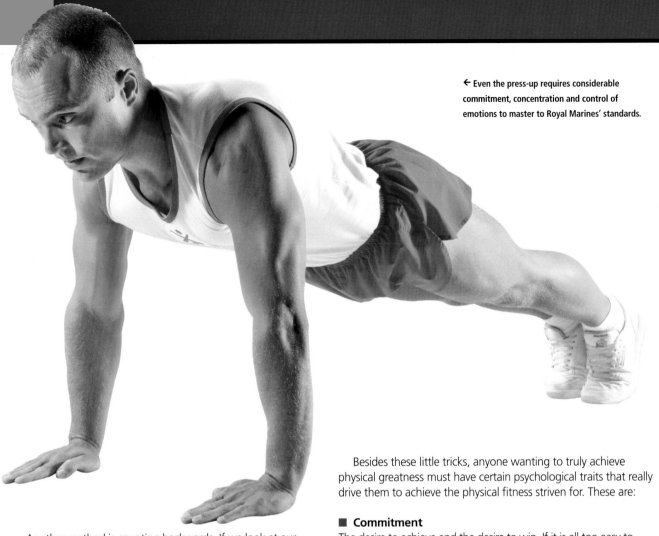

← Even the press-up requires considerable commitment, concentration and control of emotions to master to Royal Marines' standards.

Another method is counting backwards. If we look at our example above, the individual should start counting down from 25. Again, the mind is kept occupied and instead of 23 repetitions, 25 are reached. In fact the two methods can be combined: counting in fives for four lots then counting down from five to one for the last. Our 25 figure is reached.

A third method is repeating something in the mind, for example 'Don't think, just do', over and over. Whether running, or doing a repetitive exercise like press-ups, this repetition occupies the brain and stops it thinking about how hard the exercise is and convincing the body it should be in pain, which leads to fatigue. If we again take the 23-rep press-up example, if this individual does press-ups saying 'Don't think, just do' in his/her head until another cannot be performed, while someone else does the counting, 99% of the time more repetitions will be performed than if they do the counting themselves.

These methods 'trick' the brain. They are basically little mind games to play with yourself to stop you thinking about how hard an exercise is. A personal example for me is when running long distances with a Bergen or rucksack, when my legs are screaming at me to stop. I just count every time my left foot hits the ground up to ten, and then restart the counting. All this does is occupy the mind, but it stops the mind thinking about the pain in the legs, back, shoulders and lungs. People also sing a song in their head while doing this sort of running, to distract the mind from any discomfort.

Besides these little tricks, anyone wanting to truly achieve physical greatness must have certain psychological traits that really drive them to achieve the physical fitness striven for. These are:

### ■ Commitment

The desire to achieve and the desire to win. If it is all too easy to stop, to take a day off or to miss a session, then true physical fitness will never be achieved, because mental fitness is significantly lacking. This 'mental toughness' is required to never, ever quit or settle for 'that'll do'.

### ■ Control of emotions

When things get really hard, or really tough, it is the mind that will fail, not the body. It is so important to have control of anxiety, fear, anger, frustration, expectations and failure. Royal Marine training is very tough, but that means Recruits have experienced all these emotions and learnt how to control them. When faced with these feelings in real situations throughout the rest of their life, they should control them better than most.

### ■ Concentration

When the body is tired the mind is too. It is all too easy to relax and lose focus. However, a lack of focus can lead to accidents and mistakes. Focus and concentration ensure success, physically and psychologically. When tired and starting to slow, it is important to keep a 'goal' in the head in order to stay focussed and to continue to strive forward.

### ■ Confidence

With confidence and self-belief it is amazing what can be achieved. A positive attitude in any given situation can be the difference between success and failure. However, confidence should not be confused with arrogance. Being confident and believing in yourself will always give you the edge over others around you. Not surprisingly, though, confidence often comes because of sound preparation and training, as you know you will do well. In short, physical and psychological fitness training will lead to confidence in yourself, which will lead to a good performance.

## Everyone is human

Everyone has a low point at some time during Recruit training. Everyone will have a bad day, fail something, consider leaving, lose focus or commitment. That is why we tell Recruits that they will not make it through training alone; individuals cannot exist in the Corps, and they cannot make it through training – Troops will make it through by working together and for each other.

The same is true for civilian life. Even with the strongest mindset and all the best intentions, there will be occasions when everyone will have a bad day, will perform less well than expected or will let themselves down. Everyone will at some point panic under pressure; everyone at some point will falter in their training regime; everyone will at some point be distracted when concentration is required; and everyone will at some point lose confidence and have a setback.

Anyone who denies or never displays these kinds of human

emotion is either a liar or has some sort of personality disorder. These emotions are what make us humans. More importantly, by making us human they allow us to help each other, to rely on each other and to inspire each other.

The ability to self-analyse is so important at times like these – to look objectively at the situation and say 'So it looks like I'm having a bad day, I'm not performing well. Ok, but tomorrow I will rectify it.' This ability is just another form of psychological fitness controlling the mind, so it does not control you and your body. 'Know thyself' was a main theme in the philosophy of Socrates, and is very applicable in reaching true physical and psychological fitness. By knowing yourself, you can truly control yourself, and really achieve all that you want in life.

## Motivation and psychology

Everyone who is training to improve their physical fitness must be motivated by something or for something. Whether it is a Royal Marine Recruit striving for a green beret, a casual runner wanting to get a sub-40-minute 10km run time, or a bride wanting to fit into a specific wedding dress, all have specific motivations which have a huge psychological impact and, more importantly, can be harnessed to ensure that training occurs as much as possible to reach the desired goal.

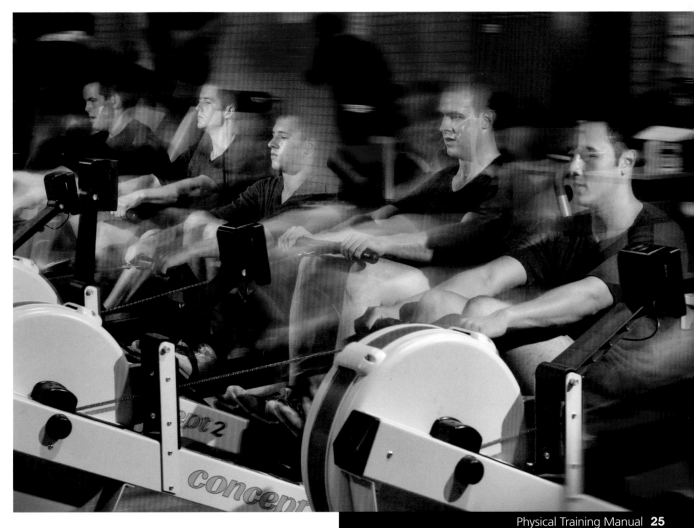

It is fair to say that we are all motivated by different things and in different ways, and whereas it is relatively simple to see what motivates someone in Recruit training, the same is not so true for the rest of society. A number of Recruits leave training along the way – clearly, for them the motivation to achieve Commando status was not there, or maybe the prize was not worth the hardship. For the casual gym-goer it is important to 'know thyself' and process what your motivation is. Whatever it is, keep it there in your mind, especially when something is hard, or if you wake up and think 'Maybe I'll give it a miss today'; use your motivation, fix it in your mind and work towards it.

The following are a number of examples of the kinds of thing that motivate people to train:

- **Goal orientated** – *ie* a desire to achieve a goal or even surpass it. This may be a certain length run or swim in a set time, a certain number of press-ups without stopping, or the ability to outperform others, such as by beating a friend at squash. All of these will provide motivation to train or to meet that goal.
- **Group orientated** – *ie* a desire to be part of a group and to achieve with that group. Examples are football teams, rowing clubs and martial arts clubs. It is often felt that the group members feed off of each other's positive energy and motivation. This does not mean all your training is done with the group, it may be that you train as an individual to improve your fitness to become more highly regarded within the group, or because your fitness will better benefit the group and what the team is trying to achieve.

- **Other people orientated** – *ie* a desire to have an impact on those around you. This may mean your fitness must improve to lead sessions for specific groups, such as a schoolmaster needing to improve fitness to take the cross-country team out for a run. Conversely it could be the vanity side of training, needing recognition for the goals achieved and physical stature attained. Although this is usually frowned upon, it is still motivation to be fit and healthy and thus is better than being lazy and unhealthy.
- **Habit orientated** – *ie* a desire to feed the habit. In truth this is an addiction of some sort, some say to the endorphins produced when training, some say to the never-ending goal of personal improvement. The habit of training may have manifested itself during formative years, such as Royal Marines' lifestyle, or from being part of a sports team at school or university, and that influence has made training part of your lifestyle.
- **Health orientated** – This requires little explanation. To get fit is to be healthy and stay healthy. A great reason to train.

## Motivation by others

Royal Marines, and in particular the PT branch, use a variety of techniques to motivate Royal Marines during fitness sessions. Whether the session is hard or not, most people find that when they train with a partner or have an instructor running the session the motivation to do well is somehow increased, which in turn leads to the level of achievement being far greater than expected. Although it is important overall to have some level of self-motivation, there is a time and a place for trainers encouraging

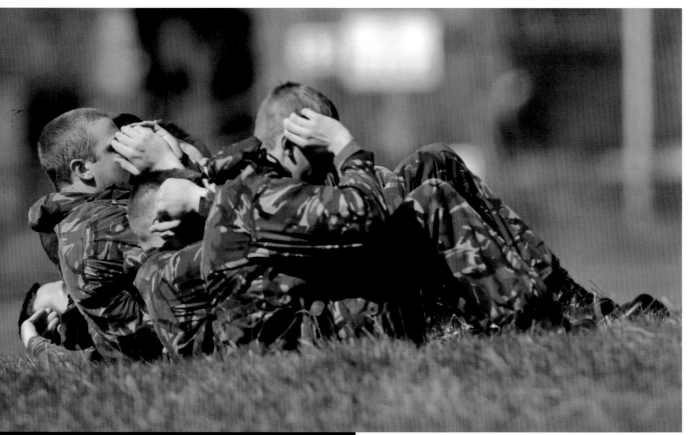

or coercing individuals to deliver more in order to attain success. Although Royal Marines are generally very self-motivated and disciplined when it comes to maintaining fitness, everyone has a low point or a bad day, and this is where a PTI really earns his money, motivating, encouraging and inspiring those around him to achieve what they are capable of.

## Habit and addiction

For many Royal Marines, myself included, physical training is not a chore, it is not something to find time for, it is part of the daily routine. A day without some sort of physical training (unless a specific rest day is in place) is quite an uncomfortable feeling. The fact that physical training is a habit means that it doesn't need thinking about, and is not dreaded but looked forward to. At this point it becomes self-motivational, it is something to be enjoyed. This is especially true when physical training has an aim, or is done as part of a group where it is also social exercise.

However, this can be taken a little too far. When the rest of the day's events are scheduled around the physical training, and slowly a person's PT starts to control their life, at this point the person is addicted. A PT addiction in itself is not too severe a problem – that is until, for some people, their social life and personal relationships start to suffer. When two or even three sessions a day start ruling your life and a rest day is never taken, the body will soon start to suffer and decline. At that stage the addiction has become more than a habit or motivation – it has become a problem.

## Lack of motivation

A lack in motivation and the following slump in training can affect us all, whether we are Royal Marine Commandos, Olympic athletes or local gym-goers. We all have things in common that lead to us losing motivation. In training, Recruits are there to help each other on the bad days – when one man is low, they pick him up as a group. Recruits have instructors there to provide that inspiration and motivation, but outside of training, and in civilian life, we don't all have that luxury, so unfortunately slumps occur and have to be dealt with when they do.

To really understand how to get over a lack of motivation and how to use the various methods that will be explained below, it is worth understanding what causes these slumps in the first place. Again 'know thyself', then you can correct thyself.

### ■ Fatigue

Fatigue is a major cause of lack of motivation. If you have trained hard for a number of days and then wake up early to go for a morning run, and your body is really stiff and achy, it is very difficult to get motivated. If the body is full of DOMS (delayed onset muscle soreness) then it is probably already fatigued and possibly on the verge of overtraining, if intense sessions continue.

### ■ Overtiredness

People often try to stick to their training programme even if they have had a very long day at work or, worse still, have been out for the night, have come back in the early hours and have woken

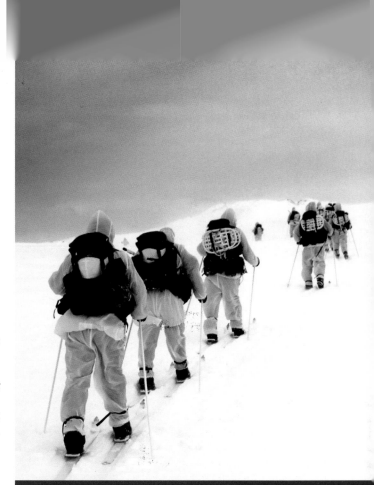

↑ Certain feats require immense psychological fitness.

up with a hangover. Believe it or not, this is not a good idea! The body is full of toxins and needs rest to recuperate. By forcing it to work when it is in dire need of fuel and rest does not help fitness gains, it just puts pressure on the heart and can lead to injury.

### ■ Overtraining

If the training is very intense for a sustained period of time, especially if rest days are ignored, then overtraining-related fatigue will set in. If this occurs the body and mind will demand rest, often by causing injury or illness. A serious consequence of overtraining is the lowering of the immune system, meaning that the body will eventually fall victim to the flu or perhaps something worse. Additionally, when the body is overtrained it is susceptible to injury, be it a torn muscle or, worse, an over-use injury such as patella tendinitis.

### ■ Repetitive training

By repeating the same session or exercising the same muscle groups session after session, with the aim of seeing vast improvements in this area, the body is never allowed time to rest and repair. Effectively this causes overtraining-type issues within the muscle groups consistently exercised, which can ultimately lead to injury.

### ■ Illness and/or injury

Illness or injury can result in lack of motivation, and so they should. It is not wise to train when ill – the body is busy fighting

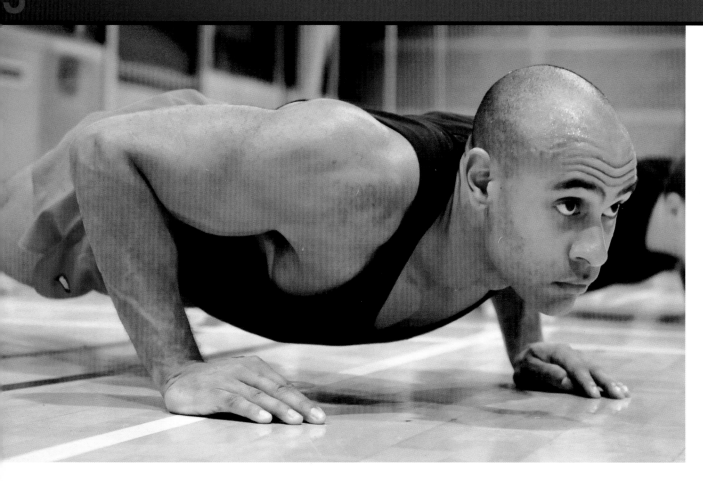

off infection, and by training it is put under further stress, which is bad for the heart. Injury can be slightly different, depending on the injury. For example, a pulled hamstring will mean no lower limb activity, but an upper body session could still take place.

Whenever an injury or illness occurs it is worth trying to figure out why. Is it because the body is run down from overtraining, or because training has taken place when overtired? Sometimes illness or injury is a sign that things need to change.

### ■ Environment
A change in climate or environment will have an adverse effect on motivation and training. Certain environments can affect the body and decrease performance; this is true for very hot and very cold climates. The Royal Marines always try to acclimatise to the environment for a few days prior to any hard training.

People often find motivation is lacking in the winter when it is cold and raining, as opposed to the summer when the good weather is inspirational and makes people want to get out and exercise. In winter, try to focus on your end goal and self-motivate beyond that day's training. Concentrate on that elation you feel following a session knowing you have trained hard, even if that elation is only because the session is over for another day!

### ■ Diet
In the Royal Marines we often say 'food is just fuel' – a car cannot go anywhere if it has no petrol, and the body will also come to a stop without fuel. If you are struggling for motivation ensure you have eaten well, and are not lacking energy. Training when energy is depleted is both bad for the heart and body, and can also lead to injury. Remember, certain environments, such as very hot, suppresses the appetite, so it may be necessary to work really hard on getting the calories in.

### ■ Reaching a plateau
At some point or another most people find that they reach a point where no more improvements can be made. If the goal/goals have been reached then this is not a problem, and 'maintenance' PT can now be performed. However, if the goal is still some way off, and yet a plateau has been hit, motivation can take a real dive. If nothing obvious is causing this plateau – such as overtraining, diet, illness or the need for rest days – then the best method of overcoming the problem is to change the regime and vary sessions.

### ■ Psychological factors
There are too many psychological factors that could influence your training to list them here. If a motivational problem exists, or a plateau continues despite trying a number of different approaches to get past it, then a psychological problem may be to blame. Again, it is important to 'know thyself', to be self-critical: is there something in your life taking your focus away from your training? Common causes are family problems at home or a love interest, both leading to a lack of focus and drive. It is important to consider what the true goal of your physical training is. It may be that the family problem or love interest should be put before fitness.

## Aids to get past failure or lack of progress

### ■ Visualisation

Visualisation is a method adopted by top sportsmen all over the world. It can be used in many guises, but in short it involves going through the sequence of events in your mind and 'seeing' yourself performing whatever you are struggling with and being successful at it. It is usually necessary to do this before a session to ensure you are relaxed – doing it during or at the very start of a session will probably mean the heart rate is already raised, as the mind knows what is about to occur, and it will be difficult to concentrate on the visualisation.

Imagine and go through in your mind what you are going to do and how you are going to succeed. When utilising visualisation it must be remembered that the visualisations must be realistic – for instance, we would all like to fly, but imagining yourself flapping your arms and taking off will not make it happen. However, if you consistently fail at ten pull-ups and only make eight, visualise yourself breezing through the first eight and then staying on the bar and struggling through the last two, but, importantly, completing all ten.

For a long-term training goal, one which is realistic but consistently evades you – for example being able to complete the splits – it may be necessary to adopt regular mental and physical practice whenever possible. There is no substitute for real-time training, but visualisation is a key to success, especially during rest periods and as an aid to regular training.

### ■ Self-study

This is usually used for sports techniques, for example a golf swing. It involves recording yourself performing the technique and then watching and analysing your performance. Not only does this allow you to review your performance and make any notes as to where improvements can be made, but it also allows you to reinforce the technique by watching it. We know that 'mirror neurons' exist within our brains, which mean we fire the correct pathways when we watch others perform activities; obviously, watching yourself also provides the same stimulus and allows analysis to take place. Watching others performing perfect techniques may also help reinforce your own performance.

### ■ Rest

Rest is incredibly important. It is so easy to get overly habitual with your physical training and let it become an addiction. When this occurs rest days are often ignored, and this is when fatigue and plateaus in training are frequent. If something that should be achievable remains unobtainable despite consistent hard training, then perhaps a rest week is what is really needed, to enable you to come back and attack the same problem refreshed and fully refuelled.

### ■ A new angle

Often when a training goal is out of reach, we get so fixated with it we cannot see that another method of getting there may be an option. A varied programme is better for the body and

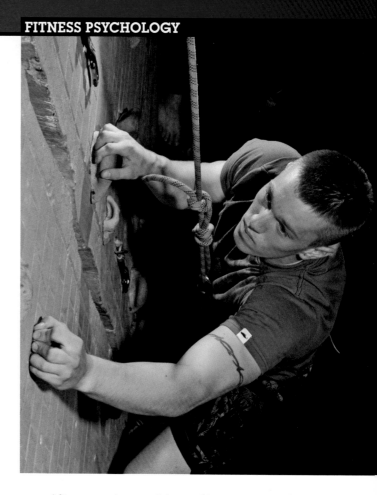

general fitness, so when a training goal becomes so specific that training is too focussed it is not as good as an all-round fitness programme. If rest has been tried it is often an idea to take a few weeks or even a month and try another type of training that improves the same area of fitness but in another way.

## Conclusion

**Psychological fitness is a very open subject with a number of areas to look at. There are hundreds of students all over the country studying for degrees in Sports Psychology, and the psychology of fitness covers a large part of their course. It is becoming recognised across the world to be just as important, if not more so, than actual fitness training itself. For Royal Marines, the mind is arguably the most powerful and potent weapon with which to achieve success. For the casual gym-goer, using the mind requires no extra resources or finance and is therefore a great place to begin getting fit.**

**It is important, especially when injured or unable to train, to stay focussed and to use the mind where possible to aid recovery and performance on your return. Whether you are a Royal Marine Recruit, a would-be Olympic athlete or a casual gym-goer, once you have realised that the mind controls the body and not the other way round then confidence, concentration and commitment will automatically increase, and so, of course, will performance and fitness.**

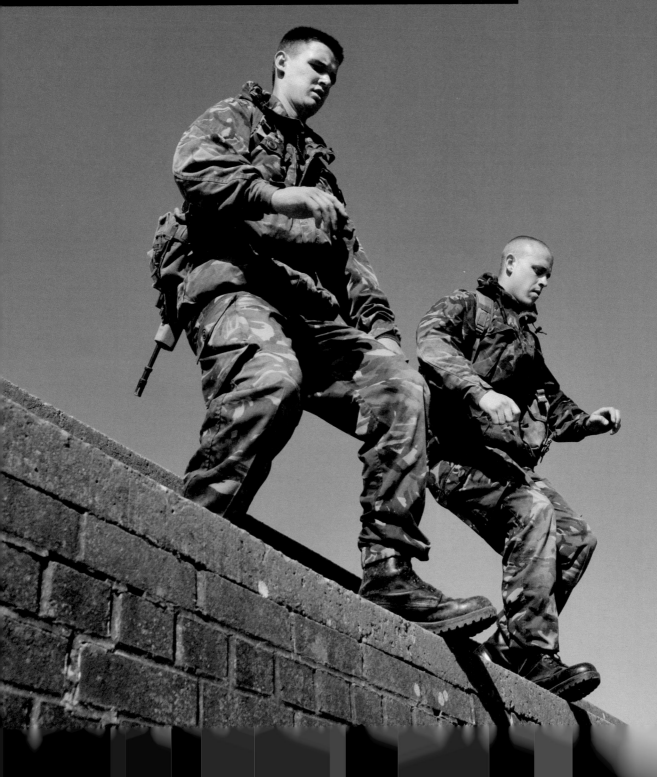

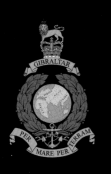

# CHAPTER 4
# ETHOS AND LIFESTYLE

The Royal Marines' ethos is a combination of the Commando spirit and the Royal Marines' key values, both of which are outlined below. There is an underlying need, stemming back to Recruit training, for Royal Marines to remain fit; for them to train in their own time to ensure that they do not let themselves or their peers down. This psychological need to train is not confined to fitness. The Royal Marines have developed their very own language, thought processes, tactics, teaching and learning methods to achieve it, to name but a few. Once exposed to this approach, even a Recruit at week 4 finds himself starting to speak and think like his instructors. Even wives and girlfriends tend to get caught up in the culture, using the odd bit of 'Bootneck slang'.

There are a number of key values or characteristics that all Royal Marines should aspire to: examples include adaptability, humility, fortitude, and a sense of humour. Furthermore every Royal Marine is expected to show great courage, strength of character, integrity, selflessness, cheerfulness in adversity, an appreciation of high standards, and a strong sense of discipline. The following chapter will look at all of these traits, and what the Royal Marines call the Commando ethos and Commando values.

## Why have an ethos?

Too much can be made of a group's ethos at times, and this is probably true even of the Royal Marines' own. Because of the way the media – and therefore the public – view the military, the Corps' ethos is often wrongly interpreted, but it is not actually difficult to explain or comprehend. It is certainly not complicated.

An ethos is most simply defined as what a group does and how it does it. Consequently the ethos of the Royal Marines refers to their role and the way it is fulfilled. As outlined in a previous chapter, since the Second World War the Royal Marines have developed a specific role as the United Kingdom's Commando and amphibious force, undertaking Operations in all harsh environments, whether mountain, jungle, cold weather or desert. The difficult and unique role of the Royal Marines means that every individual Royal Marine requires specific personal characteristics. These values are nurtured at the Commando Training Centre during training and then maintained and developed throughout a Royal Marine's career. It is because of these individual qualities that Royal Marines are able to fulfil their role successfully; and it is this ethos that sets apart all Royal Marines Commandos.

## The Commando spirit

If you ask any Royal Marine what are the four elements of the Commando spirit, he will tell you that they are:

- **Courage**
- **Determination**
- **Unselfishness**
- **Cheerfulness in the face of adversity**

By the time they have completed Commando training these elements are well known to all Recruits, not just as words but as things they have seen in their friends and themselves.

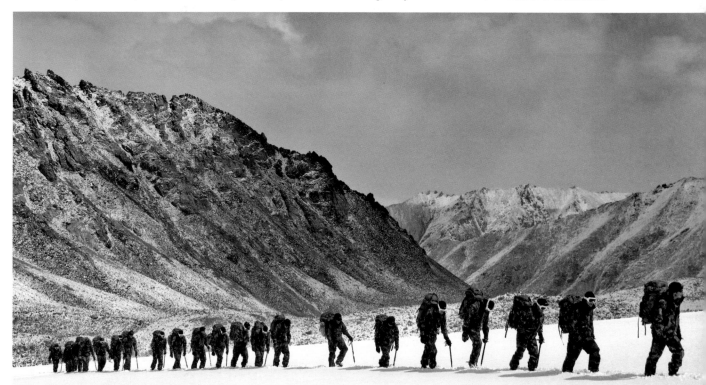

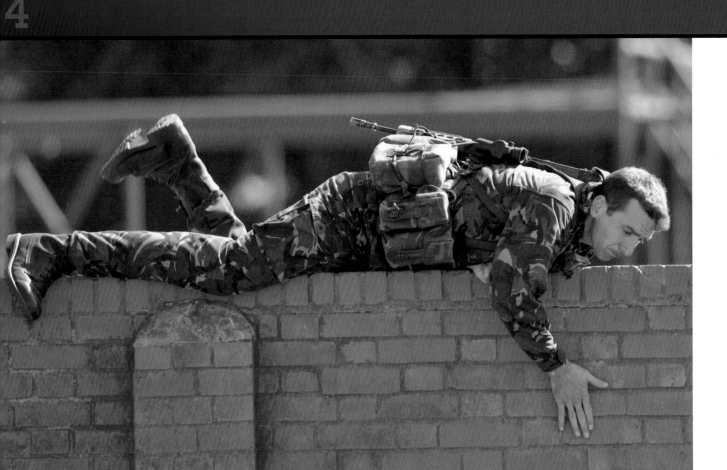

## The Corps' values

- **Courage**
- **Unity**
- **Determination**
- **Adaptability**
- **Unselfishness**
- **Humility**
- **Cheerfulness**
- **Professional standards**
- **Fortitude**
- **Commando humour**

Of these, courage, determination, unselfishness and cheerfulness are the special personal qualities contributed by the Royal Marines themselves. The rest are what might be termed collective values.

### Unity

The unity within the Royal Marines is unique in that it crosses all ranks. It draws its strength from an obvious yet very important outward sign: the green beret, which everyone equally earns the right to wear. Unity is bred into Recruits and Young Officers alike as they train side by side at the Commando Training Centre. The shared hardship of the Commando Course not only sets this unity going but also sets it in concrete. Unlike other military organisations, where officers and other ranks train in totally separate locations, the Royal Marines ensure that every single Commando trains at CTCRM. Furthermore, Commando training

stresses the importance of the *team*; the 30-Miler must be completed as a syndicate and the Nine-Miler must be finished as a whole troop. No one completes Royal Marines training as an individual: only unity will complete the course. The Royal Marines then takes this unity, learned in training, wherever it goes – different ranks, a variety of jobs, but the overriding factor is the unity we share because we all wear the green beret.

### Adaptability

Unity provides solidarity and trust across all ranks – which means that Royal Marines can be open to opinions from every person, angle and rank, and are able to adapt to new knowledge. Going back to its formation in the Second World War, but still relevant today, the Corps' Commando role requires Royal Marines to be adaptable and able to respond to new developments at very short notice. Early in training Recruits learn to expect the unexpected, and during the Commando phase exercises they become very accustomed to the phrase 'dislocation of expectation'; constant uncertainty is part of operational life in the Corps. Uncertainty breeds a 'can do' attitude, and an ability to innovate and improvise that becomes second nature to all members of the Royal Marines.

As a self-sustaining unit the Corps is able to maintain itself with little external support; as a consequence, Royal Marines often multi-task, being able to juggle a number of different roles at any one time. Consequently the Royal Marines remain open to external institutions while ensuring that they stay adaptable and flexible.

### ■ Humility

As an elite organisation, outsiders often expect the Royal Marines to be arrogant, but this could not be further from the truth. In fact the Royal Marines are often criticised for their understated approach by those in the know. This is not just false modesty. The Royal Marines strongly believe that arrogant organisations are never prepared to learn from others for fear of looking weak. The Royal Marines by contrast are always looking for new approaches and ways of doing things; warfare, soldiering and, indeed, physical training are forever developing, so why not keep an open mind when working with other forces and organisations? Anyhow, it is no secret that arrogance leads to inflexibility and rigidity, which does not fit in with the Royal Marines' adaptable nature. In addition, its humility has enabled the Corps to operate with considerable success when interacting with civilian populations and non-combatants.

### ■ Professional standards

Professional standards in the Royal Marines encompass so much, from keeping fit as an individual to ensuring 'admin' is up to date (see page 40), and from personal appearance to soldiering skills. For a Royal Marine, it is a surprise to see anyone, from any organisation or walk of life, acting unprofessionally, and it is perhaps this adherence to the highest professional standards that ensures the success of the Royal Marines as a military force. In a wartime context, it is being professional that will keep the individual Royal Marine and his fellow Royal Marines alive.

The wartime environments in which Commandos operate are complex, dangerous and uncertain, and being successful and staying alive calls for the highest professional standards. In training, all Recruits are taught the same 'core skills', so that they become second nature. These standards are then able to generate an individual and collective response to any situation, where everyone knows their role, has their responsibilities, and has the correct and workable kit and equipment, and no one lets the team down.

### ■ Fortitude

It is a common misconception that elite forces are made up of super-fit athletes. They are not, and the Royal Marines are no exception. We do not actively recruit super-fit or super-athletic individuals, but such is the mystique surrounding elite forces that people imagine they could take their place in Olympic teams or match Olympian performances whenever they feel like it! However, although the Royal Marines have indeed delivered, and still do deliver, a number of athletes of international standard, and although there are some incredibly fit individuals in the Corps, this is not the case. Although all Commandos are robust, fitter than average and strong-minded, most are by no means Olympians.

Fortitude guarantees the achievements that are made possible by physical fitness, while physical fitness alone cannot always ensure success. Unlike athletes, Royal Marines must be fit in all areas. It is essential, for instance, that along with strength they possess endurance and stamina. Nor can such fitness depend on a good night's sleep and a specific diet. Instead,

lack of sleep, uncertainty, apprehension and hostile weather conditions often add to the physical challenges faced by Royal Marines. They have to be comfortable operating at −30° in the Arctic, and equally comfortable patrolling at altitude on rugged terrain in Afghanistan. And it is *fortitude* that ensures these feats are possible – the ability to endure, no matter what the conditions and no matter how tired the individual. The 'yomp' across the Falkland Islands, the altitude of Afghanistan, the heat of Iraq, all were overcome by individual physical fitness and collective fortitude; mental will that builds upon, but goes beyond, professional skills and physical fitness.

### ■ Commando humour

Royal Marines are known throughout the British military as having a very broad sense of humour. As long as it does not affect their professionalism, how better to endure hardship than with humour? One of the four individual Commando spirit characteristics – 'cheerfulness in the face of adversity' – is made possible only by humour, which although apparently superfluous to operational effectiveness is actually fundamental to the way that Royal Marines operate. A sense of humour allows individual Royal Marines to come to terms with demanding and sometimes devastating situations, whether physical hardship or the apprehension and uncertainty of Operations. Though such humour can seem incomprehensible to an outsider it is second nature to us after just a few weeks of training. It is the only way that Royal Marines have been able to attempt, complete, succeed and put behind them some of the Operations they have had to deal with. Commando humour is very unique. It is not to everyone's taste but it allows Royal Marines not only to endure hardship but to actually find enjoyment while enduring.

## Dits

'Dits' are stories that are told to describe anything that has happened. They can be work or pastime-related, but usually have a specific moral or joke behind them. 'Spinning dits' is so fundamental to life in the Royal Marines that it has become an important way of sustaining the RM ethos. Royal Marines have a dit for every occasion, and consequently dits about operational experiences are fundamental during all stages of training, where recent operational experience is invaluable. Dits are a crucial means of ensuring that the history of the Corps and the memory of specific characters is maintained. They are essential to communicating new methods, knowledge, skills and, most importantly, the attitudes necessary to the performance of the Corps. Furthermore, when any free time becomes available while on Operations, and any necessary physical training has taken place, dits are the only entertainment to while away the hours. For many Marines, a dit session is far better than watching TV or listening to the radio!

# P.T. Branch

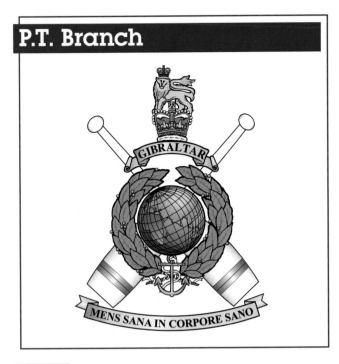

GIBRALTAR

MENS SANA IN CORPORE SANO

## Lifestyle

The motto of the Royal Marines Physical Training branch is *mens sana in corpore sano*, meaning a healthy mind in a healthy body. With a sound, exercised and healthy body comes a sound, relaxed, focused mind able to concentrate and perform at the very top level.

There are many thousands of different lifestyles found across the world. Often external factors affect and direct the way we live our lives, or make us choose a specific type of lifestyle. Except for those living in extreme poverty or in war-torn countries, most of us have the opportunity to do something about our lifestyle and to make a conscious decision to improve it. For Royal Marines, however, lifestyle is entirely dependent on the role being undertaken at the time: when training or on Operations, their lifestyle is very different from that of a unit based back in the UK. It must be said, though, that in any walk of life a small amount of exercise or physical activity can lead to vast improvements in lifestyle.

## Physical activity and lifestyle

Physical training can lead to huge lifestyle improvements and a feeling of fulfilment, health and well-being. During and post-exercise, specific chemicals (such as endorphins) are released into the body, which often give the exerciser a feeling of elation. Although this is a positive effect, and leads to training pattern, it can also lead to an addiction to physical training, which can be dangerous to your health long-term. Most people, however, do not get to this addictive stage (it often requires very hard training sessions to continually get an elated feeling); for most of us, following a training session simply provides a feeling of contentment, either at what has been achieved or that the session is over for the day!

Lifestyle-wise, the benefits of physical fitness go much further than just the release of chemicals during and following the session. Obviously there are a number of improvements to health, from a lower resting heart rate and lower blood pressure to a loss of body fat and increase of toned muscle. Furthermore, beyond the natural improvements to health, incorporating a fitness-training schedule into a lifestyle can also improve mental focus and confidence, and – with the vast number of members in some of the large gyms today – can even increase social interaction.

## Lifestyle in the Royal Marines

As stated above, lifestyle in the Corps depends heavily on the role being undertaken – obviously, a steady fitness regime is not easy to schedule when operating in Afghanistan. However, the Royal Marines have created a culture, and therefore for most a lifestyle, in which arduous physical activity plays a large part wherever Royal Marines may find themselves. Regular and varied exercise helps keep Royal Marines physically and mentally effective. Most Royal Marines find – whether they have been patrolling the barren lands of Afghanistan, sitting behind a computer at the MoD in London, or teaching Recruits all day at CTCRM – that a physical training session not only keeps the body healthy but also helps to clear the mind, and to de-stress and help refocus for the next day.

In addition, a lifestyle containing regular physical training also contributes to Commandos being relatively free from illness – it is very rare for Royal Marines to take 'sick days'. Of course, everyone gets sick at some point, but in general a sensible fitness regime helps ensure a strong and active immune system.

For most people, and certainly for Royal Marines, a routine containing regular exercise also leads to an overall positive, healthy and well-balanced lifestyle. It is important to do everything in moderation, and often a busy lifestyle means individuals are tired and do not find time to exercise. However, a few sessions of exercise a week actually lead to most people being more energetic and finding more time for hobbies and socialising.

## Lifestyle in Recruit and Young Officer training

While in training a Recruit's lifestyle is very hectic. When on camp, if he is not in lessons or physical training periods he is eating or writing up his notes, working through his personal 'admin' (as in tasks that must be completed – see below) or performing group admin tasks in the accommodation building. He will most likely be sleep-deprived and fatigued from his very active lifestyle. However, every corridor of every Recruit Troop's accommodation has at least one pull-up bar on the wall. Irrespective of whether or not they are told to perform pull-ups due to a weakness revealed in structured PT sessions, each Recruit will eventually succumb to the Commando habit of continual physical development and perform a few pull-ups every time he passes the bar! If you can adopt this habitual nature, your physical goals will soon become a reality.

## Lifestyle on Operations

An operational tour is arguably the most difficult time for any Royal Marine to perform constructive physical training. Despite the rigours of operational life – long arduous patrols, potential combat situations, sleep deprivation, extremes of climate, an unusual diet and the like – most Royal Marines will nevertheless still find some time for it. This training is often performed in groups, which encourages social interaction and combined effort. As explained below, physical training is an excellent tool for combating stress. Furthermore, group exercise sessions can enhance these de-stressing effects with a spice of humour. When very arduous physical training is performed it is often humorous for the group to watch someone else suffering, even though they will themselves have to endure the same exercises minutes later!

## Lifestyle in a unit

Day-to-day life in a Commando Unit often revolves around training, be it tactical training, field training, specific environment or operational training. Whatever the focus is, Royal Marines will always find time for physical training, be it first thing in the morning as part of the Troop or Company daily routine, or in the evening in their own time. All Commando Units are blessed with superb gyms, local running routes and an infectious enthusiasm for training that encourages them to continue striving to improve the fitness that they gained during Commando training. Again, it becomes habitual, and often Royal Marines living on the camp only go home at weekends, and hence have plenty of time to train together in the evening. Even those who live locally or in married accommodation seem to stay late to join in. Again, this attitude is inbuilt, habitual and infectious.

## Habit

If physical training is made part of a daily routine it becomes a lot easier to maintain. For Royal Marines this 'habit' is instilled relatively easily during the initial stages of Commando training, when Recruits have no choice but to take part in PT sessions unless they become injured. Even then it is possible to continue training with some types of injury, by utilising alternative exercises that will not cause further harm. So, as Recruits have no choice but to exercise this 'habit' is slowly ingrained into them during training. The majority then take this habit – and the need to improve on the fitness already achieved – on into their careers as Royal Marine Commandos. Furthermore many Royal Marines also take the habit with them into their life outside the Corps when they leave.

Once self-motivation is created – especially for a specific reason – there is a mindset that leads to Royal Marines thinking 'I must train, I must improve, I must be fit'. Consequently every Royal Marine will strive to find the time to train. Such a habit must be created, but once it is it will become part of a daily or weekly lifestyle. It will become something to look forward to and get through the day for. This is why it is so important to create such a habit.

## Finding time

It is often hard to find time to train during a busy lifestyle. However, it is important to stay motivated and to *make* yourself find time. Royal Marines cannot always be prescriptive in their training, especially when on Operations or when performing particularly important tasks. These other commitments must be fulfilled in priority to personal physical training. This is true for most people during their daily lives. Nevertheless, it should not stop anyone finding opportunities to maintain a level of fitness.

Although books such as this will help you, it is important to have a few quick training sessions in your head, which will help you to maintain fitness when only a limited amount of time is available. It may be hard to do it, but if time is tight set the alarm clock for half an hour – or even an hour – earlier, and squeeze in a quick body-weight circuit or half an hour run before the day starts. Remember, if you do set the alarm early for training it is all too easy to switch it off and go back to sleep. Do not allow yourself to do this – be strong and stay motivated!

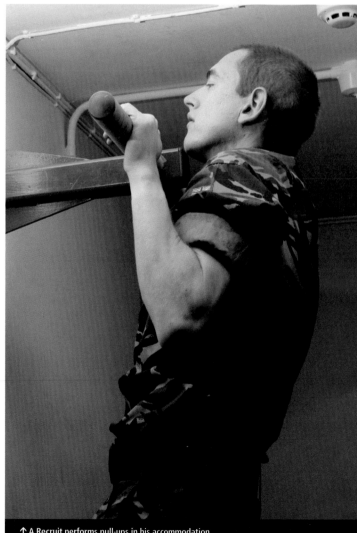

↑ A Recruit performs pull-ups in his accommodation.

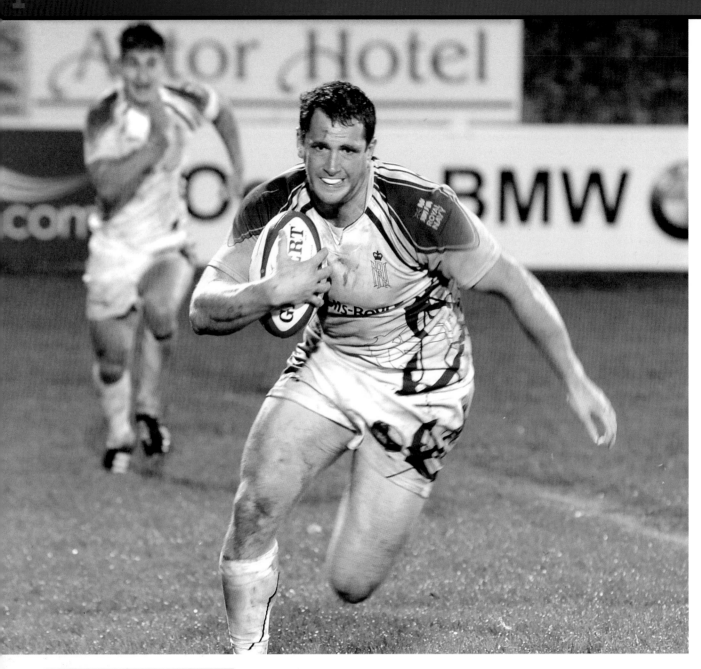

## Combined effort and competition

Training with others, particularly in a sports team, is a great way to keep fit if you do not particularly like fitness training. By playing or training for a specific sport the mind is taken off the fact that exercise is being undertaken, which often makes it easier. Furthermore, being part of a sports team or club is a great way of meeting people and socialising away from the pub. In the Royal Marines and in the forces in general, we use team sports and other team-related activities to foster a collective team spirit and to create healthy competition. Every year the Army and Navy play rugby union at Twickenham, with a large number of Royal Marines playing for the Navy. Each Commando Unit sends coach-loads of supporters and the Corps makes a real day of it. The Royal Marines and the Parachute Regiment play rugby league against each other

every year too. Again, this fosters a great collective unity and team spirit amongst players and supporters alike. Team sports are also a great way of unwinding and de-stressing, both individually and collectively, be it while playing or when chatting afterwards.

## Team building

Competition and team building is very important in the military and certainly in the Royal Marines. However, this is equally true in any walk of life, company or industry. More and more these days, businesses are spending money on corporate team-building days, but playing a team sport can often be just as valuable. Competition is a great asset to the Royal Marines and could prove so for any company or business. Despite this, competition must be handled correctly: there should be no malice or aggression, just determination and a will to win.

Team activities and competitions are not restricted to organised sports competitions or games on the playing field. Give a group of Royal Marines a golf ball or a table-tennis ball and they will soon be bouncing it across the room and into a mug or someone's empty boot in some form of competition.

## Stress reduction

Stress reduction is an important part of life these days. It seems that whatever we are doing, it 'stresses us out'. Exercise and physical training is an excellent stress combatant. As stated above, exercising can in fact reinvigorate you when you are feeling tired, low or unmotivated. On top of that it is also a great de-stressor, which is ironic considering that stress is often a cause of individuals feeling too tired to train! It is thought that any form of physical activity can contribute enormously to reducing stress levels; whether you are a high-flying businessman in London, a local policeman doing his rounds or even someone who has recently ended a marriage, it is believed that exercise can help to refocus the mind, provide time to think and help to de-stress the body overall.

For many people, even the anticipation of physical activity takes their mind off whatever is worrying them. I personally used this with great success during exam periods at university, where an hour's run in the sun gave me time to think and got me away from the books. When I returned I was relaxed and ready to refocus. Many people find that while training they have time to think and consider things, and post-training have better clarity of thought regarding decisions and pressing issues. I have found that when faced with a difficult work or social situation a long run, on my own with my thoughts, has often led to me making a good decision.

## Repetition and routine

When exercising we often get into a routine, and soon enough we are doing the same session on the same day of the week, every week. This is not a problem, and if it helps with motivation and ensures that you keep to your exercise routine it can be a very positive thing. However, it is also easy to slip into an easy routine, where you can complete every session easily and are never pushing the boundaries. If you have reached your required level of fitness and are just looking to maintain, this is fine. However, if you are striving for improvement this comfortable routine probably needs breaking. Mix it up a bit, train with others or try something new.

Training outdoors is a superb way to remain motivated, especially in the summer; it is not only a great way to see and appreciate the environment, it is a great way to break up a routine. For example, even when a specific running route is done frequently, it will vary significantly depending on the time of day it is run – you will pass different people and encounter different weather. Furthermore, if you are aiming at a specific time, something I call 'the people effect' means that you tend to speed up when people can see you, and you will surprise yourself with the times you achieve! In some ways the same can be said for a busy gym: a half-treadmill run will be varied by the people around, the music listened to, etc. Personally I use these changes to take my mind off what I am doing when it is really hard. Trying to run a certain speed for a certain time can be very challenging on the mind, with it constantly telling you to slow down; so look around, take notice of your surroundings, listen to the words of a song intently, anything to avoid feeling bored or thinking too deeply about what you are doing.

In general running and training outdoors can have more positive effects – it is certainly more inspiring in the summer. Another great benefit to training outdoors is the feeling of freedom. This is especially important if de-stressing is a real motivation for undertaking training. Getting out in the fresh air, forgetting about all the worries of your job, can be a great way to end a hard day's work. Lastly, training outdoors is an excellent thing to do if you are away from home in a new area. By going for runs in different directions from where you are staying you can explore the area quickly and get a good feel for where you are.

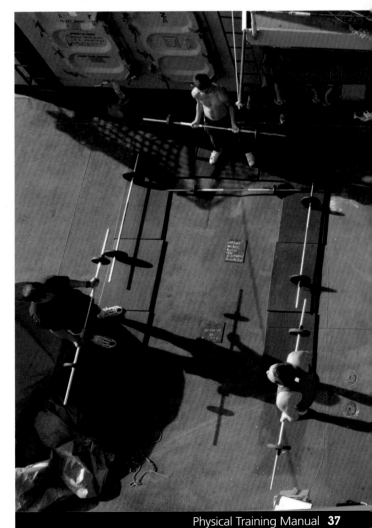

## Negative effects on lifestyle

Although physical training is very important for a healthy lifestyle, it can also be detrimental in some circumstances. The following are examples of negative effects that can occur when training is undertaken, or if you train too much. Though many of these are also mentioned elsewhere in this book it is worth reiterating them here, since it is important that you can recognise them in your own lifestyle:

### ■ Fatigue

The body and mind can become fatigued by continued, intense exercise over long periods of time. This will obviously have lifestyle effects, as it causes a reduction in your ability to participate in other activities – there is no point, for instance, in doing a ten-mile run before a date at the cinema and then falling asleep during the film!

### ■ Injury

Everyone will experience injury at some point in their training. If you are injured it is important to rest the affected area. There are too many factors that contribute to injury to name them all. However, if you remain sensible and ensure a varied training programme injuries should be kept to a minimum.

### ■ Overtraining

As stated throughout this book, overtraining is the main problem for most fitness enthusiasts. Not only can overtraining lead to injury and fatigue, it can also be detrimental to any fitness gains long term.

### ■ Repetition injuries

If the same session is repeated and the same muscle group is exercised day after day, it is basically being overtrained in an individually specific way.

### ■ Increased temperature

A good training session, especially cardiovascular, can often raise the core temperature and cause profuse sweating during and also for some time after the session.

## Positive effects on lifestyle

I would hope that by this stage you are already sold on the fact that physical training is a good thing and will have a number of positive advantages in your lifestyle. However, the following are some of the major positive effects:

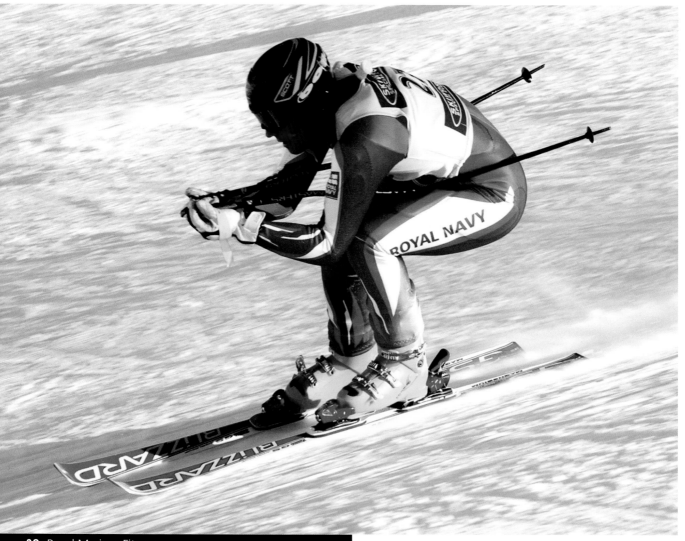

### Feeling good/self-confidence

In improving your physical fitness, whether in terms of strength, endurance or stamina, there is a real feel-good factor. You will feel good about yourself and your achievements. This in turn increases self-confidence in all areas of life, be it in work, sports or attracting a partner.

### Social effects

Physical training can have a positive social effect on your life, especially if your fitness revolves around a team sport. There is a sense of belonging that occurs within any team (often coming from shared hardships, be they hard training sessions or losing a hard-fought match). Furthermore, joining a gym also leads to a new social circle with a shared fitness goal.

### Talking point

Appearing physically fit or being seen doing a fitness session is something to talk about with friends, family or maybe even a future partner ('Check out my biceps' does not always work, however). This talking point goes hand in hand with the social effect of meeting new people, as completing a hard session or doing a challenging exercise will often lead to others asking about it.

### Concentration

As was mentioned earlier, the Royal Marines PT branch motto of *mens sana in corpore sano* means (translated literally) a healthy mind in a healthy body. Looking at this in context, it is saying that with a sound, exercised and healthy body, the mind is also sound, relaxed, focused and able to concentrate and perform to the best of its ability.

### Social barriers broken

Physical training and exercise puts everyone on a level playing field, and therefore breaks all social and economic barriers. Royal Marines are recruited from a cross-section of society in this country and abroad. Despite different cultures, thought processes, motivations and social backgrounds, during any physical training everyone finds themselves on the same level. The same can be seen when exercising in the local park or at the local gym.

### Guilty pleasures

A good friend of mine who is a Navy Commando is quite happy to admit that one of the main reasons he trains with me and trains so hard is so that he can enjoy all the cakes and brownies that the local coffee shops provide! As Chapter 6 will explain, a healthy all-round diet is important to all-round physical fitness, but the odd indulgence is important for keeping a fresh and happy outlook on life. By training hard it can feel 'earned', and therefore more easily justifiable! It is not good to be so rigid as to starve the body of all treats. However, it is equally important to avoid eating junk food.

### Earned rest

In today's fast-paced culture rest is often viewed as being lazy. Many of us feel guilty and feel that we should be working, studying, or visiting relatives – or just doing *something*. The

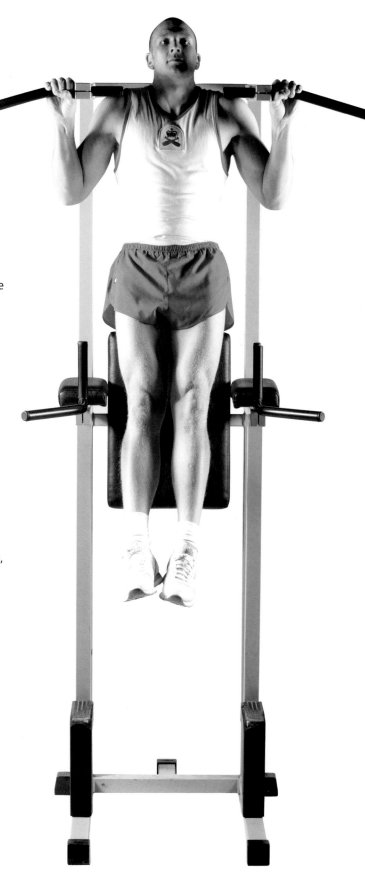

mantra 'you only live once' makes us believe that we should be active all the time. However, if you perform regular exercise and train hard, the physical activity allows you to enjoy your relaxation and de-stress without feeling guilty; you feel as if you have earned it.

### Personal administration

The term 'admin' is used throughout the military but probably even more so amongst Commandos. It is used to refer to affairs or things that need to be done and the ability to manage them. Personal administration is just as essential to a healthy lifestyle as physical training, as it applies structure and discipline to a chaotic world, from very specific military tasks such as maintaining your rifle and other equipment to looking after your uniform and possessions. It includes maintaining a good standard of personal hygiene, phoning your family, writing letters and organising your personal finances. In short admin covers everything that an individual must do individually, from daily tasks to yearly mortgage meetings.

### ■ Weapons and equipment

A Royal Marine without his weapon is next to useless, hence when on Operations or on exercise the most important admin task is the cleaning and maintenance of the Royal Marine's individual weapon. This is drilled into every Royal Marine at

## Concurrent activity

**These two words are drilled into every Marine during his first few weeks in training. When doing any admin, whether on camp or in the field, concurrent activity can really cut down on the time that a large amount of admin would take, the idea being that while waiting for something, something else can be done. Cooking in the field is a great example: it is easy, especially when tired, just to sit and watch some water boil for ten minutes and let the mind wonder. However, during those ten minutes a weapon could be cleaned, some blisters could be dressed or a button could be sewn back on to a shirt. Concurrent activity is a must in the fast-paced world of a Commando.**

a very early stage in his training. On all field exercises the Recruit's equipment is inspected first thing in the morning to ensure that they have cleaned and maintained their kit and, most important of all, their weapon.

It is while they are still Recruits that Royal Marines also learn the order in which admin occurs, whether in the field or when returning to a camp or secure location: 'your weapon, your kit, your self' – meaning that his weapon will be addressed first, split down, cleaned, oiled and reassembled; then he will clean his kit,

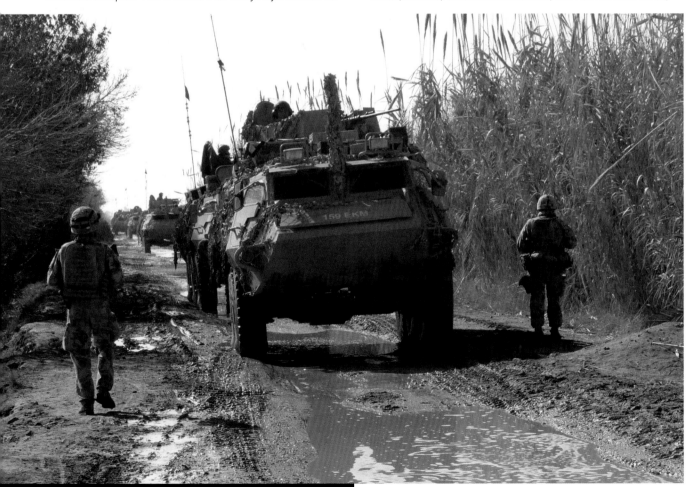

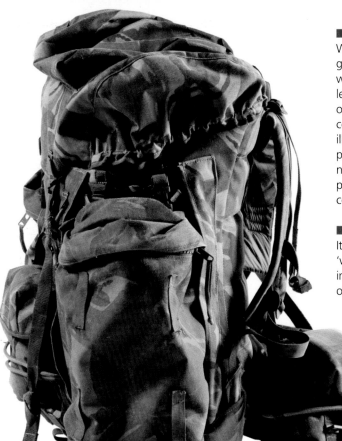

### ■ Personal hygiene and appearance

Whether in the field, on ship or on camp, Royal Marines take great pride in their personal hygiene, and have a reputation within the Armed Forces of perhaps taking it to extreme lengths! It is not uncommon for Royal Marines to have three or four showers a day, which some people find hard to comprehend. However, if one man gets an infection or illness because of his poor hygiene, the close working proximity of Royal Marines to each other means that it would not be long before everyone was affected by the same problem. Soon enough a whole troop or company would be combat ineffective.

### ■ Family admin

It is well known that a Royal Marine who has issues at home or 'welfare' problems does not do his job to maximum effectiveness in the majority of cases. Therefore, from their time in training onwards, all Royal Marines are given time and facilities to write and call home. Today, with mobile phones, this is much easier, but keeping in touch with your family is still considered to be part of personal admin, both to prevent the Royal Marine from worrying about those at home, and so that those at home know that the Royal Marine is safe. Again, this family admin is started early, with family and close friends invited to CTCRM at week 3 of training, to see the Recruits in their new environment. This relationship between Royal Marine, family and the Corps then exists as long as the Royal Marine wants it, throughout his career and beyond. The Royal Marines family is a very large and far-reaching one.

ensuring his magazines are clean and working correctly, and that any metal kit, such as his bayonet, is free of rust; and then lastly he will address himself, taking a wash, changing his socks etc, and seeing to any minor medical issues such as blisters or grazes.

When in the field it is imperative that each Royal Marine cleans and maintains his equipment, his weapon and himself. If anything is broken, he does his best to fix it with whatever he has (spare boot laces, needle and thread etc) but also makes it known to his hierarchy that he needs a replacement. This will either be sent to him, depending on what it is, or he may have to wait until his return to camp.

Once back on camp every Royal Marine must give all his kit a deep clean. This is again learnt during Recruit training, where a full kit inspection is carried out following every field exercise. Whether Recruit or trained Royal Marine, his weapon will be stripped down as far as legally allowed and then washed, dried and checked. His Bergen and webbing is emptied scrubbed clean of all mud and dirt, the same going for all the rest of his kit. Everything is stripped, cleaned, dried and checked. If anything is found to be broken it must be exchanged as soon as possible. This is because all Royal Marines could be deployed at very short notice, and if kit needs cleaning or exchanging because of laziness this could have dire effects on that individual's effectiveness, which could in turn have a knock-on effect on his section or troop.

## Conclusion

**The RM ethos can be applied to physical training and the way individuals go about their training to meet any challenge. Coupled with a solid motivation and a strong willpower is a real road to success. The same Commando qualities may provide the ethos of the Royal Marines, but they are not just for use by Commandos; the qualities can be embraced by anyone who wants to be successful in work, life or in the pursuit of being physically fit. Tied in strongly with this ethos is the Royal Marines lifestyle. This chapter has shown that physical fitness and disciplined self administration are essential constituents of a healthy lifestyle. Whatever your goals or lifestyle, physical fitness can help overcome stressful problems and difficult situations. Royal Marines have to operate effectively under substantial levels of stress, often far from home. Although physical fitness helps them manage this stress, it also enriches and enhances their lives.**

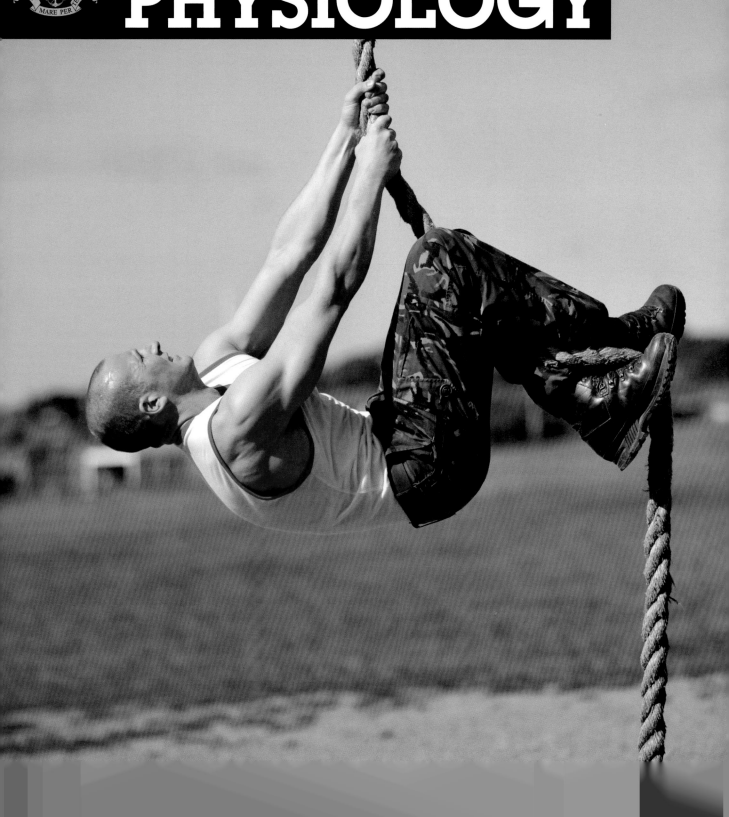

To improve the overall physical fitness of individuals there is a need to understand the fundamental components of physical fitness, which is why Royal Marines PTIs study anatomy and physiology during their PT course. However, physiology, let alone anatomy, is a huge subject, and going into too much depth will do nothing but confuse the casual reader and casual gym-goer. Therefore this chapter will do no more than touch briefly upon those important areas in physiology that will make your training more beneficial, all of which fall under the banner 'exercise physiology' – the study of the function of the human body during exercise conditions. But it should be understood from the outset that the effects of exercise are significant, whether at low or high intensity, in short bursts like a 100-metre sprint or prolonged endurance events such as the 30-Miler or marathons.

## Energy

As you will already be aware, our bodies need energy for everything we do: movement, growth, repair, and to keep our hearts beating. Humans have a high capacity to expend energy for many hours doing sustained exercise; and in the process we burn energy and therefore calories, both during and after exercising. The amount of energy expended by the muscles at rest or at work varies with size, gender and age, but will aid weight loss and fitness regardless.

All of our energy comes from the food we ingest, as described in Chapter 6. We can get all our energy requirements from a good all-round diet containing the carbohydrates, fats and proteins that our bodies require to produce it. Once the food has been ingested and broken down, our bodies can store this energy in a number of different ways, ready for when it is required. However, this energy can only be used when it is in the form of the chemical compound ATP (adenosine tri-phosphate). Unfortunately, our muscles can only store small amounts of ATP at a time, so for all the activities we undertake our bodies have to keep making it. If the level of activities being undertaken means that our muscles use up this ATP faster than it can be produced, then we will get tired and have to slow down or stop what we are doing.

## Energy systems

To provide our bodies with more energy (ATP) as we use it up, we have three different energy systems: the creatine phosphate system, the lactic acid system (or anaerobic glycolysis system) and the aerobic system. The three systems work together to maintain the muscles' energy in the form of ATP at all times.

### ■ The creatine phosphate energy system
### (0–30 seconds of hard/explosive work)

This is the body's system for generating energy for immediate maximal efforts, more quickly than the other two. However, due to the nature of the way it works, it can only provide energy for very short periods of time. Examples of activities that a Recruit would go through to use this energy system would include climbing a 30-foot rope, and sprinting to take cover during an exercise battle or on the assault course during a BPT session (see Chapter 8).

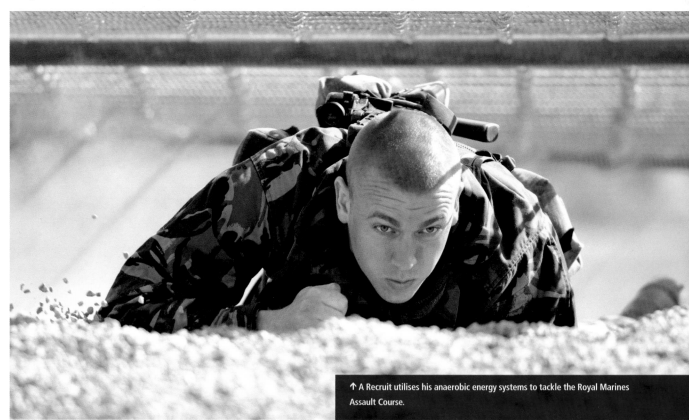

↑ A Recruit utilises his anaerobic energy systems to tackle the Royal Marines Assault Course.

### ■ Lactic acid (anaerobic glycolysis) energy system (1–2 minutes of hard work)

This system can provide energy relatively quickly, but is not long-lasting, so the muscles tire quickly as waste products build up in them, causing fatigue and pain. Examples of situations in which a Recruit may find himself using this energy system are the Tarzan Assault Course or a normal IMF (Initial Military Fitness) session, for which see Chapters 8 and 9.

### ■ The aerobic energy system

This system can provide energy indefinitely, providing sufficient fuel is available. However, it must have oxygen to work and therefore requires the energy expenditure not to exceed a certain level. Recruits would use this energy system when doing the 30-Miler, general yomping or undertaking a speed march. (Again, see later chapters regarding these.)

### ■ Energy systems interaction

Obviously, when performing a 30-Miler almost all the energy provided will be from the aerobic system; but when throwing a javelin the creatine phosphate system will be used. However, if a session involves various activities – such as in a football match or a Royal Marines training period – all three systems will be used in conjunction with each other. The amount each system is used will depend on the intensity of activity at any particular point, as well as how long that intensity needs to last.

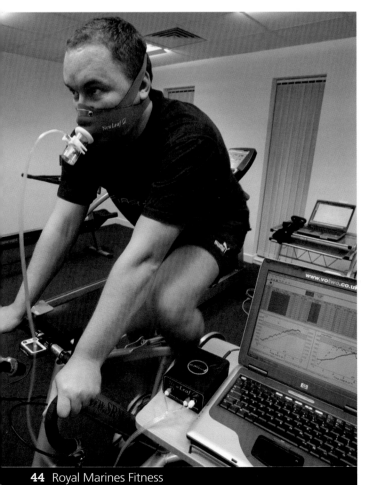

The following table shows the sources of energy for different sport/activities in which you may be engaged:

| % aerobic | Events | Primary energy sources |
|---|---|---|
| 0 | Weight lifting, 100m/200m sprint. Sprinting for cover in battle. | Creatine phosphate and lactic acid system. |
| 10 | 100m swim, 400m sprint. | Creatine phosphate and lactic acid system. |
| 20 | Tennis. | Creatine phosphate and lactic acid system. |
| 30 | Football. | Creatine phosphate and lactic acid system. |
| 40 | 800m run. Assault Course. | Creatine phosphate and lactic acid system. |
| 50 | Boxing. | Creatine phosphate, lactic acid and aerobic systems. |
| 60 | 1,500m run. Tarzan Assault Course. | Creatine phosphate, lactic acid and aerobic systems. |
| 70 | 800m swim. | Aerobic system. |
| 80 | 1.5-mile run (BFT). | Aerobic system. |
| 90 | Cross-country running. Speed marching. | Aerobic system. |
| 100 | Jogging. | Aerobic system. |

### Aerobic exercise

Performing aerobic exercises involving oxygen consumption overtime helps improve the body's utilisation of oxygen. Examples of aerobic exercise are vast, but simple examples are walking, running, cycling and swimming, each of which would be performed for a considerable length of time – eg running a long distance at a moderate pace is an aerobic exercise, but sprinting is not. To ensure these types of activity remain aerobic, each should be performed at low to moderate levels of intensity for an extended period of time.

During aerobic exercise the first thing to happen is that glycogen (a carbohydrate stored in the body) is broken down to produce glucose, which is then in turn broken down to generate energy; oxygen is needed to do this. In the absence of glycogen and therefore glucose, fat can be used for energy instead. Fat metabolism is a slower process than carbohydrate (glucose) metabolism, which means there is usually a dip in performance.

### Health benefits of aerobic exercise

■ Toning muscles throughout the body.
■ Strengthening the muscles involved in respiration.
■ Strengthening and enlarging the heart muscle, to improve its pumping efficiency.
■ Reduction of the resting heart rate.
■ Improved circulation efficiency.
■ Reduction of blood pressure.
■ Increased total number of red blood cells in the body (more transport of oxygen).

- Improved mental health, including stress and depression reduction.

Beyond its fitness gains, aerobic exercise can reduce the risk of death from cardiovascular problems. In addition, higher impact aerobic activities like running (not swimming or cycling) stimulate bone growth and reduce the risk of osteoporosis.

### Performance benefits
- Increased storage of energy molecules (fats and carbohydrates) within the muscles, allowing for increased endurance.
- Increased blood flow through the muscles.
- Increasing the speed at which aerobic metabolism is activated within muscles, allowing a greater portion of energy for intense exercise to be generated aerobically.
- Improving the ability of muscles to use fats during exercise, preserving glycogen (important in weight loss).
- Enhancing the speed at which muscles recover from high intensity exercise.

### Anaerobic exercise

Aerobic and anaerobic exercises differ by the duration and intensity of the muscular contractions required when exercising. Another major difference is how the energy is generated within the muscle. Generally, anaerobic exercise is the initial phase of any exercise, or any short burst of intense exertion. During this type of activity the glycogen stores in the muscles are consumed without oxygen, which is a faster but far less efficient process than that of aerobic exercise. As suggested, exercise must be considerably intense to trigger anaerobic metabolism; it is therefore non-endurance sports athletes that use it most, often for activities requiring power or to build muscle mass. However, a possible downside (or upside, depending on the individual's goal) is that muscles trained under anaerobic conditions develop differently, leading to greater performance in short duration, high intensity activities, which last up to about two minutes, but result in fatigue setting in very quickly during endurance events.

During prolonged anaerobic training, when lactic acid is produced faster than it can be removed, muscles will fatigue and eventually cease to work. This point is referred to as the anaerobic threshold. Exercising below this level is fine, as the body can remove any lactate produced by the muscles before it builds up. The anaerobic (or lactate) threshold is a useful measure for deciding exercise intensity and can be increased greatly with training.

For most people, the anaerobic threshold is thought to be between 90% and 95% of maximum heart rate. This type of training not only allows more effort to be exerted before fatigue sets in but also burns more calories than exercising at a constant continuous pace. It goes without saying that to train the aerobic system, long duration training below the lactate threshold is recommended.

### ■ VO2 max or aerobic capacity
The amount of energy used during exercise is directly related to the amount of oxygen consumed, as the breakdown of fat and glycogen requires oxygen. By comparing the oxygen content of

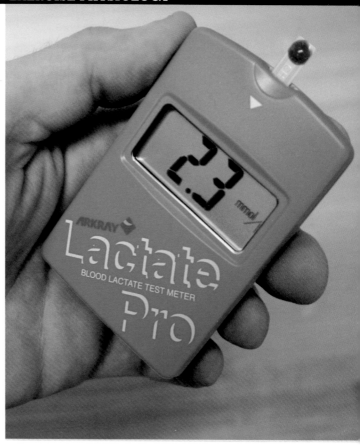

expired air with that of atmospheric air, the amount of energy used can be estimated.

At rest we consume 0.2–0.3 litres of oxygen per minute. This is our resting VO2 (v = volume, O2 = oxygen).

During maximal exercise this can rise to 4–6 litres of oxygen per minute, which would be the VO2 max.

For all of us our VO2 max can be improved by training, as it is determined by the efficiency of our cardiac, respiratory and muscular systems, which can all be improved with training. It is thought that the ability to improve varies vastly from person to person. Although an average improvement following training is thought to be an approximately 17% increase in VO2 max, it is thought that some 'high responders' can vastly improve their capacity, perhaps even doubling it. Conversely it is thought that some 'low responders' could see little or even no benefit from training. It is believed that this ability to improve by training is inherited and hence is a genetic trait.

To test a person's VO2 max it is necessary to make them perform progressively more strenuous exercise. This can be done a number of different ways. For potential Recruits and Recruits in training this is done using the Multi-Stage Fitness Test (or 'bleep test') – basically running between two points 20m apart in time to a bleep that gets faster and faster. The level at which the person drops out equates to their VO2 max score. Research exists showing that this method is not very accurate, but for Royal Marines training we are more interested in having a measurable test that can be repeated to ensure progress, rather than the actual VO2 max score. For Recruits level 10.5 must be reached, which equates to a VO2 max of 48.0.

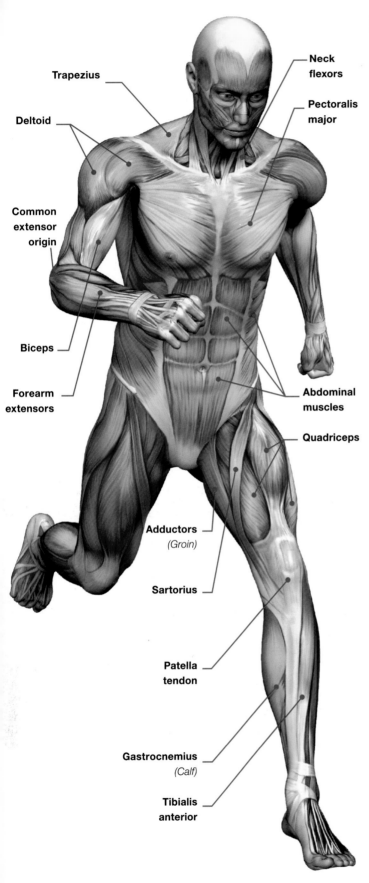

**Trapezius**

**Deltoid**

**Common extensor origin**

**Biceps**

**Forearm extensors**

**Neck flexors**

**Pectoralis major**

**Abdominal muscles**

**Quadriceps**

**Adductors**
*(Groin)*

**Sartorius**

**Patella tendon**

**Gastrocnemius**
*(Calf)*

**Tibialis anterior**

## Muscle types

Every single movement every day of your life relies on muscles. We already know that our muscles require energy to move: they convert the chemical energy from our food into the mechanical energy of movement by shortening and lengthening themselves. There are three types of muscle – cardiac, visceral and skeletal.

### ■ Cardiac muscle

Called myocardium muscle, this is found only in the heart. All the muscle cells/fibres act as a single sheet of muscle acting in unison. This muscle is totally involuntary (*ie* we cannot control it) and has its own blood supply. The heart is myogenic, meaning it generates its own impulse/beat.

### ■ Visceral muscle

These are also involuntary muscles, as they are controlled by involuntary parts of the nervous system. Associated with the viscera – internal organs such as arteries, stomach and bowel – the muscle cells/fibres are very fine, so appear smooth. Visceral muscles often form circular or longitudinal coats, so that when the (for example) artery/stomach muscle contracts blood/food is moved along.

### ■ Skeletal muscles

Connected to the skeleton either directly or indirectly, these are controlled by voluntary parts of the nervous system. These muscle cells are generally large and are bound together to form bundles or sheets. They have insertions and origins that attach them to the bone by white fibrous tissue called tendons or aponeuroses. To move the muscles, the origins remain fixed while the insertions move. Each muscle fibre is served by a nerve (motor unit), the contraction of the whole muscle being proportional to the number of fibres stimulated simultaneously.

Muscle tone is maintained by a small number of fibres being constantly stimulated, which is why being toned is so important for weight loss. By toning the muscles they will require and therefore burn more energy/calories all the time.

### ■ Skeletal muscle arrangements

Our muscles are normally arranged into pairs, so that as one contracts the other relaxes and vice versa. A simple example is the movement of the lower arm: when the biceps contracts, the triceps must relax and the lower arm is raised. To reverse this the triceps contracts and the biceps relax; if they do not the lower arm will not be lowered.

During these movements, we have different names for the muscles doing different jobs – in very basic (and not entirely accurate) terms, muscles that cause a joint to move are called 'flexors', whereas muscles that cause the joints to straighten are known as 'extensors'. Furthermore, the muscle that shortens to move the joint is referred to as the 'prime mover' or 'agonist', while the muscle that relaxes is called the 'antagonist'. If a muscle is an agonist for one movement, it will be the antagonist for the opposite movement. Muscles can also be called 'fixators' and 'synergists', as they stabilise the origin so that only the insertion moves.

## Types of muscle fibre

As has been said above, muscle fibres are grouped together in bundles, since as bundles they are powerful and strong compared to individual fibres. There are two types of muscle fibres:

### ■ Type 1: Slow twitch fibres

Slow twitch fibres contract around 20% slower than fast twitch fibres. They are physically smaller than the latter and generate force comparatively slowly. However, they do not fatigue easily like fast twitch fibres, meaning that they are excellent for low-level activity.

### ■ Type 2: Fast twitch fibres

These are faster acting than slow twitch fibres, but fatigue quickly. There are two sub-groups: Type 2a, or fast twitch high oxidative glycolytic (FOG), used for longer sprint events; and Type 2b, or fast twitch glycolytic, used for short sprint events. Type 2a have a greater resistance to fatigue than Type 2b. However, the fibres are believed to be able to adapt, so the number of each at any given time is down to endurance training.

All of our muscles are made of a mixture of fast and slow twitch fibres. It is believed that our percentage of each is a genetic trait and pretty much set. Although training can change the number of type 2a and b fibres, it is believed the number of fast or slow twitch fibres cannot be altered.

## Human thermoregulation

Thermoregulation and the ability to sweat make humans very evolutionarily advanced animals. Humans are specifically adapted to take part in prolonged strenuous endurance activities, such as long-distance running. This ability evolved to allow humans to run down (rather than hunt) game animals, by chasing them relatively slowly but persistently for many hours if necessary. This is only possible due to the ability of the human body to effectively remove muscle heat waste.

The majority of animals' bodies (many with thick fur coats) allow for a temporary increase in body temperature that enables them to escape from animals sprinting after them for a short duration, as is the case with most predators. But by removing heat using sweat evaporation, we have become very effective over *long* distances, exercising at a moderately high intensity even in heat. This ability to avoid fatigue from heat exhaustion has meant that humans chasing an animal will eventually catch it when it is itself forced to stop from fatigue brought on by heat exhaustion.

### ■ Dehydration

Thermoregulation is the body's way of ensuring that it remains at a relatively constant temperature, in order to avoid heat injuries or even death. The body combats the heat generated by exercise by sweating (or perspiration), producing water on the skin's surface

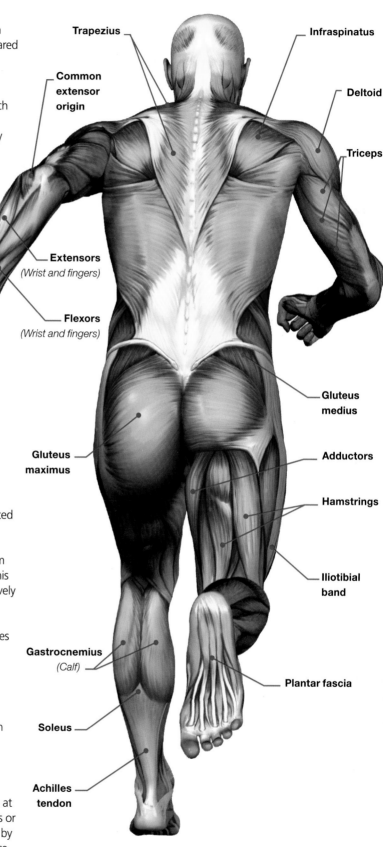

Trapezius

Infraspinatus

Common extensor origin

Deltoid

Triceps

Extensors
*(Wrist and fingers)*

Flexors
*(Wrist and fingers)*

Gluteus medius

Gluteus maximus

Adductors

Hamstrings

Iliotibial band

Gastrocnemius
*(Calf)*

Plantar fascia

Soleus

Achilles tendon

that evaporates and cools the body as it does so. Although it is a relatively simple process, sweating is particularly effective, especially when exercise is undertaken. Studies have shown that a male running a marathon will sweat around 0.8 litres in cool weather and up to 1.2 litres in warm weather. Furthermore, hard exercise sessions can lead to two and half times more fluid being lost in sweat than as urine.

A small percentage of dehydration can have profound effects on the body's ability to function. Exercising moderately hard with little water intake for around two hours in the heat (35°C) leads to a body mass decrease of around 5%, and more importantly a decrease in blood volume by up to 6%. Low fluid intake over a long exercise session also leads to a noticeable body temperature rise (as less fluid can be lost to sweat, so the system becomes less effective). A higher heart rate is seen as the body becomes dehydrated, which makes any exercises undertaken less effective. Furthermore, as the body sweats important electrolytes (such as sodium and potassium) are removed from the body along with

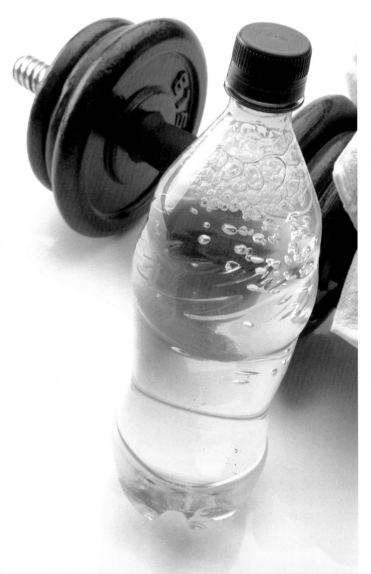

the water, and disturbances in the body's electrolyte balance lead to a loss of function in muscle contractions and in nervous impulses. As sports drink manufacturers regularly remind us, replacing the lost fluid and electrolytes counters these harmful effects, hence the importance of drinking and remaining hydrated when exercising.

Royal Marine Recruits have to keep a notebook, pen and water bottle with them at all times. Carrying the water bottle encourages them to drink and remain hydrated. It is a good bit of advice for everyone: carry a water bottle wherever you are and you will drink more.

### ■ Over-hydration

Despite the need to remain hydrated, it is also important to understand that drinking too much water can have a negative effect on salt (sodium) levels in the body, which can lead to issues such as encephalopathy, a swelling of the brain. Any issues such as this can be prevented by an awareness of the risks of drinking excessive amounts during prolonged exercise, something which I experienced when leading a YO 30- Miler across Dartmoor on a particularly hot day. One Young Officer started to have problems at around the 22-mile mark and by mile 24 had dropped out, collapsing about 20 metres from the checkpoint where the medical team were based (luckily for me). Due to the hot weather (around 25°C) he had been so keen not to become dehydrated that he had drunk too much and flushed all the electrolytes out of his body, which in the end was just as detrimental as being dehydrated.

### Changes in the body during exercise

A number of changes occur during exercise that the body has to cope with. The major ones are:

- ATP levels decrease.
- Creatine phosphate levels decrease.
- Glycogen levels decrease.
- Oxygen levels decrease.
- Carbon dioxide levels increase.
- Lactic acid levels increase.
- Body temperature increases.
- Fluid levels decrease.

### Short-term effects of exercise

Various areas within the body also change as we exercise. Those of interest to us here are the heart, lungs, blood and muscles.

### ■ Heart

Exercise starts adjusting the chemical balances within the body immediately; carbon dioxide and oxygen levels change, lactic acid increases, and of course body temperature increases. Our bodies have sensors to detect such changes and thus produce responses in our heart's pacemaker, which is told to increase the heart rate. Adrenaline is also released into the blood stream, increasing the heart rate even more. The overall effect is that cardiac output (the amount of blood pumped out of the heart in one minute) is increased as the heart is forced to make more frequent and stronger contractions.

### ■ Lungs

Changes in the proportions of oxygen and carbon dioxide are detected by the body, leading to an increase in the number of breaths and the tidal volume of the lungs (the amount of air breathed in or out with each breath). The lungs use their spare capacity (inspiratory and expiratory reserve volume) and the respiratory muscles, intercostals, diaphragm and scalene become more active, all of which increase the volume of the chest cavity and expels breath more forcefully.

### ■ Blood

Changes in blood composition are flagged very quickly by the body and initiate changes in heart rate and ventilation. Blood starts to become thicker as sweating leads to a lower volume of plasma. Furthermore, glucose levels in the blood drop as they are used to supply energy. The acidity of the blood increases due to lactic acid, which if not reversed leads to a detrimental effect on muscle activity.

The oxygen content of the blood drops dramatically, but blood flow speeds up, and more blood is directed to the muscles and away from other organs. Blood pressure also increases.

### ■ Muscles

Exercise leads to an increase in the intensity and frequency of contractions, leading to a greater use of energy. The need for extra energy means that the energy stores of creatine phosphate, glycogen and fatty acids are used up. Carbon dioxide and lactic acid levels increase in the muscles and need to be removed by the blood to avoid adverse effects on the muscles. Energy production in the muscles is actually quite inefficient, with a vast amount of energy (around 80%) being released as heat, thus increasing body temperature.

### Long-term effects of exercise

As with the short-term effects, some long-term effects are also seen with a good exercise regime. Obviously there will be an improvement in the individual's VO2 max when a continued programme containing sensible cardiovascular training is undertaken. This also markedly improves overall fitness, as the majority of the time an individual's muscles rely on the aerobic system of respiration.

Anaerobically, continued training – particularly if anaerobic training is included – leads to individuals being able to train for longer at high intensity. Type 2a and 2b muscle fibres (see above) grow in size and strength and stores of ATP, creatine phosphate and glycogen increase. Lastly an increased tolerance of lactic acid develops and, due to its better removal, an improved recovery system.

The following are also seen:

### ■ Heart

The muscles of the heart wall grow in size and strength, allowing more forceful contractions, pushing more blood around the body per heartbeat. This has an effect at rest, as the heart's stroke volume (the amount of blood pumped out of the heart in one contraction) will be greater as a result of the greater heart size. This means the heart has to beat less times per minute to push the same amount of blood, leading to a lower resting heart rate. Also, due to the large heart and stroke volume more oxygen is delivered to the muscles, meaning more efficiency and a potential increase in VO2 max.

### ■ Lungs

The respiratory muscles become stronger and more efficient, making respiration more efficient and easier, whether training or at rest. The maximum lung volume is increased, again making respiration more efficient at rest or during exercise. Lastly maximum lung capacity is also increased, allowing a greater area of the lung to be utilised.

### ■ Blood

The overall volume of the blood increases, plus more red blood cells are created leading to a greater oxygen-carrying capacity. The acidity (from carbon dioxide and lactic acid) of the blood during low-level exercise is also decreased, as the aerobic system is far more efficient. Furthermore, at high levels of exercise blood acidity is measured as far higher. This is down to training having given the individual an increased tolerance to its effects. Other changes are seen in the capillaries around the lungs and muscles, which mean that diffusion of oxygen is greater and more efficient.

### ■ Muscles

As you would expect, the muscles grow larger and stronger when a long-term exercise regime has been conducted. The muscles store larger amounts of glycogen and other energy-providing chemicals. A number of other changes also occur, such as an increased number of mitochondria in cells and more efficient enzymes, all of which lead to improved cellular respiration.

## Conclusion

**This chapter provides a basic outline of the most important aspects of physiology that apply when you exercise, and should have helped you to understand how your body works. There are plenty of books available on both exercise physiology and general physiology, and if either interests you I implore you to go and read further, to develop your understanding of your body, which will in turn further aid your training. Whatever your goals or fitness level at present I am sure there will be at least one area where you can improve yourself or your training methods by a better understanding of how to train, or how your body will respond to training.**

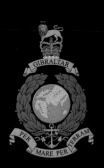

# CHAPTER 6
# DIET AND NUTRITION

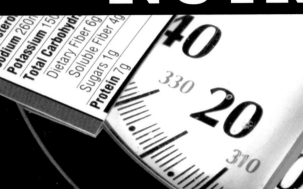

## Nutrition Facts

Serving Size 19 Crackers (31g)
Servings Per Container About 8

**Amount Per Serving**

**Calories** 140    Calories from Fat 35

| | % Daily Value* |
|---|---|
| **Total Fat** 4g | **6%** |
| Saturated Fat 1g | **5%** |
| Trans Fat 0g | |
| Polyunsaturated Fat 1.5g | |
| Monounsaturated Fat 1.5g | |
| **Cholesterol** 0mg | **0%** |
| **Sodium** 320mg | **13%** |
| **Total Carbohydrate** 22g | **7%** |
| Dietary Fiber 1g | **5%** |
| Sugars 5g | |
| Protein 2g | |

| Vitamin A | 0% | • | Vitamin C | 0% |
|---|---|---|---|---|
| Calcium | 0% | • | Iron | 2% |

*Percent Daily Values are based on a 2,000 calorie diet. Your daily values may be higher or lower depending on your calorie needs.

| | Calories | 2,000 | 2,500 |
|---|---|---|---|

## Nutrition Facts

Serving Size 1/6 box (28g)
Servings Per Container 6

| Amount Per Serving | Dry Mix | 1/2 Cup Prepared Stuffing |
|---|---|---|
| **Calories** | 110 | 160 |
| Calories from Fat | 10 | 60 |

| | %Daily Value** | |
|---|---|---|
| **Total Fat** 1g* | **2%** | **11%** |
| Saturated Fat 0g | **0%** | **8%** |
| Trans Fat 0g | | |
| **Cholesterol** 0mg | **0%** | **0%** |
| **Sodium** 250mg | **10%** | **14%** |
| **Total Carbohydrate** 22g | **7%** | **7%** |
| Dietary Fiber <1g | **4%** | **4%** |
| Sugars 2g | | |
| **Protein** 3g | | |
| Vitamin A | 0% | 8% |
| Vitamin C | 0% | 0% |

**N**utrition is a very complex subject which has been written about extensively. This chapter will give the reader an idea of how nutrition is seen in the Royal Marines, both for Recruits in training and for Royal Marines on Operations; how this differs from that of normal gym-goers; and lastly the Royal Marines' own answer to nutrition for general fitness. It must be remembered that although there are a number of specific guidelines regarding nutrition, it is an ever-evolving, ever-changing science, and while a piece of advice might work for one individual, a piece of contrary advice may suit someone else better. This is especially true for nutrition in the Royal Marines, where we try not to be too specific, preferring to offer some overall guidelines to ensure that everyone remains healthy with sufficient energy for Royal Marine life.

The Royal Marines' view of Nutrition, especially when considering Recruits in training, is a little different to what might be expected. In short, in Royal Marines training a Recruit is so active, taking part in such a vast amount of activity and exercise, that it is important to simply take on enough calories to ensure that he has sufficient energy for everything he is doing. When on Operations a similar sort of attitude is adopted, dependent on the operation and the job being performed; the nutritional/calorific intake of a Royal Marine in a fighting company patrolling in Afghanistan will be slightly different from

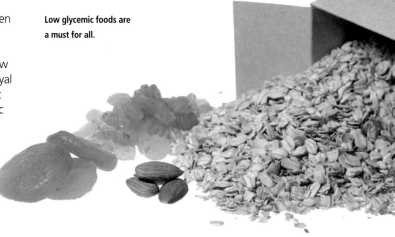

Low glycemic foods are a must for all.

that of a staff officer sitting behind a desk in the rear echelon. Additionally, the use of ration packs while on Operations must be mentioned, and although not pertinent to the fitness agenda of most people reading this book, is perhaps something that will interest even a casual reader when considering calorific intake vs serious exercise.

### Nutrition in the Royal Marines

Nutrition can be viewed very simply, and often is in the Royal Marines, in terms of calories (or energy) in and calories (or energy) out. It can be done without even breaking down what types of food make up the different calories. Realistically, however, this is not advisable, and all Royal Marines Recruits receive lectures on nutrition in their first few weeks of training, encouraging them to eat a lot, but to eat the right sorts of food wherever possible. Going back to my original point of calories in and calories out, this can be explained thus:

- If calories in is equal to calories out (*ie* energy expenditure from all daily activities), then the individual should neither lose weight nor gain weight, as nothing has been gained or lost.
- If calories in is larger than calories out then the individual should gain weight, as energy has been gained.
- If calories in is less than calories out, the individual should lose weight, as more energy has been burned performing tasks than has been gained in food.

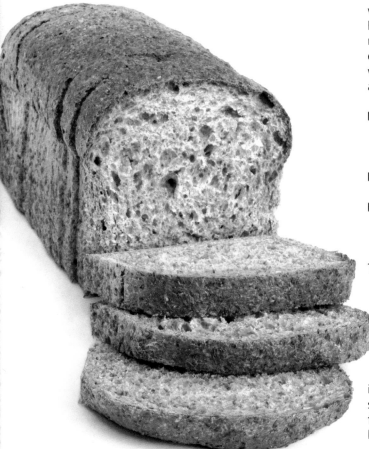

This makes it sound simple, but there is actually a lot more to nutrition than losing and gaining weight via calorie control. In the long run it is more important to choose a varied all-round diet that provides all the necessary types of food, minerals and vitamins than it is to worry about numbers of calories. It is somewhat of an old wives' tale that someone who is obviously overweight can still be significantly fitter than someone who is seen as 'skinny', but it is actually true. If someone is underweight because they are skipping meals, not eating a varied diet and lacking in proteins, fats and essential vitamins and minerals, it can be just as harmful, if not more so, than being overweight.

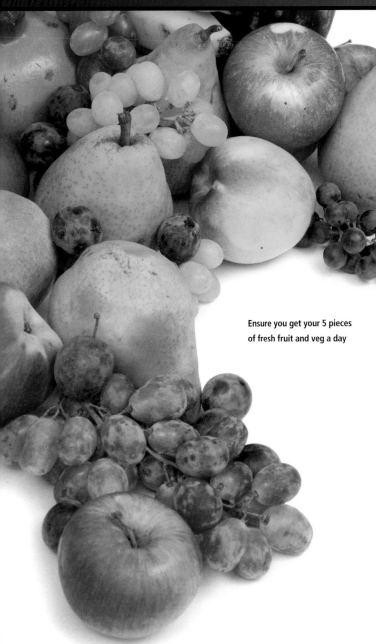

**Ensure you get your 5 pieces of fresh fruit and veg a day**

It is not necessary to eat all of these in every meal, or even every day. As long as the main foodstuffs are sourced adequately every day – that is, protein, carbohydrate, fats, fruit and vegetables, plus plenty of fluids – then most of us will have nothing to worry about.

### ■ Carbohydrates

Carbohydrate is our main source of energy. Whether it is ingested as raw 'simple' sugars or as 'complex' carbohydrates such as potatoes or pasta, it is a must if we are to perform well in our everyday tasks, let alone our exercises. Carbohydrate is stored in the muscles as glycogen. When the muscles run out of glycogen the individual will fatigue and performance will drop. Hence it is imperative to replenish carbohydrate stores in between training sessions, and ideally, for best results, to eat as soon as possible after training (ideally within one hour) – something we refer to in the Royal Marines Physical Training Branch as the 'window of opportunity'. Replenishing within that one-hour window really does enable the body to refuel much quicker for the next training session.

For Recruits, who are in need of a lot of glycogen stores due to the high tempo nature of Royal Marine training, we suggest they snack on high carbohydrate foods such as cereal bars, bread, bananas and other fruit. However, this would not be good advice for someone trying to lose weight. Additionally, we suggest that Recruits have large portions of carbohydrate foods at every meal, such as pasta, rice, potatoes, bread and cereals. Obviously, low-carbohydrate diets are not suitable for Recruits in training – diets such as the all-protein, no-carbohydrate Atkins may be suitable for celebrities in Hollywood, but would lead to lethargic and fatigued Recruits likely to injure themselves because their muscles cannot perform the tasks their bodies need them to.

### ■ Protein

Muscles are made from protein, and the body needs protein to help it to grow and repair itself. Proteins are made up of amino acids, the individual building blocks that make up all our proteins. Unfortunately the human body, unlike those of some animals, cannot synthesise all the amino acids required, so we have to get ours from ingesting proteins from elsewhere. This need can easily be met by eating a diet of meat, fish, eggs or chicken every day. We advise Recruits to do this for at least two meals a day, due to the amount of protein they will need to ensure optimum muscle growth from the physical training they are being put through by their PTIs. However, for an average person one meal of protein a day should be sufficient, unless they are significantly active or training for something specific. This will be elaborated on later.

However, we do advise Recruits in addition that eating more protein than necessary will not increase muscle mass, or improve physical performance. Although protein supplements do have their place in sports nutrition, we are not trying to build Olympic athletes, and therefore do not see protein supplements as

### A balanced diet

A balanced diet is something we all think we eat naturally, without really worrying about it, but in reality humans are creatures of habit, and we tend to stick to what we like without paying much attention to options outside our normal preferences. In truth, a balanced diet should consist of the following:

- ■ **Carbohydrates**
- ■ **Protein**
- ■ **Fats**
- ■ **Fibre**
- ■ **Fruit and vegetables**
- ■ **Dairy**
- ■ **Fluids**
- ■ **Vitamins and minerals**

necessary if a healthy diet of protein is ingested naturally. If too much protein is ingested the excess that the body cannot process ends up down the toilet, and with the high cost of most protein supplements that is just a waste of money.

### ■ Fats

It is a commonly held belief that fats are bad. They are not – we need some fat in our diet to keep healthy. But, having said that, we do not need *large* amounts. It is still important to eat a diet that is low in fat, something that in today's fast-food society can be hard to manage. We therefore advise Recruits to limit their intake of fried and processed foods (*eg* chips and burgers) and to eat a diet that is low in saturated fat. Furthermore, although protein is very important as explained above, it is as important to limit our intake of fatty meats, meats in pies and meats surrounded by pastry. Lastly, fats in oily fish (*eg* salmon, sardines and mackerel), nuts and seeds are all good for all-round health (especially for the skin and joints) and should be eaten quite regularly.

### ■ Fruit and vegetables

Fruit and vegetables are important to a balanced diet in a wide variety of ways. Unfortunately they are often the main food type missing from the average person's diet in today's society. They are an important sources of antioxidants, which help combat free radicals which can cause cancer and premature ageing. Vitamins and minerals are also found in abundance in fruit and veg, which have a wide range of functions from allowing our blood to carry oxygen to helping to stop us getting simple illnesses. Lastly fruit and vegetables provide a source of fibre, which helps keep our digestive system running smoothly.

In short, eating a plentiful diet of fruit and veg could help enhance performance, physically and mentally, reduce the chances of getting ill or injured, improve wound healing, improve long-term health and prevent constipation. All that can be achieved just by eating at least five portions of fruit and veg a day, keeping in mind there should be at least three different types amongst the five for maximum benefit. Sounds simple, doesn't it? It is.

### ■ Vitamins and minerals

A compound that cannot be synthesised in the necessary amounts by an organism is called a vitamin (this does not include essential amino acids, however). Although the majority of the essential vitamins and minerals required by the human body are provided by a healthy diet – especially if the five fruit and veg a day recommendation is stuck to rigidly – vitamin supplements can be beneficial. Royal Marine Commandos often take vitamin and mineral supplements when on Operations or exercises when their diet is out of their control (which obviously includes ration packs). Supplements such as multi-vitamins ensure that the body is supplied with everything it needs to keep all bodily functions working correctly, and additionally ensure that the immune system is at top performance.

The following is a list of the essential vitamins, their scientific names and an example of where they can be obtained:

| Vitamin A | Retinol | Cod liver oil |
|---|---|---|
| Vitamin B1 | Thiamine | Rice bran |
| Vitamin C | Ascorbic acid | Citrus fruit |
| Vitamin D | Calciferol | Cod liver oil |
| Vitamin B2 | Riboflavin | Eggs |
| Vitamin E | Tocopherol | Wheat germ oil, liver |
| Vitamin B12 | Cyanocobalamin | Liver |
| Vitamin K | Phylloquinone | Alfalfa |
| Vitamin B5 | Pantothenic acid | Liver |
| Vitamin B7 | Biotin | Liver |
| Vitamin B6 | Pyridoxine | Rice bran |
| Vitamin B3 | Niacin | Liver |
| Vitamin B9 | Folic acid | Liver |

### ■ Fibre

Eating enough fibre helps with digestion, keeps the stomach healthy and prevents constipation and some forms of cancer. Sources of fibre are fruit and vegetables, as explained above, but more often fibre is sourced from wholegrain cereals such as bran flakes, porridge and muesli, or from wholemeal bread, brown rice and wholemeal pasta.

### ■ Sugar

Besides a balanced diet it is also important to ensure certain foodstuffs are not overdone. Sugar is a prime example. Everything produced today seems to have sugar in it. Often things that are produced to be 'fat free' contain a lot of sugar instead, and a high intake of sugar is obviously not ideal for anyone, especially if a fat-free diet is being followed as a means of losing weight. For Recruits in training it is not the end of the world if they ingest a high amount of sugar, because, as has been discussed above, they need the energy. Unfortunately, however, sugars are just empty calories, basic energy but no nutrients – excellent when a quick burst of energy is needed, but not great as part of a balanced daily diet.

### ■ Salt

Salt intake goes hand in hand with sugar intake. We all seem to think salt and pepper must be used at every meal before we have even tasted the food. Actually, there is enough salt in normal food for all our needs – in fact, much like sugar, there is often too much, especially in crisps, some soups and processed food. Unless the day's activities have caused profuse sweating or cramps are occurring, when extra may be required, the addition of salt to food should always be avoided.

### ■ Dairy

Dairy foods are a difficult subject these days and are often surrounded in controversy. For Recruits in training (many of whom are 16–18 years old and still growing) we advise two to three portions of dairy foods per day for calcium, which is important for healthy bones. Due to the risk of stress fractures in Commando training it is imperative that we do whatever we can to avoid losing Recruits to these injuries, hence the advice.

However, it is still a fact that humans do not have all the correct enzymes for breaking down dairy products. In fact many of us are lactose intolerant, a high majority of us without even realising it. The advice here would be that for anyone taking on a high-impact and very active lifestyle – such as that of a Recruit in Royal Marines training – a diet plentiful in dairy products may be beneficial in avoiding skeletal issues. However, calcium can also be found in many other foodstuffs, such as fish and eggs. Additionally these days, milk substitutes such as soya milk come with added calcium, and bottled water providers have started to add calcium to their water as well.

## Calorie consumption

As stated at the start of this chapter, the number of calories ingested and the number of calories burnt has a direct impact on weight gained or lost. The average civilian male needs 2,500kcal per day, though this figure does vary depending on his size, activity and muscle tone; a short man and a tall man who are roughly the same build (despite their height difference) will still have slightly different calorific intake needs, as the tall man will tend to be heavier and, due to the length of his body, have slightly more muscle, requiring in turn slightly more energy. This is where muscle tone is important. The more muscle an individual has, the more calories they need to ingest – even if they are inactive their muscles still burn a considerable amount of calories. This is why it is so important to take part in resistance-style weight training and not just cardiovascular training when trying to lose weight.

The average RM Recruit needs 4,000 to 5,000 kcal per day, almost twice as many as the average civilian male. Firstly, it has to be said that this is not because every Royal Marine Recruit is a muscle-bound body-builder! Although some Recruits' body shapes do change considerably throughout the course of training, the main reason for this higher calorific need is the amount of activity undertaken throughout the day. Recruits often start each day as early has 0500hrs and often do not stop to rest until about 2200hrs. To ensure they can effectively take on enough calories they are therefore provided with four meals throughout the day: breakfast, lunch, evening meal and an extra nine o'clock meal. In fact, the Commando Training Centre is the only base in the British Armed Forces funded to provide four meals a day to its trainees. Many Recruits will supplement even this with their own snacks.

For most people 4,000kcal is very difficult to imagine. The following menu equates to approximately this figure:

### ■ Breakfast
Orange juice sweetened, 55kcal/100ml = 165kcal (250ml)
Muesli (average), 378kcal average serving = 378kcal
Banana, 108kcal in average banana = 108kcal
Milk semi-skimmed, 47kcal/100ml = 141kcal (250ml)
Bacon grilled, 520kcal/slice = 520kcal (one slice)
Egg poached, 80kcal = 160kcal (two eggs)
Average brown bread, 82kcal/slice = 164kcal (two slices)
Baked beans, 80kcal/100g = 80kcal
**Breakfast total 1,716kcal**

### ■ Snack
Alpen Fruit and Nut Cereal Bar, 110kcal
Can of Coke, 139kcal (330ml)
*Snack total 249kcal*

### ■ Lunch
Tuna (tinned), 186kcal/100g = 242kcal (per tin)
Baked potato, 100kcal/100g = 200kcal (average potato)
Cheddar, 415kcal/100g = 249kcal (60g)
Sweetcorn, 24kcal/100g = 36kcal (150g)
Nestle KitKat, 2 fingers of Kit Kat 107kcal (21g)
*Lunch total 834kcal*

### ■ Dinner
Chicken roasted with little oil, 265kcal/100g = 530g (200g)
Whole Wheat Fuselli pasta, 322kcal/100g = 290kcal (90g portion)
Broccoli, 32kcal/100g = 48kcal (150g)
Carrot, 32kcal/100g = 48kcal (150g)
Chocolate Cake, 390kcal/100g = 203kcal (52g average slice)
Cup of Coffee, 15Kcal (220ml)
*Dinner total 1,134kcal*

### ■ Snack
Apple, 47kcal/100g = 59kcal (125g apple)
*Snack total 59kcal*

*Day total 3,992kcal*

## Ration packs

While in training, Royal Marines Recruits must learn how to operate in field environments, living for days on end on Woodbury Common training area, Dartmoor and areas in Wales. Of their 32 weeks' training (15 months for a Young Officer) around half this time is spent living outdoors off military rations. A 24-hour ration pack provides 4,000kcal, but the average Recruit needs around 4,000 to 5,000, so for some there may be a deficit when surviving on ration packs. Of course, the 4,000kcal produced by the ration pack are only ingested if *everything* in the ration pack is ingested, including all the sachets of sugar to be used in tea and coffee and each and every boiled sweet! Often this is not practical, so where possible Recruits and trained Royal Marines alike try to subsidise their ration packs with noodles, oats bars and other forms of carbohydrate. However, when on Operations these extras are sometimes impossible to source, and many Royal Marines tend to lose a little weight when on rations alone for a long period.

## Water

Although touched on in the previous chapter when discussing dehydration, fluids are so important to health that it is worth providing some additional details here. Fluids are arguably more important to humans than food, as two-thirds of human body weight is composed of water. Water is required for circulation and respiration, it is also necessary in the process of converting food to energy. For dehydration to occur, more water must be lost than is taken in. The human body can survive for about two days without water (depending on the temperature), but can survive for many weeks without food (dependent on the size of the person and the amount of reserves they have). For this reason water is actually said to be the most important nutrient for the human body besides oxygen. Furthermore, dehydration of just 2.5% of your body weight can lead to a 25% loss in efficiency.

In terms of today's conflicts, the Middle East often requires considerable acclimatisation due to the high temperatures reached during the summer months. However, dehydration can occur at any time, and it is often during colder periods that people become dehydrated, as they do not realise that they still need to drink constantly. For this reason Royal Marines Recruits are told to carry a water bottle with them at all times. This is mandatory for physical training, but is also advised for all classroom-based teaching. This allows small sips of water to be taken constantly throughout the day, instead of relying on a drink only with the main meals.

Recruits are also taught how to spot dehydration in themselves. Water is not only lost when in hot climates and taking part in hard exercise. Nor is it expired from the human body only as sweat, being also lost during respiration and through the kidneys as urine. The most effective method of catching dehydration early is by looking at the colour of urine. The clearer it is, the more hydrated the individual is; a slight yellow tinge is acceptable, but a dark yellow or orange indicates the beginnings of serious dehydration.

## Supplements

Supplements are big business these days. From the sponsorship of top sportsmen and women, to advertisements in the majority of gyms, sports nutrition supplements can be found everywhere. The main focus of these is on protein supplementation and carbohydrate supplementation. With a balanced diet, and specifically with two good meals of protein a day, protein supplementation is unnecessary, and the body will

excrete the excess protein anyway. However, in times when the body is short of protein – for example when Royal Marines are on Operations abroad, and protein is scarce – a supplement can be a beneficial addition. For sportsmen and those training for something specific, protein supplementation can also be beneficial, to ensure that the body is getting the right amount of protein. The average person (around 95% of the population) is said to need 0.8g of protein per kilo of body weight per day, ie an 80kg male will need 64g of protein every day (0.8 x 80 = 64).

However, 0.8g per kilo of body weight is not suitable for everyone. Due to the high intensity of their training, endurance athletes will often start to burn their own proteins during training and competitions, and therefore require additional protein. Research suggests around 1.2g of protein per kilo of body weight per day is needed by them. Furthermore, research suggests that a very muscular athlete – say, perhaps, a rugby player or a sprinter – may require as much as 1.4g of protein per kilo of body weight. For a 100kg rugby player this can be as much as 140g of protein, over twice that needed by the 'normal' population, and this is where protein supplementation can help. The downsides are that it can become expensive and the calorific content can be considerable, not to mention that it could be a waste of time and with some individuals could lead to dehydration. Consequently it is not recommended for Royal Marines Recruits.

Carbohydrate and protein supplementation can be combined, and is certainly the thought process of a lot of leading companies. However, with Royal Marines Recruits avoiding protein supplementation, the basic carbohydrate drinks are most beneficial. The big brand sports drinks claim to rehydrate and provide energy via carbohydrate. There are three types available:

### ■ Hypotonic

These sports drinks contain a greater proportion of water, and a lesser proportion of carbohydrate than the human body. As the drink is less concentrated than body fluids, it is claimed that they increase the speed of water absorption by the body (compared to plain water), thus preventing or alleviating dehydration.

### ■ Isotonic

These contain proportions of water and other nutrients similar to the human body, and are typically about 6% to 8% carbohydrate. As the drink is the same concentration as body fluids, it is absorbed at the same rate as water.

### ■ Hypertonic

These sports drinks contain a lesser proportion of water, and a greater proportion of carbohydrate than the human body. As they are more concentrated than body fluids they are absorbed more slowly, meaning the energy will be released over a long period of time. It is therefore claimed that such drinks can give an energy boost and also replace lost energy over the entire session.

Energy drinks are a good form of energy boosting and rehydration. However, they should still be viewed with caution. The advice given to Recruits is that there is no substitute for water. If energy drinks are to be used, always ensure that plain water is also at hand just in case the energy drink causes dehydration or, worse, an adverse reaction. Additionally, it is always worth testing that an energy drink is compatible with your own body prior to using it for a specific event or competition, where an adverse reaction could have dire consequences.

## Diets

Diets are not something that crop up all that much in Royal Marines training. However, we do occasionally have Recruits who could do with losing some weight to make their training experience a little easier. Rather than issue a diet specifying what can be eaten when, the 'calories in and calories out' explanation is reiterated. Specific diets tend to take out certain foods at certain times, which would be contrary to any balanced diet. In short, rather than dieting, a controlled balanced diet should be maintained, plenty of fluids taken on (as they make people feel full), and a well-structured physical training plan adhered to.

## Alcohol

A few other things should be considered when looking at nutrition, the first of which is alcohol. We all know alcohol impairs reaction speed and judgement, but does it offer any nutritional value? The simple answer is no. Alcohol is actually very calorific, for example there are 184kcal in a pint of beer – compare this to 127kcal in a Mars Bar or 149kcal in a Snickers bar. However, someone might go out and drink five pints, but would anyone eat five Mars Bars in one night? For anyone reading this book who wants to lose weight, cutting out alcohol would be my first piece of advice.

Apart from its calorific content, which is used by Sumo wrestlers in Japan to increase their body weight, alcohol offers little to no other nutritional benefits. Yes, there are the supposed health benefits that red wine can provide for the heart, but the same could be argued for smoking where studies have shown that it could protect you against Parkinson's disease. So if alcohol is going to be part of your diet, as it is for most people in the Royal Marines, let it be for enjoyment reasons, and use it safely and sensibly. But do not pretend to yourself that it is doing you good. Overall, it is not.

### Vegetarianism

In the Royal Marines, it is very difficult to be vegetarian. Although vegetarian options do exist and vegetarian ration packs are available on request, it is a fair statement that vegetarian Royal Marines do not get the amount of protein they need. Outside the Royal Marines, of course, it is entirely possible to get all the necessary protein, minerals and nutrients, specifically calcium, without eating meat. The meat substitute options available in supermarkets these days are excellent and are actually often cheaper and offer more protein than their meat alternatives.

### The glycaemic index

Royal Marines Recruits are not educated in the use of the glycaemic index, as it is not necessary when eating a balanced diet and trying to ingest enough calories during meals. However, an understanding of the glycaemic index, or GI, is very advantageous for supporting most training programmes. The GI is basically a measure of the effects of carbohydrates on blood glucose levels, *ie* how the carbohydrate ingested affects the level of sugars in the bloodstream, which will in turn have effects on physical and mental capability. Some carbohydrates break down rapidly during digestion, releasing glucose into the blood stream very swiftly. These are said to be high GI. Conversely, carbohydrates that break down slowly, releasing glucose gradually into the bloodstream, are said to be low GI. Furthermore, foods that are low GI generally have some additional health benefits. There are a number of books and websites that outline whether foods are low or high gylcaemic, and if this is something that interests you I suggest that you investigate it further.

Using the glycaemic index for better sports performance is a matter of knowing what to eat and when. There are many different trains of thought, and, again, entire books have been written on the subject, so what follows should be regarded only as an example and not as *the* way forward. Basically, it is important to eat low GI foods throughout the day – this will keep the blood sugar levels in the body at a constant, rather than eating lots of high GI foods and causing sugar spikes and lows, which cause fatigue, loss of concentration and irritability. A good idea is to ensure something low GI is eaten at breakfast. Examples are porridge, muesli or wholemeal bread. It is not a problem to have something high GI with them, such as fruit, raisins or jam, but the main bulk of the meal should be low GI. Protein such as bacon or eggs can of course be eaten as well. Any snacks throughout the day should be low GI wherever possible – oat-based cereal bars, muesli or granola bars, or wholemeal bread are again good examples. Fruit snacks are good, but are in general high GI so can cause a sugar spike and subsequent low. This does not mean fruit should be avoided (we need our five a day) but should be eaten in conjunction with low GI foods.

Any main meal should be eaten with a healthy portion of low GI carbohydrate. Examples are wholemeal brown pasta, brown rice, wholemeal bread and potatoes (boiled or baked where possible). High GI foods should not be avoided altogether; on the contrary, they can be used very effectively. A glass of orange juice (full of natural fruit sugars) can be ingested first thing in the morning to kick-start the metabolism. GI foods are perfect for replenishing glycogen stores during the 'window of opportunity' following exercise, as described earlier. Just prior to exercise is also a good time for a quick sugar-spike energy boost, and if necessary during the exercise itself. However, if a low GI meal has been eaten a couple of hours prior to the exercise sessions, then sufficient energy should still be available within the body. Examples of high GI foods to use prior to, during and after exercise are glasses of orange juice, bananas, dates, sports drinks and even chocolate bars.

## Conclusion

**Sports scientists' and nutritionists' thoughts on best nutrition are forever evolving, and the Royal Marines are always looking out for the most up-to-date approach. Rather than make bold statements regarding the best way forward, I have therefore outlined the way we currently teach our Recruits, and provided some additional food for thought that may inspire casual readers to find out more for themselves. There are, however, a few key messages to remember:**

- **Eat every meal – never skip a meal, especially breakfast.**
- **Ensure carbohydrates are eaten with every meal, wherever possible low GI.**
- **Eat five portions of different fruit and veg per day.**
- **Fatty and sugary high GI foods should be treats or used prior to or after exercise.**
- **Keep alcohol consumption to a minimum where possible.**
- **Keep yourself hydrated by always carrying a bottle of water.**
- **Do not waste money on expensive supplements when a balanced diet will suffice.**

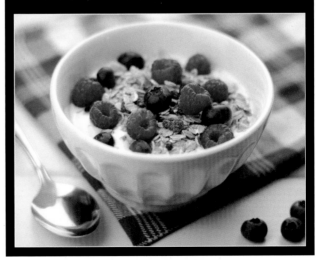

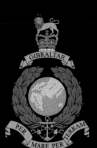

# CHAPTER 7
# ECONOMY OF EFFORT

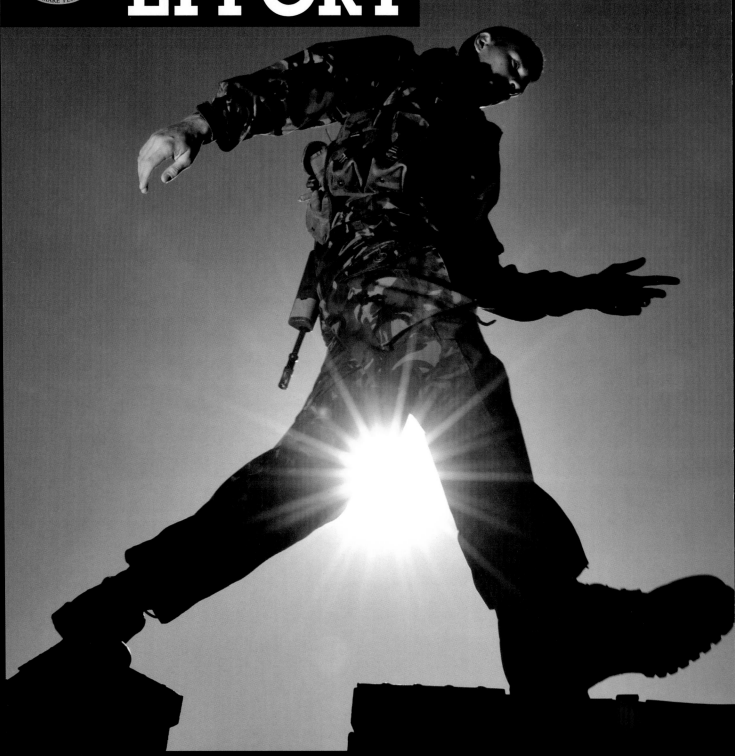

If you ever watch people exercising you may notice that they all complete the same tasks in very different ways. Whether simple press-ups or complex acts such as running, everyone has there own style. It is true that this is partly due to varying fitness levels and how hard or easy they find the activity, but actually there is far more to it than that.

## Physiological differences

If we take two equally fit individuals, they will still complete a given exercise in different ways, and this is predominantly due to their individual physiological make-up. We are all a product of our genes, taking on traits from our parents that make us who we are, give us our physical appearance, and determine our physiological make-up. Not only do our different body shapes, as provided by our genes, make huge differences, but subtle irregularities caused by old injuries and current injuries add to these.

A great example is body and limb length. I have very long arms, so although I am relatively accomplished at pull-ups I take slightly longer to complete the same number of pull-ups as some of my shorter-limbed colleagues. It is not that any of us are particularly stronger than each other, it is just that shorter-limbed people have less distance to make their body travel than I do. We all complete the exercise but it looks and seems different, somehow, due to our subtle physiological differences in body shape.

## Running

Little differences are usually at their most apparent when people are running. Years of running and training mean that I have learnt how to run in the most economic way possible, making it easier for myself and enabling me to run for long periods of time at fairly quick speeds.

This 'economy of effort' can be found in all forms of exercise, but specifically those involving endurance events (swimming, cycling, running etc). Economy of effort is especially important to Royal Marines in running and yomping, to ensure that they can complete the routes but remain relatively fresh at the end. Economy of effort usually improves with years of experience and arduous training, in which an almost perfect technique is learned that involves the most efficient movement for the least energy expenditure. Once this ability has been learnt an individual can then perform certain exercises at a very high level, but with what seems to be very little effort, often while others who appear to be equally fit struggle.

During Commando training so many different areas of physical fitness are required that, often, individuals' body make-ups and previous sporting experience mean that they each excel in different areas. Those Recruits that show a good economy of effort when running and yomping obviously have some advantage over those that do not. However, often those that are 'racing snakes' (fast runners) struggle with economy of effort in the swimming pool, or even when climbing ropes. In fact it is often the case that, despite their specific strengths, very accomplished runners and other very fit sportsmen often struggle when running or yomping carrying weight in a Bergen, daysack or webbing. Unfortunately their chosen sports provide little to assist them with running and yomping carrying weight, especially when we consider that this usually takes place over undulating terrain.

In a sense, this means that during Commando training, when it really counts during the Commando tests and while yomping in the field, everyone is on a level playing field, and everyone must learn a new running technique, the 'Commando shuffle' – a very economical way of moving across rough terrain quickly while carrying weight, in which the feet are lifted as little

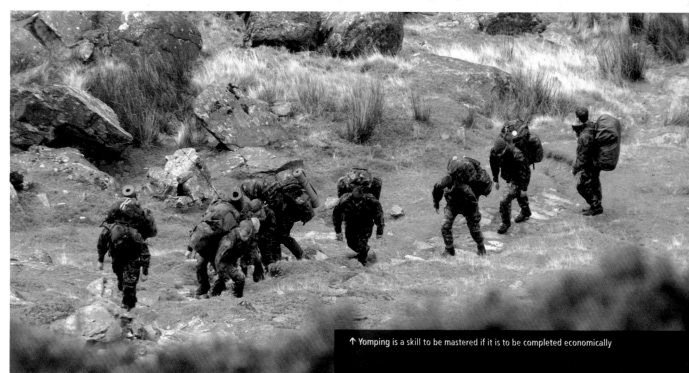

↑ Yomping is a skill to be mastered if it is to be completed economically

as possible off the ground. It must be remembered, too, that we all have our strengths and weaknesses, and must not let others' apparent ease at any task deter us from our goals. The key is to develop and maintain economy of effort in all that we do, ensuring that 100% is given at all times and never giving up or slacking off.

## The economical running gait

The following gives an idea of the best way to run in order to achieve the best economy of effort:

- **Head** – Should be up to keep the airway open and help breathing, should be looking forward to maintain good vision and avoid obstacles, and should be kept fairly still yet relaxed to conserve energy.
- **Back** – Should be kept flat where possible. When carrying a heavy pack this can be difficult.
- **Torso** – Should be upright or tilted slightly forward to maintain momentum, and should be relaxed and fairly still.
- **Arms** – Should drive forward for momentum and balance. They should not go across the body as this can cause the torso to swing and so waste energy.
- **Legs** – The quadriceps and hamstrings should drive down and backwards together. The legs should not be used to stop or brake the momentum, as this will waste energy and is not natural, although sometimes a consequence when running down very steep hills.
- **Feet** – The heels should strike the floor at the body's centre of gravity, which for most people is just in front of the body not

below it (due to forward momentum). This initiates the power in the quads and hamstrings.

## Points to note

Energy expenditure is far greater when walking or running on snow or sand than on a tarmac road. It can be beneficial to train the body on assorted surfaces and in various climates and conditions, but it is not essential. As Royal Marines we need to know we can be effective in the Arctic, and also in Afghanistan. However, if you are training for a marathon it would be sensible to do the majority of your training on roads, for obvious reasons. Furthermore, it is worth getting a good foundation of fitness in easier conditions before testing your body in harder ones.

## Footwear

The footwear worn when conducting exercises, especially running or walking long distances, plays a huge part in not only the speeds that can be produced, but also in avoiding, or even causing, injury. It is obvious that there will be considerable differences in energy expenditure when comparing walking, running or yomping in boots vs trainers. After an initial period in trainers (while Recruits become accustomed to wearing boots by walking around camp in them), Royal Marines undertake the majority of physical training wearing combat boots. All the Commando tests are performed wearing boots. Although they are certainly more draining to energy levels, training in boots is essential.

The footwear chosen for a specific function can make a huge difference to that activity. As just stated, Royal Marines wear

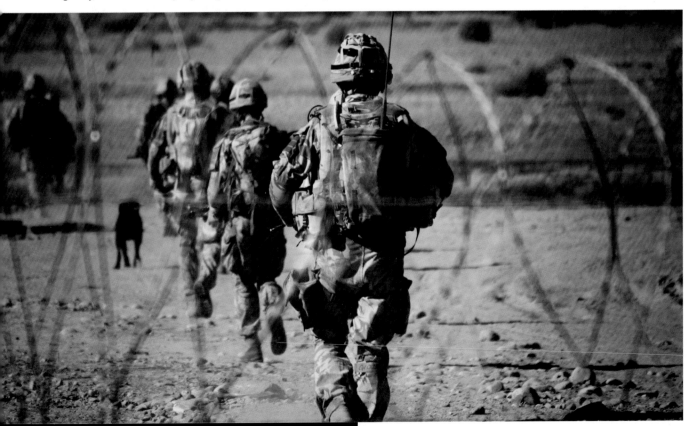

# Walking vs running

**It is thought that when walking at approximately 8kph, energy expenditure becomes uneconomical and outweighs efficiency, rendering 'economy of effort' null and void. Breaking into a run at this point therefore becomes the more economic option in terms of effort. Below this 8kph threshold, it is suggested that walking at speeds of 3–5kph is the most energy-economic speed. However, a number of factors will affect this, such as the weight carried, how it is carried, the fitness level of the individual, the terrain to be covered, weather, wind resistance and climate.**

combat boots, which adds to their energy expenditure. However, despite this seeming disadvantage there are huge advantages to wearing boots while running or yomping. Compared to trainers the wear and tear on combat boots is far, far lower, and in extended periods of constant use they will last far longer. Furthermore, the ankle protection offered by combat boots far out-weighs that of trainers, meaning that the speed a less than confident runner/walker may be able to achieve over rough terrain may be enhanced. Even if this is not so, at least the risk of ankle inversion injury will be greatly reduced.

With any footwear it is important to ensure that choice and fit are correct for the task at hand. Additionally, it is worth ensuring that they are sufficiently worn-in prior to extensive hard use.

We have already discussed the benefits of boots vs trainers, but what about different types of trainers? Unfortunately the sports market is flooded with 'fashion trainers', which due to changing styles are often only intended to be appealing to the eye, and reduce in price as fashion changes. I am constantly surprised to see would-be Recruits arrive at the Commando Training Centre for their Potential Royal Marines Course (PRMC) wearing Velcro tennis shoes or even high top basketball boots with the laces undone. Believe it or not, these are not the best choices, either for getting the best performance from your body, or for avoiding injury!

When training, ensure your footwear is correct for the task. You would not go for a run in a pair of flippers or football boots, so why is a pair of tennis shoes or skateboard shoes any more acceptable? Use equipment for its intended task, or believe me you will end up injuring yourself. A bit of money spent on a decent pair of running shoes will pay dividends in the long run (no pun intended). Furthermore, replacing trainers after a certain number of miles or every six months is also key, as they lose their shock-absorbing capacity. It is usually obvious when trainers need replacing – for Royal Marines, either by the look or the smell!

### Specific adaptation to imposed demands (SAIDs)

The SAID or 'specific adaptation to imposed demands' principle states that the body will, over time, adapt to whatever it is subjected to – *ie* the body becomes its function.

In other words, if you train your body to be able to lift big weights it will be able to do so, but will struggle with long endurance events, and, of course, vice versa. Consequently in terms of economy of effort, regularly training a specific exercise or event will naturally aid economy of effort, as the body will adapt over time and at some point find the most efficient posture, position or gait. Individuals with a background in cross-country running or the like, for instance, will already have a great economy of effort when running. Such adaptations are either acute, meaning they occur in the short term, or chronic, meaning they occur over a longer term.

### Fitness foundations

As stated, adaptations help to build on fitness, giving the body extra reserves to cope with future stress. However, as stated very early in this book, no one can maintain themselves at the peak of fitness indefinitely, so fitness levels have to be allowed to rise and fall, since once the body has reached a high level of fitness it will be easier to return to that level than it was to reach it the first time. This means that after years of arduous exercise, even if the highest fitness levels have been lost, the body will still be in a better state to cope with any physical challenges asked of it.

Establishing a good foundation of fitness and therefore a learnt economy of effort is very important to Royal Marines. As a soldier it is impossible to know exactly what threat the body will face next and therefore what it will be expected to do. The Commando tests are not only there to prepare the body and mind for those specific tests, but also to put the body and mind under stress so that it can learn and adapt to perform better in similar conditions in the future. For example, we cannot fire bullets at Recruits, but putting them under physical and mental stress in other ways will allow SAID to prepare the body as best it can. In short, for every Royal Marine the robust foundation of individual fitness set up during Commando training will quickly adapt to meet the demands of the future. Whether physically or mentally, the body becomes its function.

# Conclusion

**Economy of effort is vitally important if you are planning to compete or train in long-endurance events. It will make the whole experience far more enjoyable, as once an adequate energy-efficient style has been learned you will be able to train or compete with relative ease compared to others. Unfortunately, economy of effort cannot be learned from a book, or copied from a YouTube video. Only a progressive training programme that ensures the body has a chance to make acute and chronic specific adaptations to imposed demands will lead to a truly economic style. As always, hard work pays off.**

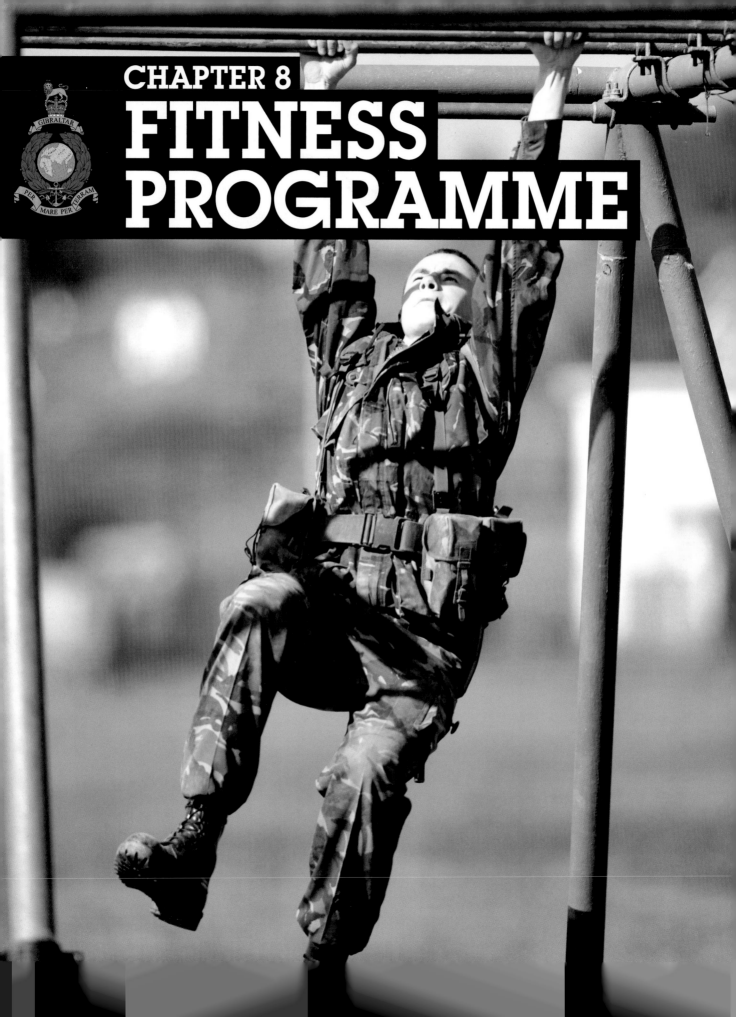

# CHAPTER 8
# FITNESS PROGRAMME

A training programme is one of the most important things to put together when setting out on a quest for fitness. This is especially true if you are training on your own. If you are training as part of a team, or, as Recruits will be, training under an instructor, then all you have to do is turn up and work hard. If training alone, without a training programme, it is easy to slacken off, to do an easier session than maybe you should be doing, or even to miss a day completely.

The second half of this chapter provides and explains a sample training programme for civilians which is similar to that undertaken by a Recruit during Commando training. Recruit training lasts 32 weeks, from the day a Recruit joins Royal Marines Training to the point when he can attempt the Commando tests, so the suggested civilian training programme is based on this same time frame. When looking at or attempting this programme, remember that it is only a fitness training programme, whereas for a Recruit the fitness sessions are only a very small part of his overall training – the rest of his programme consists of everything else necessary for him to become a trained soldier: time spent 'in the field' exercising tactics, personal soldiering skills, and the use of weapons. Furthermore, field conditions are extremely physical periods, spent carrying large backpacks and attacking and assaulting objectives, and can often add to the Recruit's fitness level while he is away from the specific fitness programme adhered to when on camp.

The civilian programme cannot include *all* the benchmark tests that Recruits must pass in order to progress on through Commando training, as for most an assault course, 30-foot rope or endurance course is not available. However, some tests can be mimicked in kind. Should Recruits fail criteria tests, re-tests will be allowed where possible, but consistent failure will result in a Recruit having to be back-trooped to repeat that part of this training. Unfortunately this means he will not continue on with those friends he has made thus far in training.

The Royal Marines Recruit training programme is divided into stages, with specific aims throughout those stages. The first nine-week period is known as IMF (Initial Military Fitness), the aim of which is to focus on building a basic level of fitness, specifically to prepare the body for the more intense physical training to come. IMF consists of callisthenic body exercises (exercises that use the body as resistance, *eg* press-ups and pull-ups) and works towards muscular endurance and cardiovascular fitness. The majority of this IMF stage is spent indoors in the gymnasium, performing circuit-style body-weight exercises rather than using weights. At week 9, some specific tests are undertaken by all Recruits. Passing these tests will see Recruits move on to the next stage of physical training.

The second stage of fitness training for Royal Marine Recruits is BPT (Battle Physical Training), which primarily takes place on the 'Bottom Field' at the Commando Training Centre using the Assault Course, the 30-foot ropes, the Regain Rope (explained in Chapter 9) and carrying exercises such as the Fireman's Carry. The aim of BPT is to condition the Recruit to the type of physical activity that could be expected in a 'battle' situation, *ie* exerting sub-maximal strength (rope climbing), agility whilst fatigued (using the assault course), casualty evacuation under fatigue (the Fireman's Carry) and the ability to perform a physical technique or skill when fatigued (using the regain). All these activities are of a very high physical intensity and therefore continue to increase cardiovascular fitness, specifically stamina, but also train robustness and the strong Commando mindset imperative to success in the Royal Marines.

Following a series of tests at the end of the BPT stage of physical training (see Chapter 9), successful Recruits move on to the final phase of their physical training syllabus: the Commando stage. During this stage the length of the physical activities is greater and a combination of military field exercises and PTI-led physical conditioning leads to more impetus on CV training, specifically running and yomping carrying weight in webbing and Bergens, and even more training to improve robustness to prepare the Recruits for the rigours of their final exercises and their Commando tests.

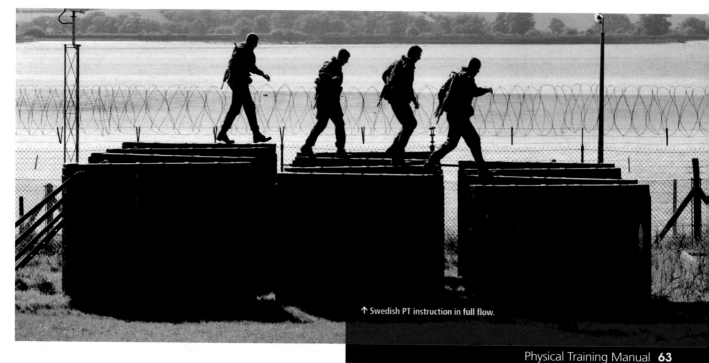

↑ Swedish PT instruction in full flow.

# Royal Marines Recruit training

### ■ IMFC (Initial Military Fitness Circuit) – 17 periods

IMFC is basically a form of circuit training that involves Swedish PT-style physical training periods led by the Troop PTI. The sessions include a warm-up, team games (like relay races), introductory exercises direct from the old Swedish PT system (basically mobilisation and core stability exercises), rope climbing, muscular endurance circuit exercises called 'the beam sequence' (involving press-ups, pull-ups, squats and dips), a sit-up abdominal strength routine called 'the main group', intervals around the 'camp circuit' (an approximately 800m sprint around the camp), sprints (the distance of the gymnasium floor), and lastly 'the run and march' as a Swedish PT means of cooling down. This will all be learnt, trained, perfected and tested over the nine weeks.

### ■ IMFS (Initial Military Fitness Strength) – 8 periods

IMFS is a slower more controlled period than IMFC, rarely involving sprints or camp circuits. It is not as rigid or regimented as the IMFC periods and does not involve any elements of Swedish PT. It still shares many of the same elements, such as a warm-up and cool-down, and there is still a set structure to the period should the PTI wish to use it.

Usually the periods will either revolve around rope climbing – sometimes with the addition of a small amount of weight in the Recruits' webbing – or around the IMFS circuit. The IMFS circuit is a set sequence of specific functional strength stations, such as a wooden mock six-foot wall (mimicking the six-foot wall on the Assault Course, which so often catches Recruits out). The Recruits run at the mock wall and get their elbows and chest up on to it, utilising the same technique that will be used on the Assault Course. Other stations include squats or kettlebell swings, deadlifts, sled pulls, back extensions, fireman's carries and the starts of a regain, to name but a few.

### ■ CQC (Close Quarter Combat) – 8 periods

The Recruits are taught basic unarmed combat such as pressure points, strikes, chokes, throws, grappling, kicks and blocks. They then move on to close quarter combat while wearing their webbing and having their rifle but being unable to use it (out of ammunition or too close to use). Lastly the Recruits are taught how to work in groups of two, three or four to disarm enemies, capture them and safely escort them elsewhere. This training is retaught and expanded at Units prior to Operations.

### ■ Swimming – 18 periods

Swimming is so important to Royal Marines because we are part of the Navy and are Britain's amphibious infantry. We must be able to swim to a high standard, and also be capable of swimming in kit and equipment should accidents happen. For this reason we must all pass the BST (Battle Swimming Test), explained in Chapter 9. Besides building up for the BST, the Troop PTI also uses the swim periods to work on the Troops' cardiovascular fitness but in a completely non-impact environment. If the troop went running every day to improve their CV, we would soon see an onset of injuries, from pulled muscles to stress fractures and tendinitis, but by using the pool we can train CV hard without the risk of impact stress injuries.

### ■ Running – 7 periods

It goes without saying that running is important for a Royal Marine. It will be performed during IMFC periods as sprints and camp circuits, and will also make up a vast majority of the DEs seen during early field exercises. Furthermore, as explained above, CV training is conducted at length in the swimming pool.

### ■ AMF (Advanced Military Fitness) – 5 periods

AMF provides the transition between IMF and BPT. It involves introductions to the Assault Course, regain and outside 30-foot ropes as well as the high-obstacle course (not the Tarzan course, a separate high-obstacle course). AMF requires a considerable amount of coaching and teaching to ensure all Recruits have grasped the techniques and developed the skills required for the 'Bottom Field' prior to moving on to BPT. As described in Chapter 9, BPT is eventually tested with 21lb of kit and a 10lb rifle. However, AMF is conducted in boots, CS95 trousers, T-shirt and combat jacket, with no kit at all. All skills are developed in 'clean fatigue' (without kit) before kit is added.

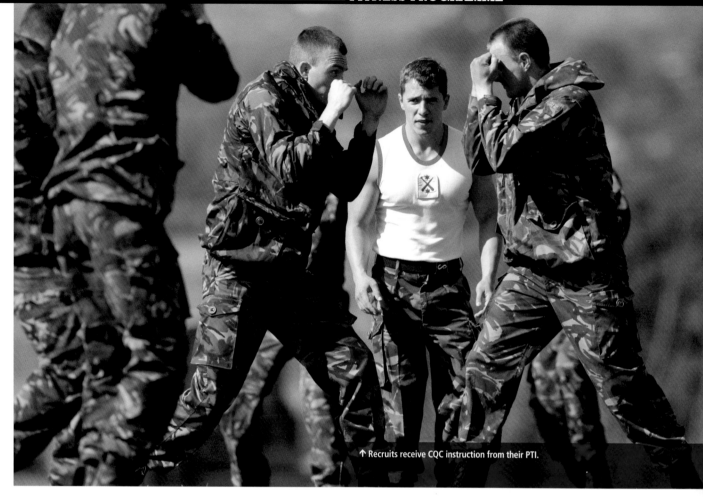

↑ Recruits receive CQC instruction from their PTI.

### ■ IMFS – 1 period

Just as the IMFS periods above. Another opportunity for the PTI to develop strength or to concentrate on a particular area of weakness he has spotted.

### ■ Speed marches – number of periods varies

Speed marching is an important skill to develop. For some it is easy, and comes naturally, as if they are just running with a bit of weight. For others it feels abnormal and never becomes natural or comfortable. During DEs while the Recruits do a two-week shooting package in weeks 11 and 12, Troop PTIs will concentrate on speed marching, aiming to have the drills, commands and techniques 'squared away' (sorted out) by the end of week 12. At week 15 the Troop will have a criteria four-mile speed march test carrying 21lb of webbing and a 10lb SA80 rifle.

### ■ BPT (Battle Physical Training) – 15 periods

The real explanation behind these periods lies in the BPT pass-out tests at week 22, which are described in Chapter 9. In short these periods aim to get every Recruit individually 'battle fit'. They must not only become physically fit, but must learn to turn their mind off when it is too cold, too hot, they are too tired or they feel sick. To use a cliché, BPT 'separates the men from the boys'. Areas of training concentrated on are the Assault Course, Fireman's Carry, 30-foot rope climbs, sprints and, of course the regain. Sounds

easy? Well all of these elements are done in boots carrying webbing and a 10lb SA80 rifle. The webbing is made progressively heavier over the periods until the target 21lb is reached.

### ■ Swimming – 3 periods

These periods allow retesting and retraining for the BST, or, if the Troop is fatigued or injury-prone, the sessions allow the Troop PTI to perform some hard CV training in a non-impact environment. These periods can also be a welcome break from the hardships of the BPT periods and the field exercises.

### Phase 3 Commando Stage – weeks 23–31

### ■ Endurance Course – 3 periods

The Endurance Course is explained in depth in Chapter 9. These periods provide an introduction to the course, a practice and a mock test prior to the real thing, and of course the added bonus of some CV fitness while performing them.

### ■ Tarzan Assault Course – 3 periods

Like the Endurance Course, the Tarzan Assault Course is described in depth in Chapter 9. Also like the Endurance Course, these periods provide an introduction, a practice and a mock test, plus the added bonus of some CV training.

### ■ 30-foot wall – 1 period

This is the last obstacle on the Tarzan Assault Course. It is a slightly under-hanging 30-foot wall with stones/bricks jutting out and 30-foot ropes hanging down its face. This period allows the Recruits a chance to practise negotiating it while fresh. It also allows the PTIs to teach or coach any strugglers, and to look out of any showing a fear of heights.

### ■ Running/speed marches – number of periods varies

As with the previous phase, this is dependent on the DEs instructed and what attention the Troop requires. At week 26 the Troop have a criteria six-mile speed march (see Chapter 9) and must be ready for this test.

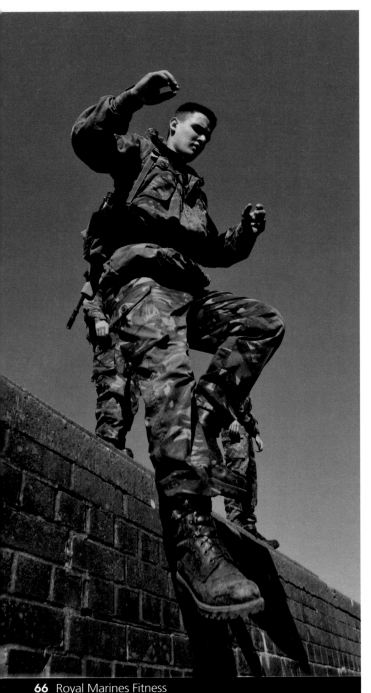

As you can see from all of the above, Royal Marines training is designed specifically to be both functional and progressive at all times. Functional training is important, as Recruit training is so short when we consider how much a Recruit must learn and how much he must improve physically – we do not have time to concentrate on non-specific, non-functional training. Progression is even more important than functionality. If we threw week 1 Recruits straight into the 30-Miler we would undoubtedly have injury problems, hence the use of IMF to prepare them beforehand. Our concerns for injuries have led to us designing a physical programme that does not involve too much running in boots early on, or too much load carrying early on, and aims to let the body adapt as the training progresses.

## Disciplined training

There is a huge difference between military physical training and civilian physical training. During military PT, and more specifically Royal Marines PT, a very high level of discipline is required in all sessions. It is important for Royal Marines to learn this discipline early in their careers, hence during the IMF stage in the gymnasium Recruits are not allowed to scratch or fidget. They are not allowed to wipe away sweat without asking, no matter how hard they have been working. This kind of self-control, once learnt, pays dividends later when performing ambushes in places such as the jungle. Furthermore, even after completing the Assault Course or Endurance Course, Recruits are not allowed to collapse on to the ground. Far from it, they must get a grip of themselves and walk away under control, all of which plays a huge part in that Commando state of mind of which we want to see potential early on.

## Mimicking Royal Marines training

The aim of Royal Marine physical training is to develop an all-round robust level of fitness to allow the body to function effectively in any scenario that the individual might encounter. Any physical training should progressively increase physical demands, and thus develop fitness slowly as the body steadily adapts. In most cases your sessions should be based on examples from Chapters 11–15 of this book.

The programme that follows is not the same as that which Recruits undertake in Commando training. It is a civilianised programme that, over the same period, would get most people to an acceptable level of fitness equivalent to that which RM Recruits reach at their various weeks of training. As stressed earlier, on top of this the Recruits have a number of others lessons, training periods and worries to contend with. Furthermore, the time they spend on military field exercises will impose physical demands on their bodies that will assist in physically preparing them for the tests ahead. These field exercises also sleep-deprive and further degrade the Recruits – something that is not mimicked entirely in the programme provided below, since for most gym-goers this would not be realistically achievable.

# Phase 1

This initial nine-week phase of training aims to develop a base level of fitness in a number of specific areas, particularly muscular endurance and cardiovascular (both endurance and stamina) fitness. Increasing fitness in these areas – a good base level for all Recruits – should allow more specific functional fitness to occur in the next phase.

If a Recruit fails the tests taken at the end of this phase – the Initial Military Fitness of IMF phase – or becomes injured he will stay in it until he is fit enough to move on. For the average member of the public trying to mimic the IMF training phase this is an important fact to remember: time spent in this phase will depend on the initial level of fitness, commitment and, of course, time available. This could take from eight weeks up to a year for some individuals, depending on their starting level of fitness, their age and the previous fitness training undertaken.

| Wk | Training | Level | Swimming | Running/CV | Other |
|----|----------|-------|----------|------------|-------|
| 1 | Various sessions. | Easy. | 1 x 20-minute session. | 3 x 1-mile runs. | 2 x muscular endurance circuits. |
| 2 | Various sessions. | Easy. | 1 x 30-minute session. | 2 x 3-mile runs. 1 x 4-mile run. | 2 x muscular endurance circuits. |
| 3 | Various sessions. | Moderate. | 1 x 30-minute session. | 2 x 4-mile runs. 1 x interval session. | 1 x muscular endurance circuit. 1 x strength circuit. |
| 4 | Various sessions. | Easy. | 1 x 40-minute session. | 2 x 4-mile runs. 1 x 5-mile run. | 2 x muscular endurance circuits. |
| 5 | Various sessions. | Hard. | 1 x 40-minute session. 1 x 40-minute pool circuit. | 1 x 5-mile run. 1 x interval session. | 2 x muscular endurance circuits. |
| 6 | Various sessions. | Easy. | 2 x 40-minute sessions. | 2 x 5-mile runs. | 1 x muscular endurance circuit. 1 x strength circuit. |
| 7 | Various sessions. | Hard. | 1 x 60-minute session. | 1 x 5-mile run. 2 x 6-mile runs. | 2 x muscular endurance circuits. |
| 8 | Various sessions. | Easy. | 1 x 40-minute session. | 1 x 6-mile run. | 2 x muscular endurance circuits. |
| 9 | Test week (see Chapter 9). For this civilianised version, download RMFA MP3s. (NB: No ropes tests are included, as impossible for most civilians.) | Hard. | Nil. | 1.5-mile run in under 10.5 minutes. VO2 max bleep tests above level 10.5 (over 20m). | Press-ups, pull-ups and sit-ups to bleep. Must get over 5 pull-ups and over 30 press-ups. |

# Phase 2

The second stage of training covers 12 weeks. It aims to increase robustness, stamina, and strength, and culminates in a series of tests of all these areas.

| Wk | Training | Level | Swimming | Running/CV | Other |
|----|----------|-------|----------|------------|-------|
| 10 | Various sessions. | Easy. | 1 x 45-minute session. | 1 x 3-mile run in boots. 1 x interval session. | 2 muscular endurance circuits. 1 x leg strength circuit. |
| 11 | Various sessions. | Moderate. | 1 x 45-minute session. | 1 x 4-mile run in boots. 1 x interval session. | 1 x muscular endurance circuit. 1 x Fireman's Carry technique circuit. |
| 12 | Various sessions. | Moderate. | Nil. | 1 x 6-mile run. 2 x 1-hour yomps in boots with 10kg of kit in rucksack. | 2 x muscular endurance circuits. |
| 13 | Various sessions. | Easy. | 1 x 60-minute session. | 1 x 6-mile run. 1 x 3-mile run in 30 minutes, in boots with 15kg of kit. | 2 x muscular endurance circuits. 1 x Fireman's Carry technique circuit. |
| 14 | Various sessions. | Hard. | 1 x 40-minute pool circuit wearing shirt and trousers. | 1 x 6-mile run. 1 x 5-mile run in boots. 1 x interval session in boots with 4kg of kit. | 1 x Fireman's Carry strength circuit. |
| 15 | Various sessions. | Easy. | 1 x 45 minute session. | 1 x interval session in boots with 6kg of kit. 1 x 4-mile run in 40 minutes, in boots with 15kg of kit. | 1 x muscular endurance circuit. 1 x leg strength circuit. |
| 16 | Various sessions. | Hard. | 1 x 60-minute session. | 1 x 6-mile run. 1 x interval session in boots with 8kg of kit. | 2 x muscular endurance circuits. |
| 17 | Various sessions. | Hard. | Nil. | 1 x 6-mile run. 3 x 2-hour yomps in boots with 15kg of kit. | 2 x muscular endurance circuits. |
| 18 | Various sessions. | Moderate. | 1 x 45-minute session wearing shirt and trousers. | 2 x interval sessions in boots with 8kg of kit. | 1 x muscular endurance circuit. 1 x strength circuit. |
| 19 | Various sessions. | Easy. | 1 x 60-minute session. | 1 x 6-mile run. 1 x interval session in boots with 10kg of kit. | 1 x muscular endurance circuit. 1 x Fireman's Carry technique circuit. |
| 20 | Various sessions. | Hard. | Nil. | 2 x interval sessions in boots with 12kg of kit. | 1 x muscular endurance circuit. 1 x strength circuit. 1 x technique session. |
| 21 | Various sessions. | Easy. | 1 x 45-minute session. | 1 x interval session in boots with 15kg of kit. | 2 x technique sessions. |
| 22 | Rest week. (Test week for Recruits.) | Nil. | Nil. | Nil. | Nil. |

# Phase 3

The third and final stage of training lasts ten weeks. Its aims are to increase endurance and stamina, especially while carrying weight, while also maintaining strength. For recruits, this phase culminates in the four Commando tests outlined in Chapter 9.

| Week | Training | Level | Swimming | Running/CV | Other |
|------|----------|-------|----------|------------|-------|
| 23 | Various sessions. | Easy. | 2 x 40-minute sessions. 1 x swim circuit in shirt and trousers. | 1 x 5-mile run. | 1 x flexibility session. |
| 24 | Various sessions. | Moderate. | 1 x 30-minute swim tests (BST – see next chapter). | 1 x 6-mile run. 1 x 3-hour yomp in boots with 15kg kit. | 2 x muscular endurance circuits. |
| 25 | Various sessions. | Moderate. | Nil. | 1 x 6-mile run in boots. 2 x 3-hour yomp in boots with 18kg of kit in rucksack. | 1 x muscular endurance circuit. 1 x technique session. |
| 26 | Various sessions. | Hard. | 1 x 40-minute circuit. | 1 x 6-mile run in 60 minutes, in boots with 15kg of kit. | 1 x muscular endurance circuit. 1 x technique session. |
| 27 | Various sessions. | Moderate. | Nil. | 2 x 3-hour yomps in boots with 20kg of kit. 1 x interval session in boots with 15kg of kit. 1 x 7-mile run in boots with 15kg of kit. | 1 x flexibility session. |
| 28 | Various sessions. | Moderate. | Nil. | 1 x interval session in boots with 15kg of kit. 1 x 7-mile run in boots with 15kg of kit. | 1 x leg strength circuit. |
| 29 | Various sessions. | Hard. | Nil. | 1 x 7-mile run in boots with 15kg of kit. 1 x interval session in boots with 15 kg of kit. 1 x 4-hour yomp in boots with 20kg of kit. | 2 x flexibility sessions. |
| 30 | Various sessions. | Easy. | 1 x 40-minute session. | 1 x 5-mile run. | 2 x technique sessions. |
| 31 | Commando tests. | Hard. | Over four days: 7-mile cross-country run carrying 31lb in under 73 minutes. 9-mile road run carrying 31lb in 90 minutes. 1-mile run off-road (fields) carrying 31lb in under 13 minutes. 30-miles cross-country carrying 45lb in under eight hours. | | |
| 32 | Rest week. | Easy. | Nil. | Nil. | Nil. |

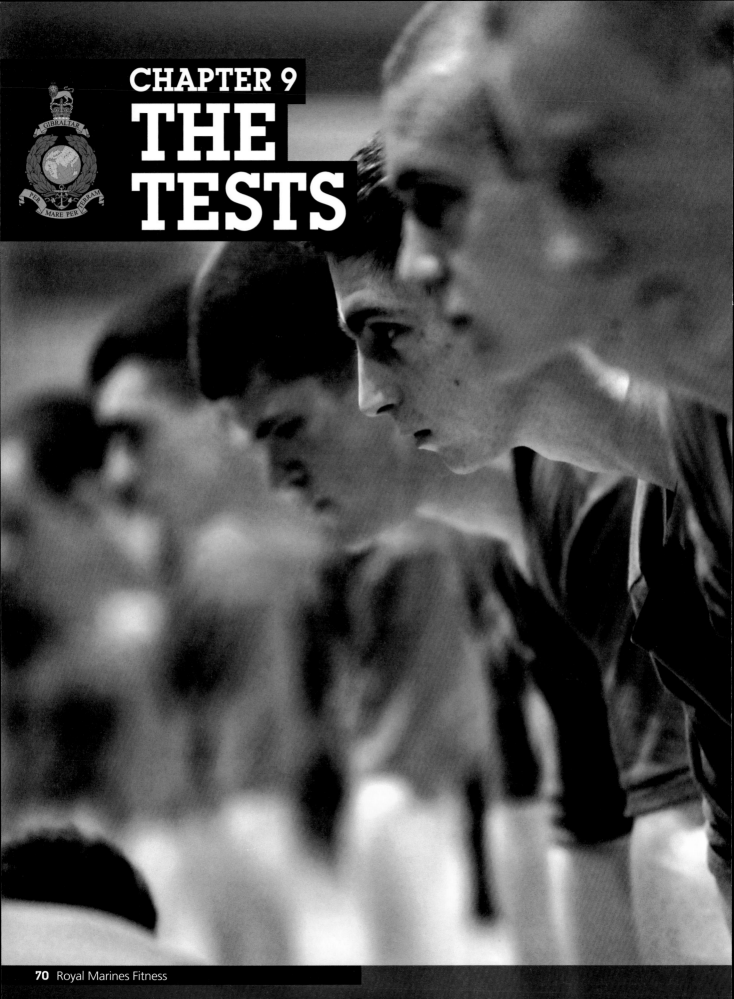

# CHAPTER 9
# THE TESTS

The Commando tests are the culmination of Recruit training, and for many Recruits their focus from day one. For the majority, whether they are Recruits, Young Officers or on the All Arms Commando course, the green beret and its Commando status is the prize they have enrolled themselves to gain. It must be remembered that Recruit training is 32 weeks, whereas YO training is now 15 months and an All Arms course lasts 11 weeks, so the benchmark tests, although the same, all take place at different times throughout the courses. For ease of explanation this chapter will focus on that of Recruit training.

The Commando tests take place at the end of the Commando phase of training, in week 30/31 of the 32-week programme. Despite being the tests that will earn them the green beret, the Commando tests are just the last in a series of tests placed strategically throughout Royal Marine training to ensure that each Recruit is picking up the necessary physical and psychological fitness along the way, to give them the best possible chance at the Commando tests.

## Week 1

Every Recruit or Young Officer will have undergone the Royal Marines Fitness Assessment (RMFA) during their Potential Royal Marines Course (PRMC) or Potential Officers Course (POC). However, in their first week at the Commando Training Centre they will repeat it to gauge current fitness levels. Due to the fact that this test assesses cardiovascular and muscular endurance it is also used extensively throughout a Royal Marine's career, whether at a unit prior to embarking on a pre-deployment fitness programme, on a PT/ML aptitude or training course, or on an SBS briefing course.

The test itself is in four parts, the first being the VO2 max or bleep test, which tests an individual's endurance and stamina when running. A true VO2 max test assesses the maximum amount of oxygen in millilitres that an individual can use in one minute per kilogram of body weight (see Chapter 5). Those who are fit have higher VO2 max values and can exercise more intensely than those who are not as well conditioned; however, for Royal Marines recruit training, we do not need to be that scientific. All we require is a level on the bleep test, which when the test is repeated can give us an indication as to whether the individual has increased or decreased in fitness.

The second part of the test is press-ups to a bleep, where the individual is required to perform one press-up, touching his chest to a 'counter's' fist below his chest, every time the audio bleep is heard. The press-up position must be maintained at all times, the knees cannot be rested or the hips raised. This gives us an indication of how much upper body strength and endurance the man has in his chest, shoulders and core. Again, it gives us something to make comparisons to at a later date.

The third part of the test is similar to the second, and involves performing a sit-up every time a bleep is heard. The exerciser's feet are held in place by a fellow Recruit who is the 'counter', and his elbows must touch the top of his knees on each repetition, and his elbows, shoulders and head return to the mat after each sit-up performed. This test allows assessment of an individual's core strength and endurance.

The last part of the test is pull-ups to the bleep, using the overhand-grip method (*ie* with palms facing away) on a wooden beam. When the bleep is heard a pull-up is performed, but the exerciser must stay with chin above the beam until a second bleep is heard, indicating he can lower. This is not an easy test if specific

**All exercises must be completed to a perfect standard.**

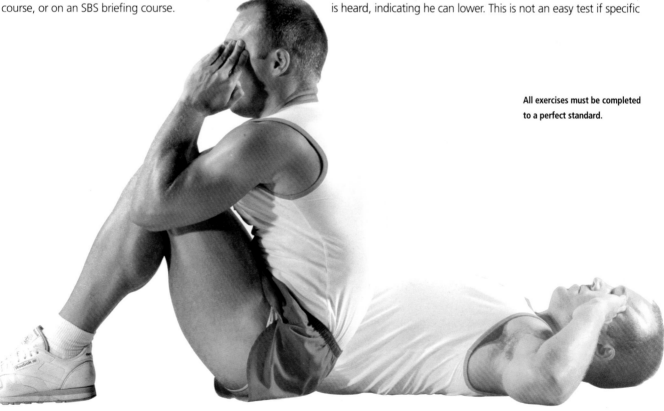

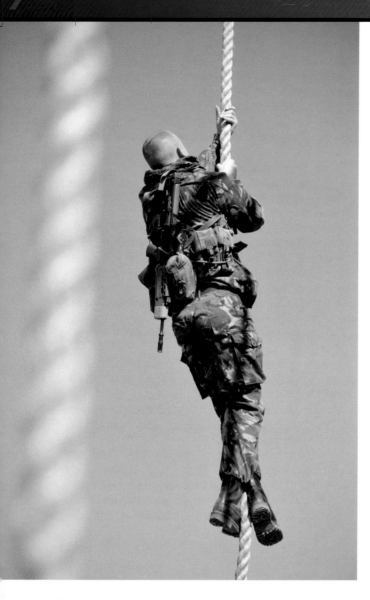

is dependent on the individual's age. For all Recruits a time of under 10 minutes 30 seconds is required. A good time is under 8 minutes. At this stage this test is performed in trainers (to avoid injury), combat trousers and a T-shirt, but later in training and as a trained Commando it will be done in combat boots, timings remaining the same.

## Week 9

Following two months of physical training, mixed in with a rapid introduction to life in the Royal Marines, which includes an extensive amount of admin and even a couple of visits to Woodbury Common for introductory field exercises, the Recruits are tested physically at week 9. These tests come in three parts over three days, including the RMFA and the BFT, which allow us to assess each Recruit individually, to ensure that they have improved enough to continue on to the harder physical training to come, and also to assess if our current methods are working. If the majority of Recruits have not improved, then perhaps it would be time to reassess our training methods.

The Friday of week 9 sees 'The Rope Test' or 'Week 9 Gym Pass Out'. This is not only a test of how well a Recruit has picked up the technique of rope climbing, but it also allows the Troop and individuals a chance to grade themselves physically from their performance. The test consists of a full IMFC (initial military fitness circuit) session including warm-up, team games, Swedish PT, rope climbing, main group, beam sequence, sprints, and run and march – basically everything they have learnt thus far. The session is graded by two senior PTIs, who can award the Troop a pass, superior pass or distinguished pass based on the effort put in, any failures at any point and any major mistakes made. Additionally, any individual Recruits the Troop PTI has noted with particularly high scores on the BFT and RMFA will be put forward for Superior PT certificates. If during the Week 9 Gym Pass Out they perform to an exceptional standard as judged by a senior PTI, they will receive a certificate to state they were a Gym Superior in their Recruit Gym Pass Out.

The most important part of the test, however, is the rope climbing. The Recruits are expected to climb a 30-foot rope three times wearing trainers, combat trousers and a T-shirt. If they can complete three climbs with a short rest between each, they have passed the Gym Pass Out. Any less than two climbs, studies have shown, could lead to injuries and failings at later stages, so usually results in the Recruit being 'back trooped' to redo the test. Anything over two climbs but not the full three (two and a half, for example) would lead to a discussion with the Troop PTI and Troop Commander to see if the Recruit should be taken on at risk. Obviously at this stage his scores on the RMFA VO2 max and pull-ups will have a major input as to his success. Additionally, it is worth mentioning that if any Recruit gets less than level 10.5 on the VO2 max bleep test or less than five pull-ups on the pull-up test he will be made to redo the test the day after his Gym Pass Out. Should he fail on either count he will again be back trooped.

pull-up training has not taken place and is a true indicator of muscular strength and stamina. If at any point the Recruit drops from the beam, the counting stops. MP3 downloads of these bleep tests are available on the Royal Marines website.

Arguably the most important tests and the most indicative of success in Recruit training are the VO2 max and pull-up tests. Without a strong VO2 max, many Recruits fail to keep up with the long yomps, speed-marches and eventual tests expected of all Commandos. Pull-ups are an excellent test of upper-body strength, and something that a high majority of civilians cannot do at all. To successfully complete the rope-climbing and 'regain' expected in some tests, a strong score on the pull-ups is very important and can save a lot of blood, sweat and tears at a later date.

All Recruits, YOs and All Arms Candidates also perform the Basic Fitness Test (BFT) in the first week of training. This is a test which should be done by all three services (Army, Navy and Air Force) every six months and involves completing a 1.5-mile run as a group in a slow time, followed by the same 1.5-mile run as an individual as quickly as possible. The time needed for a pass

## Week 15

At week 15 the Recruits have to pass a Four-Mile Speed March Test as well as a week-long Field Test Exercise. If a Recruit passes both he complete Phase 1 Training and is said to be a trained soldier (as an Army Infantryman is on leaving Catterick). He can then move on to Phase 2 training to become a Commando. Should he fail either test, he will be back trooped to allow him to redo the tests with a different troop.

A speed march is a quick way of getting a body of men from one location to another, with kit, without using vehicles, but in such a way that they are still fit to fight or operate on arrival. The speed march is basically a run but in a squadded formation, *ie* in three files with a PTI calling time (left right, left right). He will generally try to run on the flat and downhill, but use a fast-paced walk on the uphill, still ensuring everyone keeps in step. For the Four-Mile Speed March Test, the Recruits will be carrying their webbing, weighing 21lb, and their rifle, weighing 10lb. As with all speed marches, the test is conducted in boots and CS95 trousers and jacket, and the PTI aims for an exact 10-minute mile pace, meaning the four-mile speed march should take 40 minutes.

## Week 22

At week 22 all Recruits must get through the Battle Physical Training (BPT) Pass Out. This involves passing four separate tests, one immediately after the other, while wearing combat boots, CS95 trousers and jacket and carrying webbing weighing 21lb and a rifle weighing 10lb. They will have had extensive practice at all four tests, having completed all of them in 'clean fatigue' – *ie* without webbing and rifle – usually at around the week 13 or 14 stage of training. From weeks 13/14 to weeks 21/22 the Troop PTI will have progressively added weight to the Recruits to get them ready for the full weight tests at week 22.

As stated, the test is in four parts, which are basically four separate tests:

### ■ The Rope Climb

The Recruits must climb a 30-foot rope carrying the 21lb webbing and 10lb rifle on their back like a rucksack. There is no time limit. As with all the tests, it must be completed to the same standard, regardless of whether it is sunny, raining, windy or snowing.

### ■ The Assault Course

The Royal Marines Assault Course is something that many people – and media people in particular – want to attempt. For example, in the last three years alone we have had people from the *Sun*, *Blue Peter*, *Newsround*, *Extreme Sports*, *Zoo* magazine, *FHM* and numerous sports teams (including internationals) attempt it!

The Assault Course is approximately 800m long with obstacles along the way in the following order: Tank Trap, Six-foot wall, Fallen Gate, Crawl under the Cargo Net, Monkey Bars, Zigzag Wall, Chasm (including a half regain – explained later), Unstable Bridge, Five-foot wall, Gate Vault, Tunnels, and 12-foot wall.

The Recruits have to complete the course, carrying their 21lb of webbing and 10lb rifle, in five minutes or less. Young Officers and PTIs (who have to redo the tests on their PT course) must complete it in 4.5 minutes or less. A good time is around the 3.5-minute mark, but it has been completed in under three minutes.

### ■ The Fireman's Carry

The Fireman's Carry is exactly what it sounds like. All the Recruits have a partner roughly the same size and weight as themselves (wherever possible), and both men have to wear their 21lb of webbing and carry their 10lb rifle. The test involves picking the partner up on to the shoulders and then carrying him 200m in 90 seconds or less over grassy and muddy terrain. See page 176 for the technique.

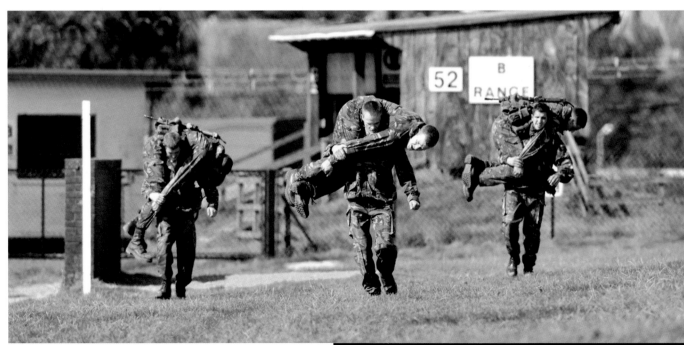

## ■ The Regain

The regain is an old technique used for righting yourself if you lose your balance whilst crossing a horizontal rope. Commando training has always taught going over the rope on the top, by laying the chest on to it, hooking one foot on top of the rope, using the lace part to push down and back for movement, and pulling hand over hand to move along the rope. This could be used to cross a rope over a large gap safely. Additionally, one of the Commando tests is the Tarzan Assault Course (see below) which involves crossing ropes in this fashion, at considerable height, while under time pressure.

Should a man fall underneath the rope, not only does the regain allow him to get back on top to continue with the test, but it also means he does not have to drop off the rope and risk injuring himself.

The regain test itself involves crossing a rope over 'the tank', a water-filled outdoor tank that breaks the Recruit's fall if he should fail to get across.

A half regain is the same thing, but without letting go with the feet to the dead hang position – ie it just involves rolling under the rope and getting back on top. This is performed on the Chasm obstacle of the assault course.

## ■ Failure

If a Recruit fails one part of the test it does not spell disaster, he can still pass the overall test – he just has to redo, and pass, the part he failed. For example a Recruit who passes the Rope Climb and the Assault Course, but then fails the Fireman's Carry, will still go on to attempt the Regain. If he passes the Regain he will then re-attempt the Fireman's Carry. However, if he then fails the Regain his test is over – ie an individual can only fail and re-attempt one part of the overall test. Two parts failed equals a failure on that day. A recruit failing the whole test will be given two further re-tests (of the whole test) with that Recruit Troop. If he fails the test three times he will be sent to Hunter Company to work on his specific weaknesses. (Hunter Company is our rehabilitation unit. If any Recruit suffers illness or injury – from a virus to a fractured leg – during training that prevents him from continuing, he will be put into Hunter Company until he has fully recovered. He then rejoins training with a different Troop, but at exactly the same point at which he left. Doctors, physios and remedial instructors see each recruit daily to ensure their recovery is as swift as possible.)

## Week 26

At week 26 every Recruit Troop completes the Six-Mile Speed March. Just as with the Four-Mile Speed March at week 15, this is completed in boots and CS95 trousers and jacket, carrying 21lb of webbing and a 10lb rifle. It is run as a troop in files, and the step is called by the PTI, who ensures a 10-minute-mile rate is kept up. As long as a Recruit can keep in step and keep the pace he should pass this test. However, if he starts to drop back or to run at his own pace it is very difficult for him to complete the test.

On successful completion of the Six-Mile Speed March in 60 minutes, each Recruit receives a 'cap comforter' and relinquishes

his blue Royal Marines beret. This signifies that the Recruits have moved into the last phase of their training: the Commando Phase. The blue beret is worn by all Royal Marines prior to being Commando-trained, and is consequently worn by all Royal Marine Recruits and YOs, and by the Royal Marines band, as they do not complete Commando training.

## The Basic Swim Test

As the Navy's infantry, the Royal Marines are amphibious soldiers and often transported on Naval vessels or smaller raider craft. In either case, all Royal Marines must be able to swim to a high standard, not just in a pair of shorts or even in clothing, but also carrying a certain amount of kit.

The BST requires a Recruit or YO to wear CS95 shirt and trousers, carry webbing weighing 10lb and carry a dummy rubber rifle weighing 10lb. He must then jump into the deep end of a swimming pool from a 3m diving board. Once he has surfaced he must swim 30m (usually 15m out and 15m back) without touching the side or bottom of the pool. Once back at the deep end he must tread water, without touching the side of the pool, and take off his weapon and hand it to the PTI on the side of the pool. Continuing to tread water, he then hands his webbing out in the same way. This mimics handing his kit back on to a boat if he has fallen into the sea. To drop his rifle and webbing to the bottom of the ocean would be disastrous, hence the test assesses his ability to remain calm, tread water and hand his kit to safety, which would then enable him to get into the boat. During the test, after handing his kit to the PTI he is required to tread water for a further two minutes. He can then get out, and has passed the BST.

## The Commando tests

It is worth mentioning at this point that prior to completing the Commando tests every Recruit Troop, YO Batch or All Arms Commando Course will spend between one and three weeks in the field, yomping very long distances with very heavy Bergens (100lb), practising troop and section attacks, undertaking Observation Posts, all the time living off Rations and having to cope with considerable sleep deprivation; all off which means that prior to the Commando tests they are highly degraded physically, and certainly not in possession of all the preparation an Olympic athlete would have before a big competition.

The four Commando tests are (in order):

- ■ **The Endurance Course**
- ■ **The Nine-Mile Speed March**
- ■ **The Tarzan Assault Course**
- ■ **The 30-Miler**

Ideally these tests should be completed over four consecutive days, and all must be completed with a single seven-day time frame. However, much like the BPT Pass Out a Recruit is only allowed to fail one test, and only once. If he fails two he is back-trooped and has to take all the tests again from the start, including the two- to three-week pre-test field exercises.

# Regain Technique

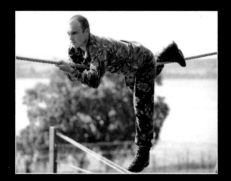

**1** At the centre of the 20-foot horizontal rope over the tank, the Recruit stops and composes himself.

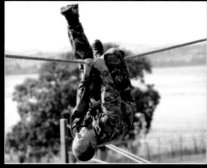

**4** He throws his head back and his hips up towards the rope, and hooks the back of his right calf over it.

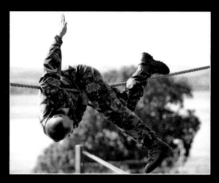

**7** Once his leg is facing down he throws it hard back the opposite way, which rotates him all the way round...

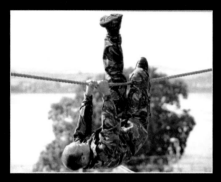

**2** He then purposely rolls himself underneath the rope so he is hanging underneath it by his hands and feet.

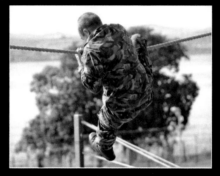

**5** Ensuring his left hand is above his right hand, he points his left leg straight up in the air and throws his right elbow over the rope (keeping hold of the rope with his right hand) until the rope nestles into his right armpit.

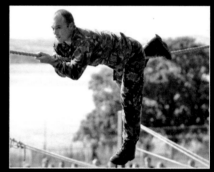

**8** ...and back on top of the rope. He then continues to the far side to complete the test. This is usually all done carrying his 21lb of kit and 10lb rifle.

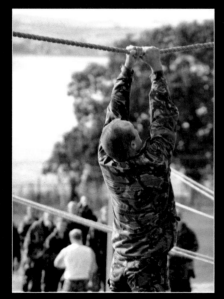

**3** He then lets go with his feet until he is hanging by his hands alone (a 'dead hang').

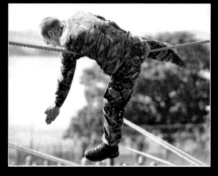

**6** He then lets go of the rope with his left hand and moves his left arm above the rope to put the rope under his left armpit, turns his left palm upwards and forces his arm back against the rope to ensure it does not slip out of his armpit.

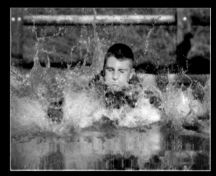

**9** For safety reasons "the tank" provides a water landing if the technique goes wrong.

### The Endurance Course

The Endurance Course test involves a 2–2.5-mile cross-country course on Woodbury Common, including crossing large ponds up to waist-deep (Peter's Pool), a completely submerged tunnel (the sheep dip), some large muddy bogs (the Crocodile Pit), and some extremely tight tunnels with water running through them (the Smarties Tubes) – all of this while wearing CS95 trousers and jacket with a T-shirt underneath and carrying 21lb of webbing and a 10lb SA80 rifle. Once the tunnels course is completed, the Recruit must then continue running all the way back to CTCRM, about 4.5 miles, carrying the kit already mentioned. Once at the camp he runs through it to the 25m firing range at the far end. He has 73 minutes to complete this test (YOs and PTIs have 71mintues).

However, the test is not complete at that point. To show that he has kept his rifle clean while completing the course the Recruit must now fire ten shots at a target and score at least six hits. If he gets less than six he will have to repeat the test. The reason for this is that a Commando without his weapon is effectively useless, therefore he must have learnt by this point to put his weapon before himself and ensure it is kept functional at all times.

### The Nine-Mile Speed March

There is not much to say about the Nine-Mile Speed March that hasn't already been said about the Four- and Six-Mile marches. It is conducted in the same kit and equipment, and the PTI again keeps to a ten-minute mile, meaning the test must be completed in 90 minutes. The test is relatively simple: stay in step and keep pace with the man in front and a pass is guaranteed. However, remember that Recruits are by now suffering the cumulative effects of being in the field for a couple of weeks and having completed the Endurance Course. The test is, for many, 90 minutes of private mind games, testing that oh so important strength of mind that every Commando must possess.

### The Tarzan Assault Course

The Tarzan Assault Course is a combination of two smaller courses: the Assault Course as explained for the BPT Pass Out and the Tarzan Course, a high-rope obstacle course that includes challenges such as the Commando Rope Slide, the Swing into the Net, the Postman's Walk, the Reverse Slide, the Jump into the Net, and a 30-foot wall to finish. The Tarzan course tests confidence at height, and the ability to move quickly while still remaining focussed at all times. Both the Assault Course and the Tarzan Course are in themselves tested: the Assault Course during BPT Pass Out (it must be completed in under five minutes); and the Tarzan course just prior to the Commando tests, to ensure that an individual can do it fast enough on its own, let alone when combined in the Tarzan Assault Course. Every Recruit must show they can complete the Tarzan Course in under five minutes.

For the Tarzan Assault Course the Recruits are expected to complete the Tarzan Course and all its obstacles except for the 30-foot wall, then sprint across the camp to join the Assault Course at the tunnel obstacle. They then complete all the obstacles of the Assault Course in a clockwise direction, finishing with the gate vault last. They then sprint back towards the Tarzan course and go up the 30-foot wall as a final obstacle. All this is done in boots and CS95, carrying webbing and weapons weighing the usual 21 and 10lb respectively. Recruits are expected to do the test in 13 minutes or under (YOs and PTIs in 12 minutes or under).

For many the Tarzan Assault Course is the worst test of all, as it requires a maximum effort for the entire time. Whereas the endurance course and Nine-Miler require a constant pace which is sub-maximal, the Tarzan Assault Course requires the pace of an 800m runner, but with obstacles on the way. It is a true heart and lung burner, and produces a lot of lactic acid in the muscles: the feeling of wanting to be sick on completion is not uncommon!

### The 30-Miler

For the other three Commando tests, the Recruits get to practise the test somewhat. For the Endurance Course and Tarzan Assault Course, the Recruits have actually run the whole course with their kit and been timed, so they know roughly where they are with the test. Before the nine-miler the Recruits have already completed a six-mile speed march, and have been on many long runs, so they know roughly what to expect. However, none of them will have done the 30-miler or anything like it before. For some, this

↑ The Commando Slide starts the Tarzan Course .

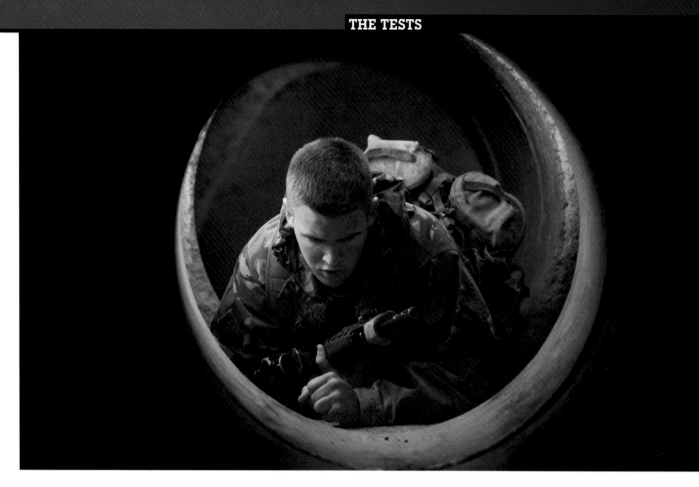

unknown aspect will be a good thing; for others, it is a real test of the mind.

The night before their 30-Miler (so on the day of their Tarzan Assault Course) the Recruits will travel to Okehampton Camp on Dartmoor, where they will spend the night. Dependent on the time of year (*ie* the light conditions and heat during the day), the Recruits will set off shortly before sunrise, which hopefully means that they will miss the hottest part of the day. They set off on the 30-Miler route in syndicates of between six and twelve Recruits. The instructors with them will know the route, but the Recruits will have received the details the day before and completed a route card, and will be expected to navigate while moving.

The 30-Miler requires the Recruits to complete 30 miles across Dartmoor cross-country in eight hours or just under. Young Officers are expected to do the same route but in seven hours or under, navigating themselves under the instructors' watchful eye, as major mistakes could lead to a failure for the entire syndicate. To complete the 30-Miler in the required time it is necessary to run on the flat and downhill and walk during the uphill elements. This may sound simple, but the Recruits are, of course, again carrying some kit and equipment. On top of their 21lb webbing and 10lb rifle each Recruit will have a daysack containing food and water, and some specific safety stores such as waterproofs, a warm jacket, a bivvy bag, flares and medical kits. The total weight of their kit is somewhere between 40 and 60lb.

For the majority of Recruits the cumulative effect of their time in the field, the three previous Commando tests and a certain amount of sleep deprivation over the last six months, means the 30-Miler is a tough test. Conversely, as it is the final test to obtain that oh so important green beret there is a certain amount of 'light at the end of the tunnel' enthusiasm. However, this cannot last for the whole eight hours! This test is the pinnacle of Commando training, being both a physical and mental test, requiring strength and endurance from both body and mind to complete.

## Conclusion

Following the Commando tests every successful Recruit receives his green beret and Commando flashes and becomes officially a trained Royal Marines Commando.

As you can see, the physical tests throughout Commando training are extensive and frequent. Although they are in place to ensure each Recruit is hitting the relevant fitness levels to give him the best chance of passing the Commando tests, they also put him under a lot of physical and mental strain throughout training. But this strain is itself a very important part of Commando training, as the mental and physical pressure it applies is probably as close as we can get to simulating the strains felt when on Operations in places such as Afghanistan.

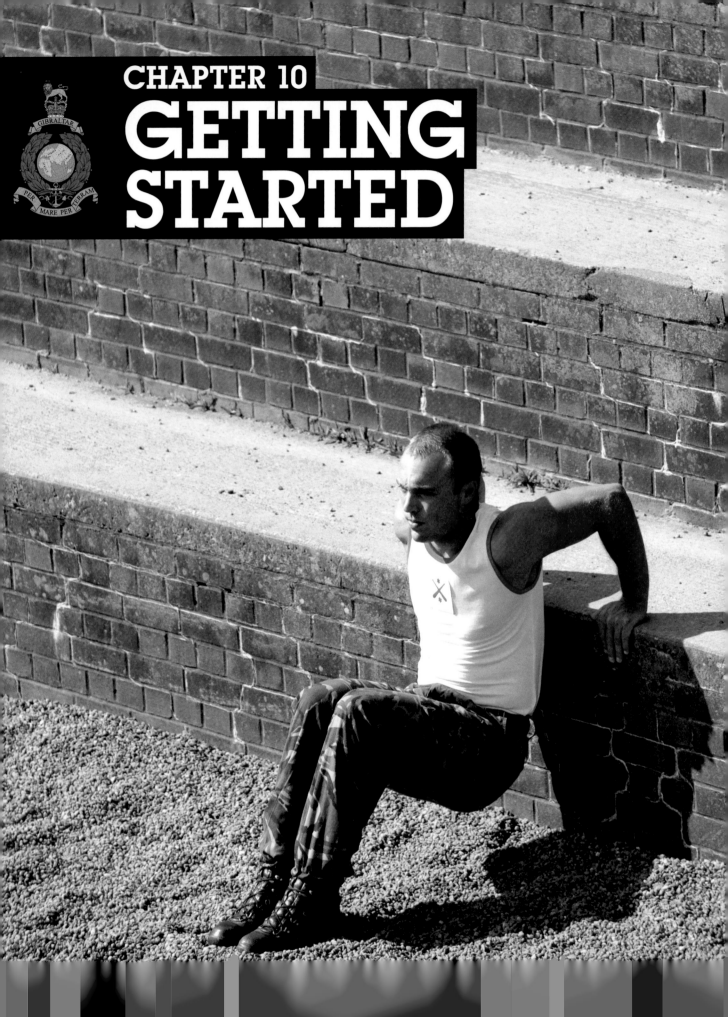

# CHAPTER 10
# GETTING STARTED

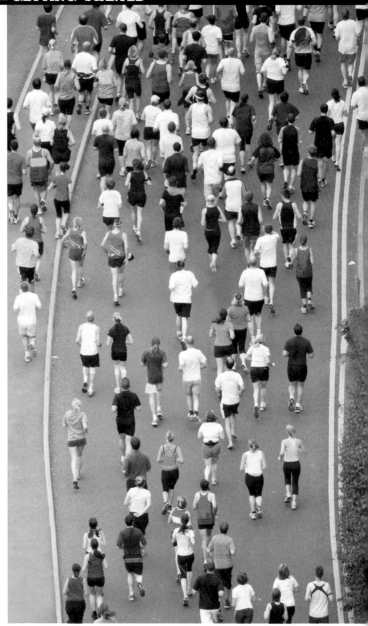

Be it a piece of course work at school, a university dissertation, quitting smoking, the first day in a new job or starting a new fitness regime, starting can often be the hardest part of all. Motivation is often the most important thing you need: keep your goal firmly in your mind and know that once you have started, once that first session has begun, it can only get easier.

If you have a specific end goal – say to lose a certain amount of weight, run the London marathon, or pass the PRMC – then setting an achievable milestone partway to this goal can help. If necessary, it is also worthwhile to set a few smaller markers or 'flags' that lead towards that milestone. Imagine your goal is to run the London marathon, all 26 miles of it: your motivation or end goal is obviously the marathon itself, but your achievable milestone may be a local half-marathon of 13 miles. Being half a full marathon it is probably achievable, but will still require significant training, just not quite as much as the full marathon. The flags leading up to the half-marathon milestone may be runs of specific lengths, either mile flags or time flags. So a flag may be four miles, six miles, eight miles etc, or a 30-minute run, a 45-minute run, a one-hour run etc. As the flags are reached it may be necessary to reassess at what point the milestone will be achievable, and to adjust your training accordingly if necessary.

The acronym 'SMART' is a good way of putting your goals, milestones and flags together. It stands for:

- **Specific** – All your goals must be specific and not general.
- **Measurable** – As stated above, it is important to aim at a certain number of miles, or a certain time, or a specific amount of weight. Just saying 'I want to be fitter by a certain date' is not measurable.
- **Achievable** – When setting a goal it must be achievable. If your goal is to run a marathon, but the race is in three weeks' time, that is unachievable for most people.
- **Realistic** – Goes hand in hand with achievable. There is no point having a goal if it is totally unrealistic. For example, not many of us could ever run a marathon in under two and a half hours, so this would not count as a realistic aim.
- **Timed** – You must apply realistic time scales to your goals, otherwise you will never reach them as there is no real pressure on you to train and improve. Even if the times have to be modified, everyone needs something to work to.

Just as with Initial Military Fitness (IMF) in Royal Marine Recruit Training, the initial focus of your training should be an overall body workout, ensuring that cardiovascular and muscular endurance is paramount. This will work on your robustness and ensure you are functionally fit for the more arduous fitness training to come. Initially it is probably sensible to exercise using only your body weight, and avoid too many weights or complicated pieces of equipment. Concentrate on pulling and pushing exercises to start with. Imagine you are stuck on a desert island and have no equipment but must stay fit. Use your body weight to exercise your muscles by performing pull-ups, push-ups, squats and lunges. You should find that initial improvement is relatively rapid, depending on your starting fitness level. Try to add one repetition to each set every time you do it. In no time at all you will be surprising yourself.

By using your imagination and improvising you will soon come up with ways to expand your exercises, such as performing your press-ups with your feet raised on a box or bench, or performing squat jumps instead of just squats. Don't forget to train your cardiovascular system; simply get out and run, cycle or swim. Set small targets (ensure they are realistic!) and try to improve each time, or each week.

Aim to make all your sessions progressive, and try to increase the number of repetitions every session or every week. With body weight exercises it is quite possible to work sub-maximally to near failure each time, then give yourself a set

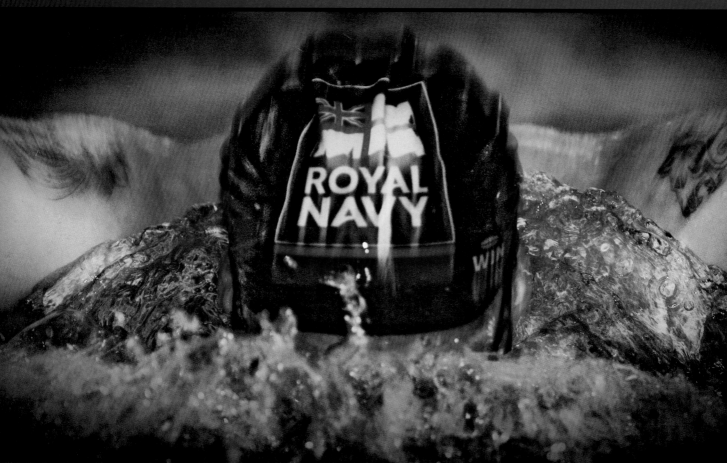

rest period (make sure you time it or you'll give yourself longer or get preoccupied chatting to someone). I usually take 30 seconds, one minute or two minutes, depending on how hard the exercise is.

There are a few more things that may very well help in the early stages of starting a fitness regime. We have spoken about motivation and having a goal, but there is also another necessity: you must have *commitment*. I have the utmost respect for every Royal Marine who gets himself through Recruit training, because I know the hardships that were involved. And the only way they did it was through *commitment*. Commitment requires you to say no to those nagging thoughts of quitting that we all have when things get really hard; it focusses us on our goals and what we want to achieve. If you stay committed, you will make yourself proud, which in turn will give you self-confidence that not only you notice but others will too. Commit to being committed now.

By purchasing this book you have already shown that you want to get fit the Royal Marines way, so in a sense you have already taken that difficult first step – you are not really 'getting started' at all, you already have started. So why stop now? Keep going, buy some good trainers, dig out some old (but usable) clothes or treat yourself to some new kit, and start training. Find yourself a goal, a milestone and some flags, and start planning your training. Remember, your body weight is your gym (press-ups, squats etc) and your environment is your treadmill, so get out there and start exercising. Stay committed, stay focussed and believe in yourself. Your mind is your only potential weakness, but it can also be your most powerful weapon and strength. Use it to ensure you reach your goal, whatever that may be.

### Medical advice

Every fitness professional is taught to advise that anyone beginning an exercise programme who has not exercised for some time should consult a doctor prior to embarking on it. Safety must always come first. For Recruits embarking on Commando Training, there a huge number of comprehensive medical checks and tests to go through prior to acceptance, and anyone undertaking a fitness regime should do the same where they can.

## Don't forget to train your cardiovascular system; simply get out and run, cycle or swim

# Kit and equipment

Once a decision has been made to commence an exercise programme, a doctor has been consulted to confirm that it is safe to do so, and some motivational goals, milestones and flags have been set out, it is time to get started! A good thing to do at this point is to ensure that you have the right clothing and kit to perform your exercises without injuring yourself. Don't get me wrong – it is not necessary to go out and buy all the latest kit from the top High Street sports shops, but it is worth spending a few pounds to ensure that your kit will not cause you problems. In addition, for some people, having spent hard-earned money on sports kit is all the motivation they need to keep training, rather than see the kit go to waste in the bottom drawer!

Many people are happy to exercise in old T-shirts and jogging bottoms and a pair of squash shoes or football trainers from about five years ago, and this is not a problem, depending on what you are planning to do. For example, I see many men running home from work or going out for a run in football (Astroturf) trainers or skateboard shoes. My very strong advice, however, would be *don't!* Use things for what they are designed for. You wouldn't go for a run in a pair of diving flippers, and you wouldn't expect to see a woman going for a run in stilettos, so why go for a long run in football or skate

shoes? They do not support the arches of the feet or provide cushioning like a specially designed running shoe, and hence over time will lead to injury. So always look for the right footwear. The Internet is a great place to start. If you have no luck there, many sports shops have sales on throughout the year.

As for clothing it is up to you. An old paint-splashed pair of jogging bottoms may be fine at first, but as you train harder you will find them hot and they will get soaked with sweat; they may even slow you down. Again, a couple of pairs of sports shorts will suffice – they do not soak up sweat so will not start to smell after washing, and they dry quickly so can be turned around day to day. In a similar vein, a baggy old T-shirt or rugby shirt will suffice at first, but will soak up sweat and soon start to smell. Rugby shirts and rugby shorts also tend to 'rub' in the wrong places due to the hard cotton from which they are made. So get a couple of sweat-wicking T-shirts or vests, which will wash and dry quickly as they are designed for purpose. The Internet is again a great place to find trainers, shorts, socks and T-shirts or vests being sold relatively cheaply, compared to the High Street.

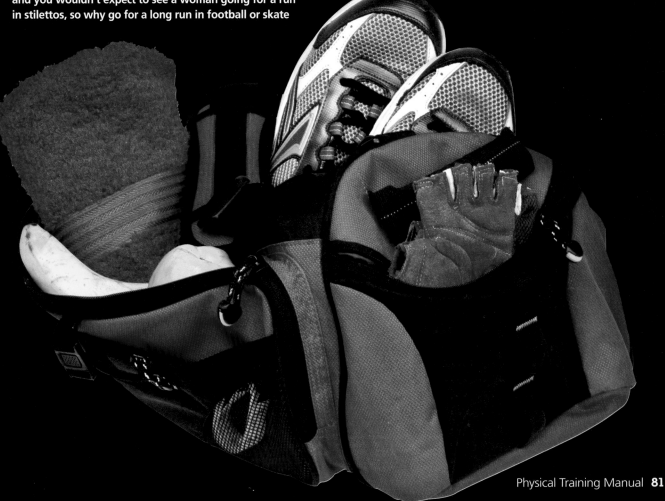

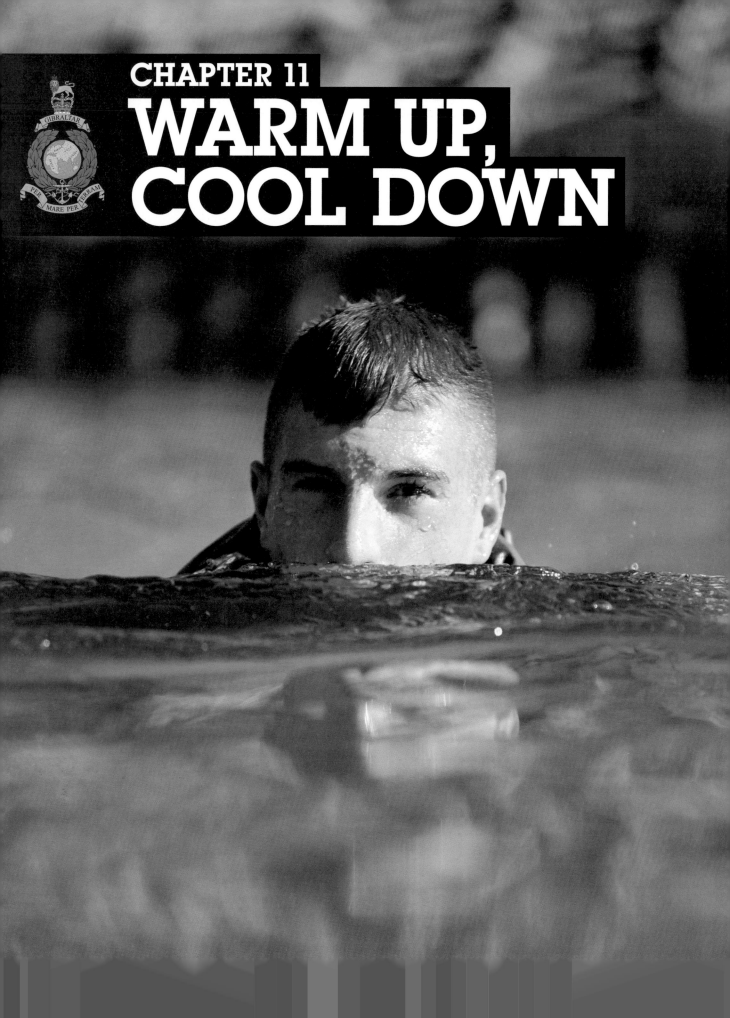

# CHAPTER 11
# WARM UP, COOL DOWN

Skipping the warm-up and cool-down is the single most common mistake people make in physical training. We have all done it at some point or another, me included. However, take it from me, skipping it is also the single most common reason why people get injured. A simple, basic, planned and constructive warm-up conducted prior to exercise is worth its weight in gold. Equally as important is the cooling-down routine at the end of a session, since not only does this again help avoid injury and aid recovery but it also allows the body time to make a steady return to normality.

The type of warm-up undertaken depends on the exercise session to follow. However, the majority of warm-ups will follow the same basic structure outlined below. During Commando training Recruits are warmed up specifically before each session. All PTIs are assessed on their PT course in a number of areas, one of which is how to conduct a warm-up, safely, appropriately and effectively. Recruits are therefore taught that a warm-up is not only necessary to avoid injury, but also has an effect on success. Warming up is especially important as part of Commando training because so much of the training inflicts large amounts of stress on the body and the connective tissue.

### Why warm up?

As well as the obvious reasons why we warm up, such as to help avoid injury, there are a number of other major benefits to taking 10–15 minutes to conduct a full warm-up:

### ■ To prepare the body for the demands of harder exercise to follow

As the cardiovascular system begins to work the blood vessels open more fully, allowing more blood to flow around the body, to warm it and to supply the major muscles and organs with an adequate supply. The increase of blood causes an increase in the rate of oxygen exchange from blood to muscle and tissue, which in turn allows the body to exercise to a higher aerobic level before the reduction of energy stores and rapid fatigue.

### ■ To warm the muscles, ligaments and tendons thoroughly

As the body temperature is raised, the muscle fibres, ligaments and tendons become more elastic as they are moved through their ranges of movement. This increases flexibility and reduces potential injury. There is also an increase in joint lubrication as synovial fluid is released into the joints, which only occurs on increased activity; hence the necessity of a warm-up.

### ■ To increase the core temperature

The increase in exercise causes an increase in energy production, which causes an increase in heat. Not only does this temperature increase allow the joints and muscles to become more flexible, but it also enables the body to start all the processes necessary in thermoregulation prior to the real session beginning. It will therefore be more efficient when needed.

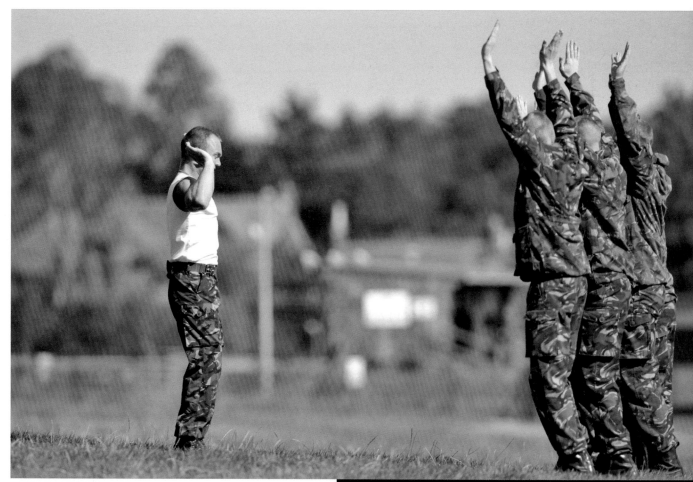

### ■ To increase mental focus and prepare the mind for physical stress

A warm-up allows the mind to start to focus on what is about to occur. It helps all the problems of the day to be forgotten and allows the brain to practise and enhance co-ordination, which helps avoid injury. If a hard session or competition is about to take place it ensures the mind is fixed on the job in hand.

### ■ To rehearse neuromuscular channels and their function

Similar to the co-ordination mentioned above, a warm-up rehearses the body for movement and function required for the session, by sending messages from the brain. This will again aid co-ordination. This is why some warm-ups, specifically for certain sports, should include sport-specific elements rather than being a generic exercise warm-up.

### ■ To prepare the body for extreme environment training

If the exercise session is to be performed in extreme heat or extreme cold, then a warm-up gradually allows the body, and more importantly the cardiovascular system, to adapt to the climate. To jump straight into hard exercise without a gradual warm-up, in either environment, would be unwise and is likely to cause problems to the body and its regulatory systems, let alone lead to injuries.

## Factors affecting the warm-up

### ■ Environment

It may be necessary to increase or modify the warm-up and cool-down periods when operating in certain environments. For example, if a session has taken place in the wind and rain, performing a cool-down outside in the same conditions may do little more than help the body catch a cold. It would be better either to seek shelter and do the cooling down inside, or to cut the cool-down short.

### ■ Timing

There is no real set time for a warm-up. It depends on the exercise ahead, time of day, activity prior to the warm-up (a ten-minute walk or jog to the gym vs just got out of bed), and the individual. However, a good warm-up should last for about 10–20 minutes, depending on the activity it is preceding. If time is short, the warm-up should last no less than two minutes, and ideally no less than five, once again depending on the activity to follow. I have conducted both two-minute warm-ups (prior to a gentle run in relatively warm conditions) and 30-minute warm-ups (prior to an important sports match).

### ■ Session intensity

The type of session will affect the type and length of warm-up necessary. For example, a very ballistic session like sprints or plyometrics can easily cause muscle pulls and tears and should therefore be preceded by a more comprehensive warm-up than, for example, a steady endurance run on a treadmill.

### ■ Session duration

A decent proportion of the time in each session should be allocated to a warm-up and cool-down. It is not wise to curtail the warm-up or skip the cool-down because time is short, but do not be unrealistic. If you have an hour for a session a 20-minute warm-up could be your way of sneaking out of doing some hard training. A quick five- to ten-minute warm-up would suffice, followed by a hard 40–45 minute session and a five-minute cool-down. Again, this will depend on the content of the session.

### ■ Session aim

Sometimes it is worth focussing the warm-up on the appropriate muscle groups that will be worked during the session. For example, a muscular endurance circuit for the upper body will still require a warm-up involving some form of cardiovascular (bike, jogging, skipping etc) to raise the heart rate and core temperature. However, a series of dynamic stretches on the legs are not really necessary, as the legs are not going to be worked. The upper body should be concentrated on. If time is a factor then the warm-up should reflect the session.

### ■ Ability level

If someone has not exercised for a long time, especially following long periods of inactivity or, worse, injury, a more prolonged and restrained warm-up may be necessary, not only to avoid further future injury, but to give the person confidence in the recovered area prior to the hard work of the session. Remember, for some people who have not exercised for long periods the warm-up itself may feel like a session.

## Psychological warm-up

It is often important to warm-up psychologically. This is more important if your warm-up is preceding a session that involves a competitive element, is particularly hard, or if you have not exercised for some time or are returning from injury. The psychological warm-up can form part of the overall warm-up or could be something you consciously do in the car, on the bus, or when walking to the session. For many people a piece of inspirational music can often help with psychological preparation.

Alternatively, during the warm-up itself go through the aims, goals and anticipated outcome of the session in your head. Keep your motivational goal at the forefront of your thoughts and – particularly for hard sessions – try to 'psych up' your mind. Some people find it helps to visualise themselves performing or competing effectively and efficiently.

### The 'psyching up' warm-up

This type of warm-up is usually reserved for professional sportsmen (especially boxers, rugby players and martial artists), but is used extensively by the Royal Marines prior to big tests. To properly 'psych up' it is necessary to bring out a certain amount of physical aggression. This can be achieved as part of a more dynamic warm-up in the form of combative games (Recruits, for instance, will sometimes wrestle prior to BPT sessions) or through certain inspirational songs that bring out the required aggression.

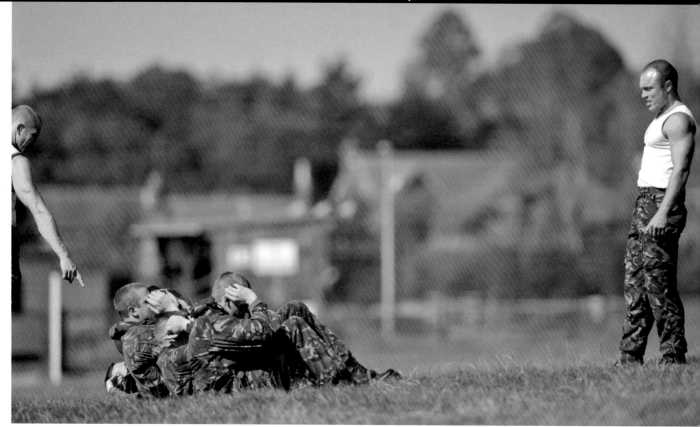

### Types of warm-up

There are two general types of warm-up:

- **The passive warm-up** – This involves increasing the body temperature using external means such as clothing (tracksuit bottoms, sweatshirts, hats etc), the sun (not always possible in the UK!) and massage (a good sports massage increases blood into the muscles in a similar way to exercise). Although these methods increase the heat of the body, they do little to motivate the body fully for increased physical activity.
- **The active warm-up** – This involves the progressive warming-up of the body and mind through exercise. This should be structured to start with easy exercise that is not explosive or ballistic, and then move steadily on to dynamic exercise.

### The phases of the warm-up

- **Passive warm-up**
- **Psychological warm-up**
- **General warm-up, mobilisation and initial pulse raiser**
- **Stretching (ideally dynamic)**
- **Second pulse raiser**
- **Sport/activity specific**

### ■ Passive warm-up

This involves wearing layers of clothing to warm the body. A good example is the 'warm-up suits' that substitutes in rugby matches often wear while waiting to come on to the pitch.

### ■ Psychological warm-up

As explained above, the psychological warm-up involves preparing the mind for the exercise to come. In some instances this involves 'psyching up' prior to a hard session or competition.

### ■ General warm-up, mobilisation and initial pulse raiser

This warm-up phase should be executed in a very controlled manner, starting slowly and ensuring that all movements are through the correct planes of the limbs. Any changes or build-up should be very gradual. This phase can be initiated by running slowly between two points, even if only five metres apart, running slowly in a circle, or running or skipping on the spot.

While running, it is important to mobilise the upper body's joints. This is done by moving the arms through a number of planes of movement. Examples are punching to the front, floor, sky, left and right; performing bench press, shoulder press, biceps curls etc in the air; or performing swimming strokes – front crawl, back stroke, breast stroke and reverse breast stroke (no, it's not a real stroke!) – in the air. This gentle mobility should be performed for one to two 2 minutes.

Whether running between two points or in a small circle, the neck can be warmed up by looking up, then down, left then right, then running backwards while looking over alternate shoulders. It is then necessary to mobilise the lower limbs further. This is done by gently flicking the toes out to the front while running forwards and backwards. Next gently bring the knees halfway up to the chest while running forwards and backwards, and lastly flick the heels halfway up to the rear, again while running forwards and backwards.

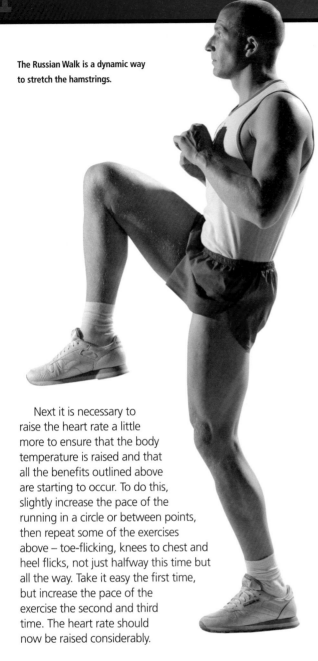

The Russian Walk is a dynamic way to stretch the hamstrings.

Next it is necessary to raise the heart rate a little more to ensure that the body temperature is raised and that all the benefits outlined above are starting to occur. To do this, slightly increase the pace of the running in a circle or between points, then repeat some of the exercises above – toe-flicking, knees to chest and heel flicks, not just halfway this time but all the way. Take it easy the first time, but increase the pace of the exercise the second and third time. The heart rate should now be raised considerably.

### ■ Stretching (ideally dynamic)

It is still acceptable to perform static stretches held for 8–10 seconds, and for many people who have been doing so for years it would seem unnatural to exercise without doing so. These days, however, it is suggested that, although static stretching is still regarded as the best practice post-exercise, it is not considered necessary pre-exercise. Dynamic stretching is now preferred instead, ie stretching the muscles via active exercises in the range of normal movement. Examples include five slow press-ups to stretch the pectorals and deltoids (chest and shoulders), five slow squats to stretch the adductors and glutes (groin and backside), five lunges on each leg to stretch the quadriceps (front of the thigh) and five 'Russian walks' on each leg (ie scraping the bottom of the shoe down an imaginary wall from as high as possible each time) to stretch the hamstrings (back of upper leg). See page 89 for examples.

### ■ Second pulse raiser

Following the dynamic stretch it is important not only to again raise the pulse but also to develop the warm-up somewhat. Now that the body has been through a dynamic stretch more ballistic exercises can be used, such as sprints, strides, hops, and jumps. These should be performed for about two minutes to ensure the onset of sweating and that the neuromuscular pathways are firing effectively. Where possible the exercises performed should reflect the exercise to come. If running, perform some sprints; if doing a martial arts session, do some kicks and punches; if weight training, perhaps some plyometric style exercises.

### ■ Sport/activity specific

At this point a football team could introduce the footballs and continue with dynamic stretching or secondary pulse raiser exercises but with the ball involved. The same can be done for rugby, hockey, rowing etc.

## Are you warm enough?

Following the second pulse raiser, you would want your pulse to be significantly high. Ideally, in fact, your pulse rate at the end of the warm-up should be around the same rate as that expected during the first exercise or part of the session to follow. In answer to the question posed, short of wearing a heart rate monitor you can only judge by how you feel. If you feel warmed up and prepared then move into the session; if you don't, then continue the warm-up. The following guidelines may help:

## Indications of a comprehensive warm-up

- **The onset of sweating** – Sweating is a true indication that the body's core temperature has risen and the muscles are expending more energy and thus are warming from the activity.
- **Increased heart rate and breathing rate** – As stated above, the heart rate should be around the level expected for the first part of the session. Breathing rate should be increased and by the end of the warm-up a shortness of breath should be developing as the energy systems are worked through.
- **Increased motivation** – For many of us, particularly prior to a hard session, there is a low, almost a lack of motivation. If this is the case then the warm-up should not only prepare the body, but should flush these feelings out of the mind and leave the exerciser feeling 'up for it' and raring to go.
- **Reduction in muscular stiffness** – In the first few weeks of starting exercise or following a particularly hard session, DOMS (delayed onset muscle soreness – basically exercise-induced muscular stiffness) may be present. A good warm-up should significantly reduce, if not rid the body of these feelings, thus allowing the exercise to take place without problems.
- **Increased concentration and focus** – Often the issues of the day cloud our minds when we start exercising. Consequently it is sometimes necessary to rid the mind

of all these issues so that you can concentrate and focus on the session. This is particularly important if the session is to involve complex or even dangerous exercises. A warm-up should focus the mind on the session in hand.

■ **Having to remove clothing** – This goes hand in hand with the onset of sweating, but can be an indicator just the same, especially in particularly cold climates where the thought of removing any layers prior to warming up may have been horrifying!

## Increasing the warm-up

As already mentioned, it is necessary to vary the length of a warm-up depending on who is training, what is being trained for, and when the training takes place. Most of this is self-explanatory, but here are a few recommendations regarding when the length of a warm-up should be increased:

### ■ Training in cold climates
It is very easy to tear or pull a muscle when it is cold. There is also a very real feeling of just wanting to get the training done and get back into the warm. However, it is well worth completing an extra-long warm-up to really ensure that the whole body is prepared, so as to avoid causing yourself any injury

### ■ Low fitness levels/returning from injury
Your muscles and body are not as resilient as those of someone who has been training for some time, hence you need to fully ensure that your body is prepared for what is to come, so as to avoid injury and also to minimise the muscular soreness that is likely to arise from the session. For injury returns, it is just not worth taking the risk of re-injuring the same site.

### ■ Training first thing in the morning or following a very static period
If you have been up and wandering around all day, then in effect you have been partaking in a very low-level warm-up (of sorts) all day. Your joints are somewhat mobilised and the muscles somewhat warm. However, if you have been in bed all night the opposite is true. It is therefore necessary to complete a slightly longer warm-up, not just to prepare the body but also to wake you up!

### ■ Attempting a new exercise or significantly harder session
If you have not been doing any weights on your lower limbs and have just performed endurance and stamina sessions using running, bikes, rowing or swimming as a medium, and then all of a sudden you attempt a weights session, the muscular soreness can be incredible. The same can be true if you suddenly up the weight of a certain exercise, or attempt to add another few miles to a run time etc. In these instances, it is a good idea to really prepare both the body and the mind with a long warm-up.

### ■ Training the same session/body part on successive days
Although I have suggested this is not advisable, as it can lead to overtraining, there are instances when it is necessary, or just part of the programme. When doing such sessions it is necessary to spend extra time warming these already tired and sore areas prior to training, so as to avoid injuries such as muscle pulls or tears.

### ■ When tired or fatigued
The Commando tests are an excellent example of the fact that rest is not always available. Recruits have to complete the 30-Miler despite being fatigued from a field exercise and the three previous Commando tests. To increase their chance of success and lower their chances of injury they are put through a lengthy warm-up prior to the test.

A final word. The current sergeant major of the Physical Training Troop, WO2 Rob 'Beau' Beauchamp, has long been the author and provider of the literature that PT courses are taught and tested upon. His words on warm-ups have stuck with me, and I feel they are just as poignant here as anywhere:

'If you haven't got time to warm-up, you haven't got time to train.'

**An explanation of the Russian Walk can be found over the page.**

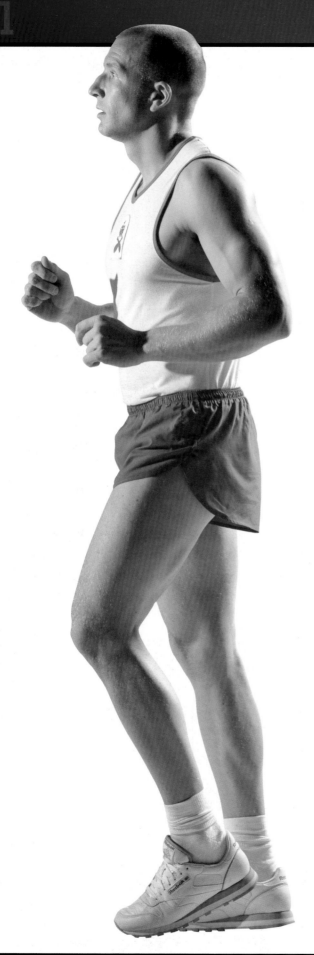

### The cool-down

As with the warm-up, the cool-down is often forgotten. If I had a pound for every time I've been training with someone and they have said they will skip the cool-down and 'stretch in the shower', then probably I could have paid someone else to write this book for me. The cool-down should *not* be skipped over. Not only will it help you avoid injury, but it also promotes recovery from the session just performed and allows development of your muscles' flexibility, which will pay dividends in the long run. Having said that, a cool-down is far more than just stretching.

Cooling down helps return the body steadily to its 'normal' state. It promotes recovery, provides time to consider the training just undergone (noting the good and bad points in your mind) and prepares the body for the next training session. Cooling down can also aid the body in removing the waste products built up during the session. It can be especially important in light of subsequent sessions on the same day or within 24 hours. Again, the example of the Commando tests is relevant.

Lastly, cooling down prevents blood pooling, as the muscles aid the heart and the cardiovascular system moving blood around the body; basically as the muscles contract they help squeeze the veins and push blood back to the heart. If a hard session is completed and then you just stop and sit or stand still, the blood pools in the lower extremities, as the muscles are no longer contracting to help it return. This can lead to a lack of consciousness (fainting) as oxygen delivery to the brain is inhibited and the body makes itself horizontal in order to ensure that blood is recirculated. The average cool-down will last anywhere between 5 and 30 minutes.

### Phases of the cool-down

The cool-down should focus on deliberate and controlled movements; there should be no need for any ballistic or dynamic movement. Hence the fact that 'bouncing' when stretching is frowned upon. The phases of a cool-down should include:

#### ■ Reduce

Keep active, don't just stop. Following a run, for instance, continue to jog or at least walk. This may be applicable to other exercise too, but for specific sports it is sensible to perform light versions of some of the sport's specific warm-up exercises. Reducing rather than stopping exercise does the following:

- Keeping skeletal muscles active ensures that blood is pumped around the body and does not pool in the legs, which can lead to fainting.
- The pulse rate is allowed to slow steadily, ensuring blood is still pumped actively round the body, which ensures that waste products in the muscles are circulated and disposed of in the liver and kidneys.
- By actively cooling down, sweating will continue, thus allowing the body to ensure its temperature is controlled adequately.
- Continuing activity ensures that the mind has something to concentrate on and can prevent the 'sick' feeling that often accompanies a hard session.
- Keeping the blood flowing ensures the delivery of nutrients essential for recovery.

# Dynamic stretch examples

Pick two points, and perhaps lay markers with cones or a jumper etc to distinguish them. Begin by running slowly between the markers, forwards in one direction and backwards in the other, ie so that you are always facing in the same direction.

- Run on the balls of the feet, flicking the toes out to the front for four lengths (ie twice forwards, twice backwards).

- Return to running forwards and backwards.
- Bring your knees half way up at the front (all the way up would be level with your waistband, so half this distance). Do this twice forwards, twice backwards. Ensure your arms move as well, but through the shoulder, not the elbow, just as in normal running – your hands should go from hip level to lip level ('hips to lips').

- Return to running forwards and backwards.
- Bring your heels halfway up at the rear (all the way up would be level with your backside, so half this distance). Do this twice forwards, twice backwards.

- Return to running forwards and backwards.
- Turn sideways, one way or the other, and continue to face in this direction (ie don't ever face the opposite way). Perform lateral sidesteps/lateral skipping as you move sideways. Ensure you use your arms for balance by swinging them up and down through your shoulders.

- Return to running forwards and backwards.
- Bring your knees fully up at the front (ie level with your waistband). Do this twice forwards, twice backwards. Again, ensure the arms move as well, hips to lips.
- Bring your heels all the way up at the rear (ie level with your backside). Do this twice forwards, twice backwards.
- Return to running forwards and backwards.
- Perform the walking lunge. Step forward with one foot (say the right) in a lunge motion – this should be a long stride to ensure that the knee of the foot stepping forward does not come above the foot of that leg. It should stay above the ankle. The knee of the static leg should get about an inch from the ground each time, while keeping the toe of the back foot in contact with the ground. Do three of these forwards and three backwards on each leg.

- Perform the walking squat. Ensure your feet are about shoulder-width apart and squat down so that your knees are at 90° and the upper thigh is parallel to the ground. Hold for two seconds, then come up, run two steps forward and repeat. Do five of these forwards and five backwards.

- Perform the hamstring (Russian) walk. Bring one leg (say the right) up off the floor so that you are standing on one foot with the knee of the raised leg bent. Straighten the raised leg as if you are trying to place the foot as high up on an imaginary wall as possible. Now scrape that foot down this imaginary wall until it reaches the ground. Run a couple of steps forward and repeat with the other leg. Ensure the foot is placed as high up the imaginary wall as possible each time to enable a good hamstring dynamic stretch. Do five of these forwards and five backwards on each leg.

- Repeat the high knees to the front and heels to the rear moves, but all the way to the waistband and backside respectively and as quickly as possible. Your feet should move as little forwards (or backwards, depending on the direction being travelled) as possible – ie you should fit as many steps as you can within the space you are using, while still performing the exercise.
- Return to normal running forward and backwards.
- Perform five controlled press-ups and five controlled sit-ups.
- Return to normal running forwards and backwards, but at an increased pace.
- Perform eight controlled press-ups and eight controlled sit-ups.
- Return to normal running forwards and backwards, but with increased pace again.
- Perform ten controlled press-ups and ten controlled sit-ups.
- Sprint one direction, walk back and repeat once more.

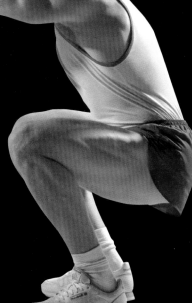

The above is just an example. There are many other dynamic exercises and pulse raisers that can be incorporated, some requiring a little more explanation and co-ordination than those above. Furthermore, though I have suggested repeating each twice, or performing five of each dynamic stretch, these numbers can of course be increased or decreased to suit.

■ Oxygen continues to be delivered to the muscles, to ensure any lactate is cleared as the body is moved closer to 'normal' levels (creatine phosphate/glycogen and ATP stores returned).

### ■ Re-dress

It is very easy post-exercise, especially when training outside or in a particularly cold gym (especially in a cold climate), to get cold very quickly. This means that the nicely warmed muscles that are about to be stretched get cold and are not as supple as you thought, and hence injuries occur. By replacing the clothes shed during and after the warm-up, your temperature is maintained and the muscles kept warm in preparation for the stretch.

### ■ Recover

Walk about ensuring good posture and keeping the head up; bending over or sitting down reduces the amount of oxygen the lungs can take in and also leads to blood pooling, whereas walking around and staying upright allows controlled deep breaths to be taken. It is important, no matter how hard the session was, to walk or even jog lightly to allow your pulse to lower slowly under control.

### ■ Relaxation

Stop and continue to take in deep breaths. Lie down on you back, as this will aid in lowering the pulse further (blood pooling cannot occur if the body is horizontal). Concentrate on relaxing – imagine yourself somewhere else, on a beach, in bed, wherever relaxes you most. Soon the heart and breathing rates will return to almost normal.

### ■ Stretch

There are two types of stretches: maintenance and developmental. At first it is probably best to stick with maintenance stretches, which should be held for eight to ten seconds. These ensure the muscles stay flexible and help improve flexibility to some extent. In time it is worth moving on to developmental stretches, which should be held for 30 seconds on each stretch. See page 92 for examples.

### ■ Eat

It is very important to eat something post-exercise. As explained earlier, there is a 'window of opportunity' to replace the energy (glycogen) stores within your muscles. In fact, research suggests that those who ingest some carbohydrates and protein within an hour of exercise will recover faster from the session and exhibit faster muscle growth compared to those who do not. However, it is not always possible to have carbohydrate and protein following a session, unless a specialised supplement drink (which can be expensive) is ingested. If this is the case, then something with a high glycaemic content is a must – a drink of pure fruit juice or a banana are great examples and will take advantage of the fact that the body can digest, process and store nutrients much faster than normal following exercise.

### ■ Treat

Prior to or while in the shower, or perhaps while drying off, assess your body for any injuries or perhaps a quick onset of muscle soreness. If any little niggles are picked up, the use of an ice pack can be a godsend. Obviously this is dependent on the severity of the injury, but either way it will certainly aid in the healing process and speed recovery.

# Ice treatment and injury

Before explaining the use of ice to treat injuries, it must be emphasised that, with any injury, it is worth seeking medical advice to ensure that serious damage has not been caused. Additionally, if your injury is to the head, neck or back you should seek medical attention immediately.

If you are certain that medical advice is not needed, or have sought advice and established that the injury is minor rather than major, the following guidelines maybe of use.

The acute phase of an injury is said to be the first 48 hours, so the important time to use ice is the instant an injury occurs. The type of injuries you can treat yourself are sprains to ligaments, strains to muscles, or impacts causing bruising. All of these injuries, if left untreated, will be dealt with by the body's natural biological pathways, but icing can speed the process up dramatically. All these injuries lead to classic inflammatory responses, *ie* heat, pain, redness and swelling, all of which are designed to protect from further injury and are characteristic of this phase, along with discolouration and loss of function.

'PRICE' is a simple mnemonic device to help you remember how to treat an injury. It stands for Protect, Rest, Ice, Compress and Elevate:

- Protect – To aid recovery and prevent further injury the injured body part must not be used in any painful activities or positions. It is sensible to immobilise it entirely. In a sense this means stopping all further activity immediately if injured; do not just press on, as there is a risk of adding to the injury.
- Rest – Arguably the most important part of injury management during the first 48 hours, which makes a direct contribution to the healing process. Anything causing pain and/or discomfort should be avoided. However, as soon as activities can be carried out pain-free, it is important to begin active recovery.
- Ice – Ice is a valuable tool for injury treatment. It reduces swelling and heat by narrowing the diameter of blood vessels, and numbs the area to reduce pain. Once the ice is removed and the area reheats, blood rushes back in, bringing all the good nutrients to aid healing.
- Compress – Some form of compression will help to control swelling by offering counter-pressure to the injured body part. There are a number of ways in which pressure can be applied: a Tubigrip-style bandage, a regular wrapped bandage, or a 'compression bandage'. NB It is important to check the circulation of the compressed area by squeezing a part of the body below it (*eg* toes or fingers) and ensuring that blood is seen to return. If it starts to hurt above and below the injury, chances are that the compression is too tight and should be removed or loosened.
- Elevate – If it is a leg or an arm, the injured body part should be elevated above heart level. This allows the return of blood and inflammatory fluids from the injury site and therefore reduces swelling. While elevated, it is important to carry out active recovery exercises in the pain-free range, *ie* static and joint mobility exercises. This enables your muscles to aid in the drainage of swelling, as they 'pump' while they contract.

We are all likely to sprain, strain, pull or bruise a muscle or joint at some point. Therefore, although a simple bag of frozen vegetables can be used, it may be worth purchasing an ice pack system from a sports shop. Most are under £10 and consist of a gelatine ice pack for the freezer (which can also be microwaved to act as a heat pack), a cover to put it in (to protect skin from hot or cold burns) and an elastic Velcro strap for applying it to the injury site. If you keep it in the freezer it will always be ready when it is needed.

Ice should be applied to the injury site until it is numb, which usually takes around 10–20 minutes. This should be done every two hours while you are awake.

It is important to protect the skin from an 'ice burn'. This is done by wrapping the ice or icing implement in a damp towel or cloth (or the cover the ice pack is provided with). Additionally it is valuable if icing a joint (knee, elbow, ankle, wrist etc) to remove the ice briefly every five minutes or so, to allow movement of the joint within its pain-free range. Due to the numbing effects this range may be greater than it would be without the ice.

If the injury is to the left shoulder it is important to seek medical attention prior to icing, due to its proximity to the heart.

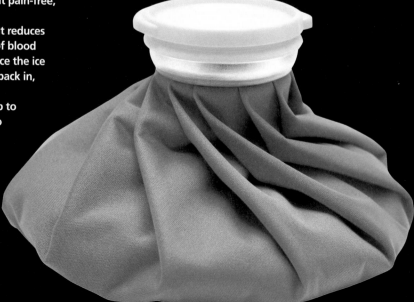

# STRETCHING

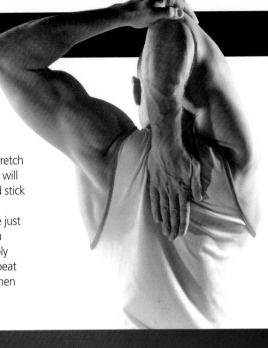

Below are a series of stretches that should be performed during the cool-down process. All can be performed as either a maintenance stretch (8–10 seconds) or a developmental stretch (30 seconds). For a maintenance stretch, take a deep breath and then breathe out as you go into the stretch, count or time for five seconds. Take another deep breath, breathe out and increase the stretch as you do so. Hold for the final five seconds. At first these stretches will feel uncomfortable, but should not be painful. Be strong-willed and stick with them. However, if at any time you do feel pain, stop.

Developmental stretches work in entirely the same way; they are just held for longer. Again take a deep breath, put the stretch on as you breathe out and then hold for around ten seconds. Breathe in deeply again, breathe out and increase the stretch, hold it for ten, then repeat one more time. Try to repeat each 30-second stretch three times when performing developmental stretches.

## Single leg hamstring stretch

Tuck the left foot into the groin, but extend the right leg so that it is straight and the left sole nestles into the inside of the right thigh. Reach forward as far as possible and take hold of part of your right leg (the bottom of the foot is your final aim, but to begin with the ankle or shin is fine). Try to bend from the lower back as you stretch and don't round your upper back too much. Keep the leg straight – the back of your knee should be on the floor. Repeat for the left leg. You should feel the stretch on the back of the upper part of the outstretched leg.

## Double leg hamstring stretch

Similar to the single leg hamstring stretch, but the double leg involves sitting with both legs outstretched and then reaching as far down them as possible (taking hold of the bottoms of the feet, ankles or shins). Again, try to bend from the lower back, not the upper back. Stretch should be felt in the backs of both legs.

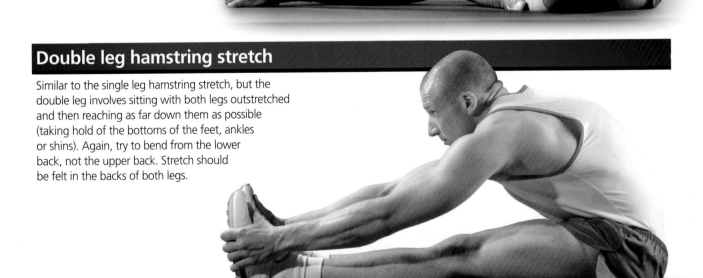

## Groin (adductor) stretch

Sit up with your legs bent as if you are going to cross them. Put the soles of your feet together (I usually remove my trainers) and pull your heels in towards your groin, keeping your soles together. Take hold of your ankles with your hands and place your elbows on to the inside of your knees. While keeping your soles together, heels in, hands on ankles, use your elbows to push down through your knees, flattening the legs out and stretching the groin. You should feel a stretch on the inside of both legs.

## Glutes (backside) stretch

Sit on the floor with your left leg outstretched and right leg bent up. Staying seated with your left leg outstretched, place your right foot over the left leg and allow it to nestle on the outside of the left thigh, parallel to it. Your right leg should now be up across your chest. Keeping your right foot on the floor, hug your right leg into your chest with your arms. Repeat with the opposite leg. You should feel the stretch in the buttock of the bent leg.

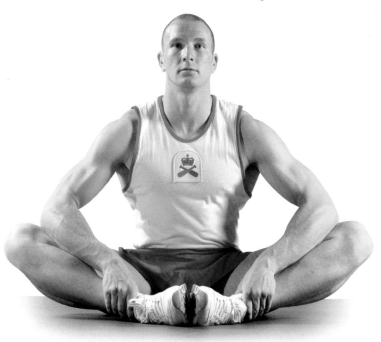

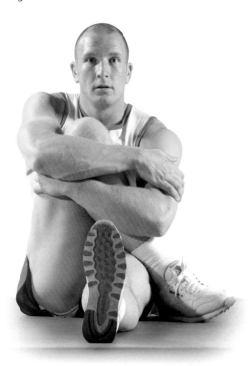

## Quadriceps stretch

Roll over on to your right side, ensuring your right leg is straight. Bend your left leg and take hold of your left foot and pull it up towards your backside. Try to keep your knees level with each other, and your shoulders, hips and knees in line. This will avoid structural injuries. To increase the stretch, pull the foot further into your backside and ease your hips in a forward direction. Repeat, lying on your opposite side, for the other leg. You should feel the stretch at the front of the bent leg.

## Standing hamstring/lower back stretch

From a standing position, with your legs just under shoulder-width apart, drop your chin on to your chest and allow the upper body to fold, lean forward and hang down. Do not bend the legs at all, but keep them as straight as possible. When coming up from the stretch be careful – ensure you do so slowly and safely. Stretch should be felt in the backs of both upper legs, and for some people in the lower back.

## Calf stretch

Pushing against a wall or a partner with straight arms, place one foot in front of the other about shoulder-width apart. The rear leg should be straight, the front leg bent, and your body should be at an angle of about 45°. Force the heel of the rear leg into the floor. To increase the stretch, move the rear leg back further, away from the body. Do not bend the rear leg. Repeat for the opposite leg. Stretch should be felt at the back of the lower rear leg.

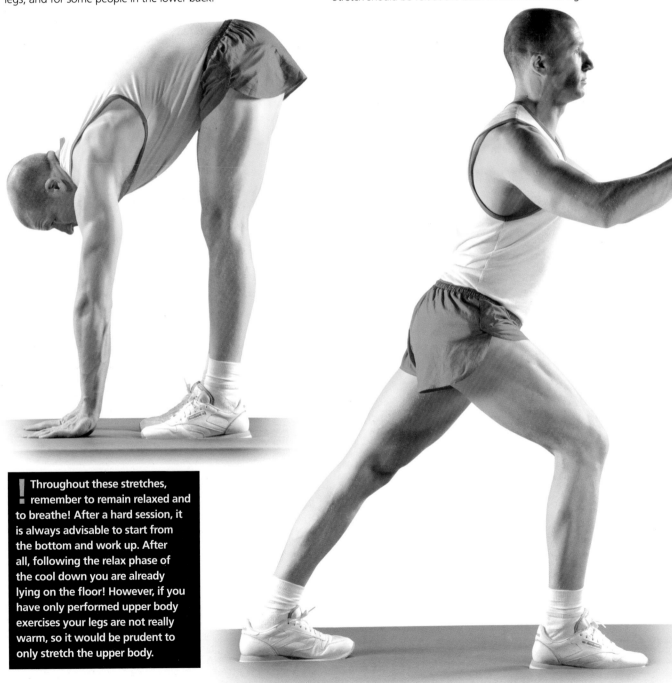

**! Throughout these stretches, remember to remain relaxed and to breathe! After a hard session, it is always advisable to start from the bottom and work up. After all, following the relax phase of the cool down you are already lying on the floor! However, if you have only performed upper body exercises your legs are not really warm, so it would be prudent to only stretch the upper body.**

## Deltoid (Shoulder) stretch

Stand in an upright position, with feet about shoulder-width apart. Put your right arm across your body at chest height. Use your left arm to pull the right arm into the body and then look over your right shoulder. Repeat with the other arm. Stretch should be felt in the shoulder of the arm across the chest.

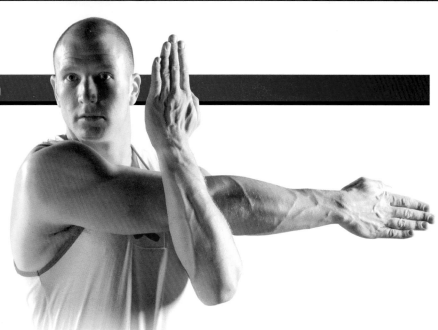

## Pectorial (chest) stretch

Standing in an upright position, with feet about shoulder-width apart and a slight bend in the knees, place the palms of both hands into your lower back with your fingers pointing down. Push the chest forward and try to bring the shoulder blades and elbows together behind you. Stretch should be felt in the chest and front of the shoulders.

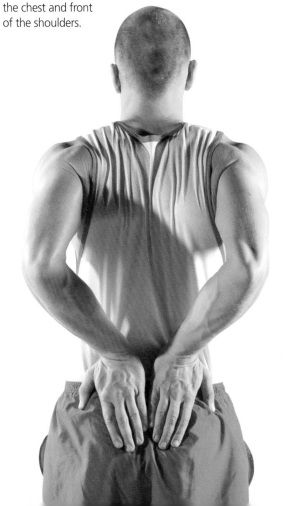

## Triceps (back of the arm) stretch

Stand in an upright position, with feet about shoulder-width apart. Put your right arm down your back, behind your head, down the line of your spine. Place your left hand on your right elbow and gently try to ease your right arm further down your back, walking your fingers if necessary. Try to keep your head up. Stretch can be increased, and partially moved into the lats (upper back), by leaning to the opposite side of the arm being stretched (ie in this example by leaning to the left). Repeat with the opposite arm. Stretch should be felt down the back of the arm behind the head.

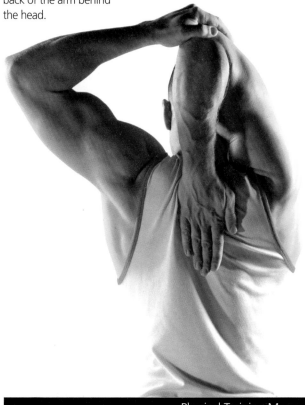

## Forearm stretch

Kneel down on all fours with your hands on the floor directly under your shoulders. Turn both hands outwards so that your fingers point back towards your knees, not away. Shift your weight backwards (*ie* move your backside towards your heels) but keep your hands flat on the floor. Stretch should be felt down the front of the forearms.

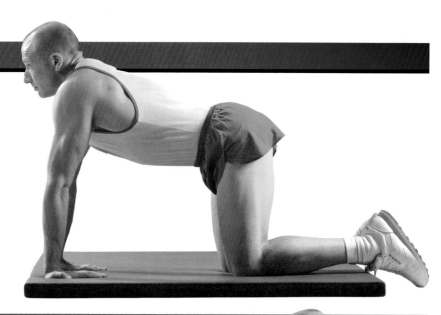

## Abdominal stretch

Lay flat on your front on the floor and place your hands under your shoulders as if you were going to start doing press-ups. Push down through your hands as if performing a press-up but do not allow your hips and legs to come off the floor (*ie* rotate through your lower back). Try to straighten the arms as far as possible without allowing the hips to rise from the floor. Stretch should be felt through the abdominals at the front of the lower torso.

## Back stretch

Lay flat on your back on the floor, arms outstretched to your sides as if on an imaginary crucifix. Take one leg across your body (say the right leg) and try to get the foot of that leg as far up towards the opposite hand as possible (in this case the right foot into the left hand). Hold for the normal time period. Repeat on the opposite side. Stretch should be felt around the middle of the spine, somewhere between the upper back and the lower spinal area.

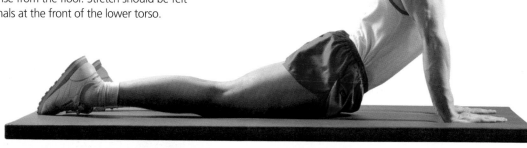

There are a number of other stretches that can be performed, the above being examples of just the major ones you could utilise for the main muscle groups you will use in general cardiovascular and muscular exercise. All of the leg stretches described on the floor also have standing versions that can be substituted if the ground is wet or particularly muddy. However, I have not included these, as the list is already lengthy enough. The standing stretches are not only available on the Internet and in other books, but are also shown in video format on the official Royal Marines website (also accessible via YouTube).

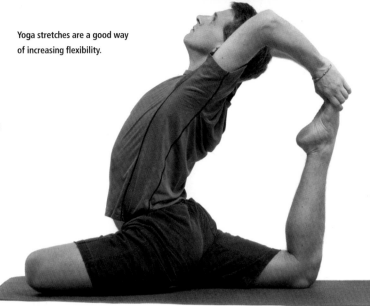

Yoga stretches are a good way of increasing flexibility.

### Stretching beyond

Ensuring you stretch after every session is a great start, especially if you can start moving into developmental stretches as soon as possible. This will not only aid your recovery, but will make your muscles fitter and healthier in an all-round sense. Additionally, flexibility will, of course, help in avoiding injury. However, to really make the most of developmental stretching it is worth planning in some specific stretching sessions. Yoga and Pilates classes at gyms are often a good way of increasing flexibility in an instructor-led fashion, especially if you are not good at motivating yourself. Personally I find that 20–30 minutes sat on the floor in front of the TV performing a number of maintenance stretches has paid dividends for my overall flexibility, strength and fitness.

### The complete session

- **Passive warm-up** – Add layers of clothing, walk or jog to your session or get out into the sun (if there is any).
- **Psychological warm-up** – Keep your motivational goal at the front of your mind. Focus on the feeling of success that awaits you at the end of the session.
- **General warm-up, mobilisation and initial pulse raiser** – As described above. Running in a circle or using a couple of markers, perform a series of drills and simple exercises.
- **Dynamic stretching** – Use realistic movements to stretch your muscles over their true range.
- **Second pulse raiser** – Some form of aerobic exercise and more dynamic exercises to get the heart pumping and the blood flowing. Focus on raising the body's temperature and inducing sweating.
- **Sport/activity specific** – If warming up for a specific sport or activity it may be an idea to include some of the games or techniques that it involves.
- **Main session** – The reason you are warming up in the first place. This should last for at least 30 minutes.
- **Reduce** – Towards the end of the session do not just stop! This can cause blood pooling and possibly fainting. Instead, reduce the activity – perhaps walk around in a circle, or perform a reduced version of the activity. Some of the early warm-up exercises could be used, performed slowly.
- **Re-dress** – Put back on the layers removed during the passive warm-up, to ensure that the muscles do not get cold prior to the stretch phase. Obviously, if training in hot climates this may not be necessary.

- **Recover** – Continue to move, but take it down to a walk, swinging the hands naturally at the sides. Continue to concentrate, think about the session. Analyse its good and bad points while walking around and allowing the body to settle.
- **Relaxation** – Lie down on the floor, or preferably a mat if indoors, and relax. Starfish your arms and legs and let gravity aid the heart. The pulse should reduce dramatically.
- **Stretch** – Perform all the stretches that are relevant to your session.
- **Eat** – Do not let the 'window of opportunity' escape you. At least have something with a high glycaemic content to replace the glycogen stores in your muscles. If possible have a full meal within the hour, preferably consisting of protein and carbohydrate.
- **Treat** – Check for any niggles or injuries while you are in the shower. These should have shown themselves during the stretch, but adrenaline can often still be high. If any issues are found, ensure ice is applied immediately.

## Conclusion

As stated at the start of this chapter, skipping the warm-up and cool-down of a session is the major and most common mistake made by people undertaking physical training. Although the young can get away with it, it will not take long before you start feeling the aches and pains that a warm-up and cool-down could have reduced. Worse still, you may be injured because no warm-up was conducted. Most people learn this the hard way – don't be one of them. If you are starting a fitness regime, build a warm-up and cool-down into it. Keep it simple and easy to remember, involving the elements outlined above, and you cannot go far wrong. Time and space should not be an issue. Remember: 'If you haven't got time to warm-up, you haven't got time to train.'

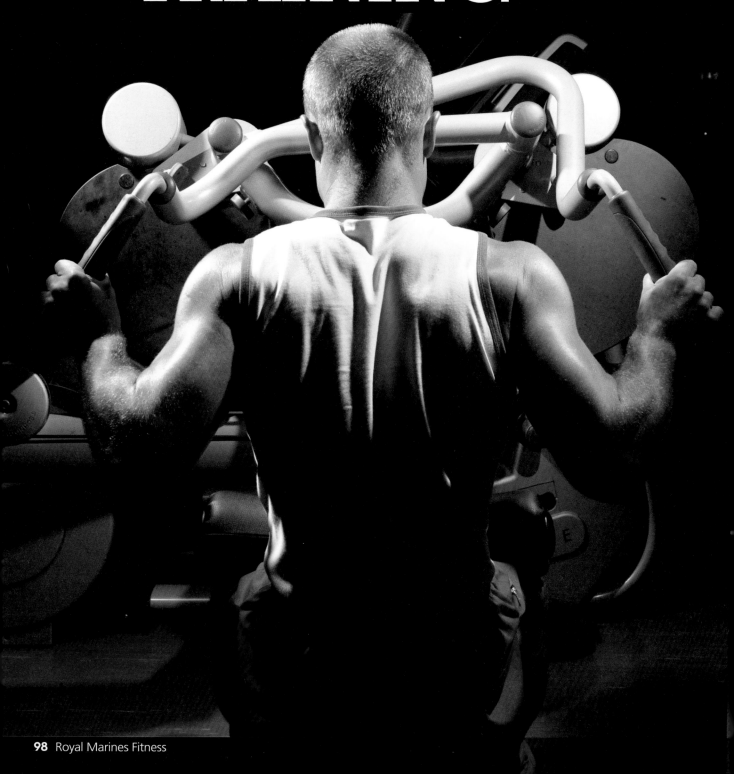

# CHAPTER 12

# FITNESS TRAINING

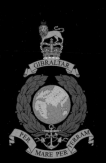

**N**ow we are finally coming to the meat of this book and what you are really here for. The next few chapters will provide the tools and methods that will allow you to start training towards your goals. This chapter in particular explains some of the ideas and processes behind fitness training and how to use the methods discussed in this book. It will also provide some specific ways of improving your fitness in the areas you want.

## The principles of training

It is obvious that to become fitter any individual must train. But how does the layman know when to train, how much to train, or if they are overtraining? Not everyone can afford a personal trainer who will explain and programme-in these elements. It is therefore important to understand the five principles of training:

- **Specificity**
- **Progression**
- **Overload**
- **Reversibility**
- **Tedium**

By remembering these five principles (which form the useful mnemonic SPORT), fitness training is made a lot easier. They ensure that training is focussed on the areas you wish to improve (specificity), ensure you increase gradually and do not overtrain (progression), ensure that you work harder every time than you would 'normally' expect to (overload), stop you losing your fitness through inactivity (reversibility), and ensure your training is interesting and engaging (tedium).

### ■ Specificity
Specificity ensures that you do not train the wrong component for an entirely different goal. In simple terms, training is very specific: if you want to see an improvement in something, you must train it – specifically. For example, if a young man wishes to increase the strength of his upper body muscles, but is continually training his legs, he will not see the gains he wants. He is not being specific with his training. He needs a training programme that puts regular stress on the muscles he is concerned with strengthening, in this case his upper body.

If we consider this in terms of muscle fibres, a sprinter needs speed, so must include speed and power work in his training to specifically develop his fast twitch muscle fibres. Conversely, an endurance runner would want slow twitch fibres that can work for long periods of time without fatigue, so needs training that involves long periods of steady stress. Recruits and Royal Marines require both fast and slow twitch fibres, so therefore have training programmes that develop both types.

### ■ Progression
Increasing the amount of exercise increases the amount of stress on the body, and causes adaptations to that stress. If this stress is added in too big an increment or too quickly, then injury or overtraining can occur. If the stress is not big enough, then often boredom and staleness can occur, and the need for a challenge will mean that interest is lost or a very large challenge is sought, which can lead to injury. Therefore any training or 'stress' must be progressive and gradual, but specific to the individual. Remember, there are lots of different parts that can become injured if stresses increase too rapidly. It is not only the muscles that have to adapt, but ligaments, tendons and bones as well. Furthermore, in general ligaments, tendons and bones take longer to adapt than muscles and hence can be more prone to injury if training is increased very quickly.

It is often very difficult to know if you have progressed too quickly or if you are not progressing quickly enough. This comes back again to 'know thyself'. If you feel drained or faint, or are particularly struggling with a new or increased session, then perhaps you need to pull back. On the other hand, if you feel bored or disinterested then perhaps a change and a progression is needed to re-enthuse and re-challenge you.

For cardiovascular training, a heart rate monitor can be a godsend. It provides feedback as you need it so that you can judge for yourself if the progressions you have introduced are a little too much, just right, or not quite enough.

### ■ Overload

To improve the fitness of any part of any body there is a necessity to overload (or stress) the various body systems. Basically, we need to make the body work harder than it normally does. In response to working harder than normal the body will gradually adapt to this 'extra work' and become fitter.

An example of this is running. If someone has been training their aerobic system and can now run three miles twice a week at the same pace, they have reached a certain level of fitness. They will not become fitter by continuing to run three miles twice a week at that pace. Their body has already adapted and is happy with this requirement. To improve their fitness this individual must increase something – either the distance (from three to, say, four miles), their speed (by completing the three miles faster), or the number of times they run (from twice a week to three or four times a week). All of these methods will overload the aerobic system so it will have to gradually adapt to cope with the chosen overload. Obviously, the chosen overload will be specific to the individual's overall goal, ie to run a marathon or to run three miles in under 18 minutes will require different overloads. This brings us on nicely to the 'FITT' overload principles:

– *Frequency*
– *Intensity*
– *Time*
– *Type*

These help ensure that the principles of training are adhered to, but more specifically ensure that training takes place often, is increasingly harder over time, is increasingly longer over time, and trains the correct areas of fitness.

#### Frequency

It is important to ensure that training takes place at least three times a week. As has already been discussed, the body needs time to rest and recover, so these sessions should be spaced throughout the week. Once the body becomes fitter, it is possible to increase the number of weekly sessions from three to four, five or even six. However, some sessions will need to be far easier than others.

#### Intensity

Fitness will not improve unless the body is worked hard enough that it needs to adapt. It is important to up the intensity enough to ensure gains, but not too much to cause injury. A heart rate monitor is an excellent tool for the job.

#### Time

To see improvements in the aerobic system, training sessions will need to gradually increase in length. By making the sessions last longer, the aerobic system is stressed for longer and adaptations are made to aerobic fitness. It is also necessary to increase the heart rate that is worked at as the body adapts and becomes fitter.

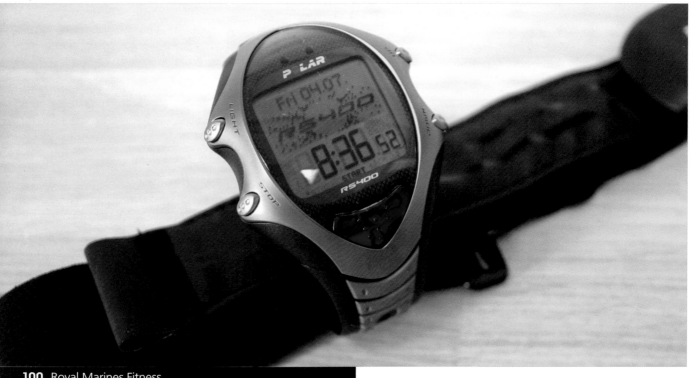

*Type*

Any training programme developed must be based in the foundations of the required fitness goals. For example, a top rugby player does not want a training programme to prepare him for a marathon. A training programme must contain the types of activities and exercises that will develop the fitness needed. It is, of course, paramount to analyse the fitness requirements in relation to the goal.

### ■ Reversibility

It is clear that our bodies adapt to an increase in stress by becoming fitter, so it makes sense that a decrease in stress will have the opposite effect. It only takes three to four weeks for the body to start to adapt to less stress and to become less fit. Studies have shown that aerobic fitness is lost much more quickly than anaerobic, as the muscles very rapidly lose their ability to use oxygen more effectively. Anaerobic fitness is affected far less by lack of training. If our muscles are not used they waste away, gradually losing strength and speed. Research has shown that strength gains are lost at about one third the rate of gain. For example, if strength training has been occurring for about four weeks, then after 12 weeks of no training all resultant gains would have been lost.

### ■ Tedium

Boredom is the route to giving up training and going to the pub or sitting in front of the TV. By having a variety of sessions and ideas at your fingertips you should never become bored. However, some training programmes do become boring and the trainee loses interest. To avoid this it is necessary to use a variety of training methods, change things frequently, and every now and again throw in a different type of session. By doing this overuse injuries are also avoided, as the methods for performing activities are constantly changed and varied.

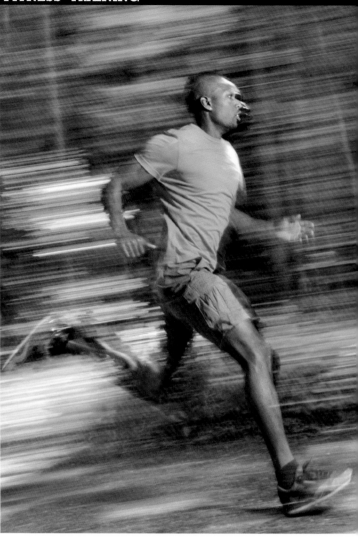

## Planning a training programme

When planning a training programme it is important to bear in mind all the principles highlighted above to ensure that the training is going to be beneficial and not detrimental to fitness, and most importantly to ensure that it is going to work.

## Training methods

There are many different methods of training. Though each develops the body in a number of different ways, each is based on how the body adapts to different types of training. Which training methods are applicable and usable by an individual will depend on the goals required. For all-round fitness like that required by a Royal Marine, all or at least most of the methods will be applicable. For specific sportsmen, some will be highly applicable but others will possibly be detrimental.

## Endurance/stamina training exercises

These are classified as either non-impact exercise (*eg* swimming, cycling), low impact exercise (*eg* walking, rollerblading), or high impact exercise (*eg* running, step aerobics).

## Continuous training

Continuous training involves exercising without rests or intervals and can be broken down into two sub-groups: long slow distance training; and high intensity continuous training.

### ■ Long slow distance training

For this type of training it is necessary to run, swim, cycle or row, or do some form of aerobic/whole body activity for a prolonged period of time. Ideally these sessions should be performed wearing a heart rate monitor and the exercise performed at a heart rate of between 60–80% of maximum. Ideally the activity should last between 30–60 minutes. However, sessions up to 90 minutes are also beneficial.

This type of training is ideal for those people wanting to train for health reasons. It is fairly easy and relaxing but still provides a workout with an end product. These types of session are also applicable to most sportsmen/women in their off season, for 'maintenance' training.

### ■ High-intensity continuous training

These sessions should also be performed wearing a heart rate monitor, with the exercise being done at 85–95% of maximum heart rate. An example would be a 20-year-old runner who runs

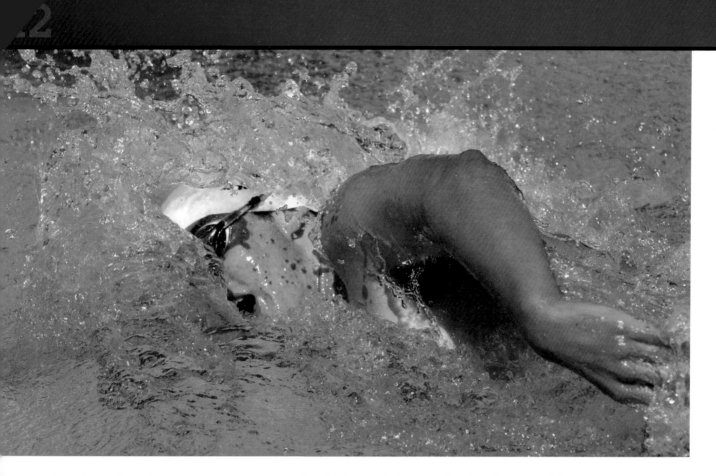

five miles at a five-minute-mile pace. His heart rate will probably be around 180bpm (beats per minute), which is very high considering his maximum heart rate is probably around 200bpm. This is very hard work and very high intensity, but it will improve his leg speed, strengthen his leg muscles, and improve his muscular endurance.

This type of training should only be one part of a training programme, as it is very high intensity, leads to considerable fatigue, and can lead to injury if overdone.

### ■ Basic continuous training intensities

| Level | % of maximum heart rate | Remarks |
|---|---|---|
| Low-intensity level. 'Fat burning'. | 50–65% | Long duration of 45–60 minutes or more. 90% fuel from fat. Unless individual is very unfit there is a negligible effect on CV fitness. |
| Mid-intensity level. Endurance. | 70–85% | Moderate duration of 35–45 minutes. 50% fuel from carbohydrates. Very effective at improving CV fitness. |
| High-intensity level. Stamina. | 85–90+% | Hard training. 90% fuel from carbohydrates. Highly effective at improving CV fitness through anaerobic means. |

### ■ An example of continuous training

Almost all of my training programmes contain continuous running sessions of both high intensity and long slow intensity, but this could just as easily be rowing, cycling or swimming, or a combination of all four.

An example of a week's continuous training that I have done many times over the years involves three runs – one high-intensity and two low- to mid-intensity, although one slightly higher than the other.

For my high-intensity session I would run at least 5km (just over three miles) and up to 8km (five miles) as fast as possible. I would be running for between 20 minutes and half an hour with my heart rate around 85-90% of my MHR.

For my very low-intensity long run I would run for between one and one and a half hours, covering between 9 and 13 miles. I would often do this completely off my heart rate (about 60% of my MHR) to ensure that I maintained a slow steady pace and did not try to push myself.

My third continuous session of the week would be halfway between the two. I would usually run between 10km (about six miles) and 12km (around seven miles) at a relatively hard but still comfortable pace. These sessions would last between 36 and 50 minutes. Again, a heart rate monitor is often used to ensure that I do not increase the pace too much.

### ■ Methods of determining endurance intensity levels

It is important that you can determine at what level you are training and how much stress you are putting your body under. The following can be used to assess this.

### Time and pace

Time trials 'against the clock' over a known distance, number of laps or checkpoints is the simplest and most efficient method of determining intensity. This simple method is the most useful for general fitness and in particular competitive endurance athletes. By cycling or driving a route you can note where the mile or kilometre markers are, and then when running you can check the time to get an idea of your pace. Alternatively, many GPS training aids are now available that will give you this feedback combined with a heart rate reading as well.

### Perceived exertion

Exertion has a direct relationship to the intensity of the exercise – the harder it feels, the greater the intensity. The level of exertion can be based on breathing rate and depth, the feel of the muscles, basic body/running co-ordination, and the level of fatigue. However, the perceived exertion method is not specific or accurate. Its accuracy will vary with the individual's training experience and the duration of the training session. However, if this method is initially used in conjunction with a heart rate monitor the perceived exertion can be 'learned' for a certain intensity and therefore judged without a heart rate monitor.

### Heart rate monitor (HRM)

There is a strong correlation between oxygen uptake (percentage of VO2 max) and heart rate. The heart rate can therefore be used as a guide to exercise intensity. Every individual has different abilities or fitness levels and, therefore, corresponding working heart rates. The traditional working heart rate zones can be inaccurate by plus or minus 10bpm or more. Additionally, the heart can be very misleading in its actual indication of exercise intensity, since it can be affected by the weather, climate, psychological state, hydration status, sleep patterns and other factors.

Out of interest, monitoring the resting pulse rate can be a good indication of recovery from previous training sessions, and thus can help prevent overtraining.

## Heart rate training zones

Research has shown that with arm work alone, such as arms-only swimming, the same VO2 max cannot be obtained as is reached when running, even though the heart rate may reach its maximum in both cases. Therefore to gain maximum benefits a swimmer will gain a greater training effect by running, as it uses a greater muscle mass and creates a greater load on the CV system than arms-only swimming at the same heart rate.

This means, then, that compared to running the heart rate will be a little lower when performing other activities such as swimming and cycling. In fact, for accurate heart rate usage the following should be noted when compared to running:

| | |
|---|---|
| Cycling | Subtract 10bpm |
| Swimming | Subtract 10–15bpm |

## Methods of measuring the pulse rate

### Manual pulse measuring

The heart rate can be measured by feeling the pulse in the wrist or the neck while timing using a watch. To minimise inaccuracies the count is taken over ten seconds and then multiplied by six.

### Heart rate monitor

This piece of kit speaks for itself, and is a great tool for improving fitness. I would advocate everybody owning one. The main advantage is the immediate feedback when training in different activities, conditions and terrain.

## Fartlek training

'Fartlek' comes from the Swedish for 'speed play'. It is a training system designed for runners, to allow them to exercise over much greater distances than they normally race and varying the pace so that it is enjoyable but still beneficial. Fartlek training can be used for running, walking, cycling or skiing. The emphasis is on enjoyment of the activity and improving your ability at it. The sessions are put together to produce aerobic and anaerobic effects, and despite having been originated for runners these sessions are also very good for sports players, as they mimic short intense bursts followed by brief periods of recovery.

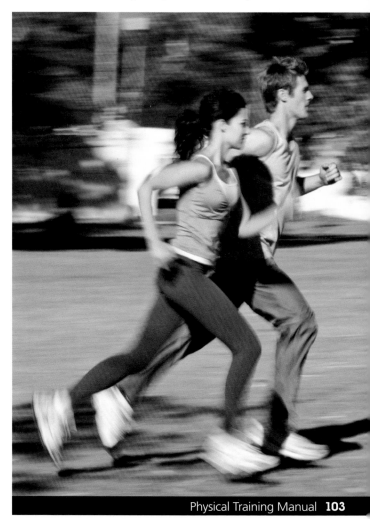

## An example of Fartlek training

A good way of performing a Fartlek session is to find a large field that has a number of sports pitches. It is then possible to divide the whole area up and do different paces and activities along the sides of the various pitches. If the sports pitches have a car park, track or road close by or around them, this is even better as the concrete, tarmac or shale provides a variant surface.

Set the different activities to be performed in different areas. It is always better to plan these, otherwise you will find yourself making the easy activities take longer and the harder ones shorter.

Following a good warm-up, you could start with high knee raises along the width of one pitch, then high heel kick along the width of the next. Then try over striding for the length of a pitch, then a steady normal running pace for three pitch lengths, before approaching a set of trees and running at a slower pace but weaving in and out of them, practising changing direction. Next sprint the side of a pitch as quickly as possible before slowing down into a recovery jog and approaching the shale track around the pitches (up until now everything has been on grass). Using the lamp posts along the shale track, sprint to one, jog to the next, sprint to the next, and jog to the next, etc. Repeat the whole Fartlek route three, four or five times.

Obviously, the above is an example in a specific area, but your own area and your imagination can also provide a fun, challenging and, most importantly, interesting session.

### Interval training

For most people interval training is the sort of training that is dreaded the most. It is a method that involves alternating between very strenuous exercise and rest, the rest periods giving the body time to recover from each exercise period. This means that the body can train for much longer periods of time than if no rest periods were included.

It is a common misconception that interval sessions can only improve anaerobic fitness, when it is actually possible to develop both aerobic and anaerobic fitness. It just depends on how the training is organised.

During interval training the following can be varied:

- Time or length of each exercise period.
- Intensity (ie amount of effort) put into each exercise period.
- Length of rest time between exercise periods.
- Type of activity undertaken during rest period.
- Number of exercise and rest periods per session.

### Intervals for aerobic fitness

To increase aerobic fitness using intervals it is necessary to exercise for relatively long periods, during which it is necessary to exercise at 75% of maximum heart rate.

### Intervals for anaerobic fitness

To increase anaerobic fitness using intervals, it is necessary to work for short periods at 85–95% of MHR.

## Rest periods

If high-quality speed training is the aim, then rest periods should be two to three minutes long each time. This gives the body time to replenish ATP and creatine phosphate stores in the muscles. Having very short rest periods simply develops the body's ability to perform or work when tired and when such stores are depleted. Again, which you choose will depend on your training aims and goal.

Studies have shown that our bodies recover better if we exercise very lightly during the rest periods as opposed to doing nothing. This is even more apparent for sports players, as it mimics what occurs in a game.

## Examples of interval training

In almost every gym you will find rowing machines (or ergos). Although these are excellent for continuous training, they are even better for intervals. Most can be set for intervals of time or distance, with specific rest times and even a boat on the screen for you to chase in order to maintain your effort. As the whole body is used during rowing, overall fitness, endurance and weight loss is seen remarkably quickly. I would thoroughly recommend the following session.

Set the rower for 500m intervals, or select 'just row' and row for 500m. You should be rowing as hard and as fast as you can for the whole 500m, which should take you between 90 seconds if you are fit and up to three minutes if you have significant room for improvement. Don't worry, improvement will occur quickly.

Following your row, have a set rest. I recommend starting with two to three minutes – any less is very difficult. As soon as the rest time is up, row another 500m as quickly as possible. When this is finished, take the same rest period before rowing again.

Try to decide how many intervals you are going to do prior to the session and keep to it. A good start is three or four, an excellent start is six. If you do not set the number of intervals before the session begins, I guarantee you will take the easy route and stop early. Once you have set the number you want, stick to it. When you can complete ten intervals with a set rest it is time to increase the stress. Either decrease the rest time, or, if you are feeling adventurous, increase the row length to 600 or even 750m.

Outside of the gym, an excellent interval training session involves a simple full-size football or rugby pitch. Start at one corner and run around the pitch as quickly as possible. This should take between 50 seconds and two minutes. Take a two to three minute rest period and then repeat. As with the rowing, try to set the number of intervals prior to starting and the length of rest period, and stick to both. For added incentive, time the first interval you do at 100% and then ensure every further interval is less than 10% more than this. For example if the first time round you get 1 minute 10 seconds, all the subsequent intervals should be done in less than 1 minute 17 seconds. This encourages you to put maximum effort into each interval. A football pitch is a good start, but half a pitch, two pitches, a car park etc could all be used as well.

Intervals are also a great way of improving swimming. Many people find, when starting out, that they cannot swim a front crawl (properly, with their head in the water) constantly for 30–40 minutes. Doing a swimming interval session not only builds fitness through intervals but also allows the stroke to be practised with rests in between. A good start is two to six lengths (dependent on the length of the pool) and one to two minutes' rest, then repeat. Over time you should up this to 8, 10, 12, 15 lengths etc. Ensure that the number of lengths and rest times are decided beforehand and kept to.

## Parlauf training

This is similar to interval training but is usually performed as a pair. The partners alternately complete one lap around a marked circuit (eg around a football pitch). This can be done on the flat or over varying terrain such as on the flat and slopes (up and downhill), or on sand, grass and shale etc. The aim is to complete as many circuits as possible within a set time. Therefore there is a need to work as hard as possible for each other to beat the previous best.

## Circuit training

A circuit is a sequence of selected exercises that must be completed in the sequences given. Generally a circuit has 6–12 exercises that are known as 'stations'. Depending on how the circuit is designed and laid out, it can work on aerobic or anaerobic fitness. By specifically choosing certain activities, the number of circuits completed and the time spent at each station, it is possible to determine which type of fitness will be improved. Additionally, by the choice of exercises and way they are conducted muscular strength and/or muscular endurance can be trained as well.

Chapter 14 is entirely dedicated to circuit training, as it tends to form the backbone of Royal Marines' group fitness sessions once a Royal Marine has passed training. This is partly due to the ease with which a circuit can be used to train large numbers, and also because circuit training has been proven to have positive effects on the CV and muscular endurance systems – perfect for the Commando lifestyle.

### Arms, trunk, legs

Although there are many types of circuits with many different aims, it is always important to allow the muscles and body parts to recover where possible. For example, if my aim is to improve leg strength and I put 12 leg exercises in a circuit, I will soon fatigue and find it difficult to complete the circuit and this will possibly lead to injury. Ideally one exercise for a specific body part should not follow another for the same body part. So if I did want to overload my legs I could arrange the exercises so that every other one is a leg strengthener. Then at least my legs will have time to rest in between. In general, however, for basic aerobic/anaerobic fitness gains and muscular endurance improvements 'arms, trunk, legs' circuits are perfect – ie the 6, 9, 12 or more stations are laid out in the order arms (an upper body exercise), trunk (an abdominal/lower back exercise), legs (a leg/ overall body CV exercise).

## Rowing technique

When rowing ensure your technique is correct: keep your back straight, drive with the legs first and then pull the arms into the abdomen. When returning to the start, allow the bar to return all the way to the machine before repeating the technique. As you get tired it will become more difficult to maintain the technique.

As fitness is improved, it is possible to make circuits more difficult and thus stress the body into adapting again. To make a circuit more difficult:

■ Increase the number of stations.
■ Increase the time at each station.
■ Increase the number of repetitions at each station.
■ Increase the number of completed circuits.

### Plyometrics

Plyometrics is a technique that uses the stored up elastic energy of a muscle to make the contraction more powerful. Using running as an example, the strong muscles in the upper leg are slightly stretched prior to contracting to drive the body forward. As the muscles are slightly stretched, elastic energy is 'stored' within them. When the muscles contract, this elastic energy is released, which makes the contraction that much more powerful.

Surprisingly, this extra power does not take up much extra energy; in fact it provides more power without any extra effort, and this principle is the same whenever a muscle is stretched prior to a contraction. Any training method that uses this principle to develop power is known as plyometrics.

Examples of these types of movements include moving from down to up when jumping or the switching of leg position during running as described above. By training, it is possible to reduce the time needed to make these changes in direction, which in turn will mean speed and power are increased. It is because of this ability to improve speed and power that this type of training is so beneficial for certain sportsmen, such as sprinters, volleyball players, rugby players, basketball players and, of course, gymnasts.

Plyometric training uses a series of exercises, repeated after each other, to increase this speed and power. Exercise examples are bounds, hops, jumps, leaps and skips. The major downside with plyometrics is the incredible strain that is put on the muscles and joints. A good warm-up is therefore imperative. Furthermore, for beginners it is worth starting slow and steady rather than jumping (excuse the pun) straight into the more advanced exercises. Additionally, starting on grass or using gym mats is a good idea until the muscles, joints, tendons and ligaments have had time to make initial adaptations. (See page 198 for examples of Plyometric training).

## The Plyometric pull-up

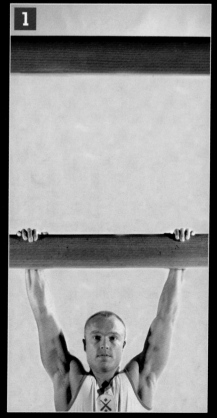

↑ From a normal start position . . .

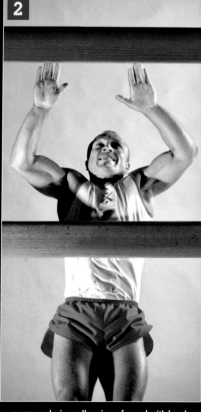

. . . a very explosive pull-up is performed with hands leaving the first bar . . .

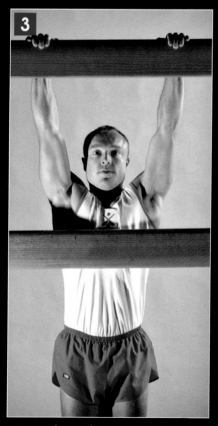

. . . to grasp the upper bar.

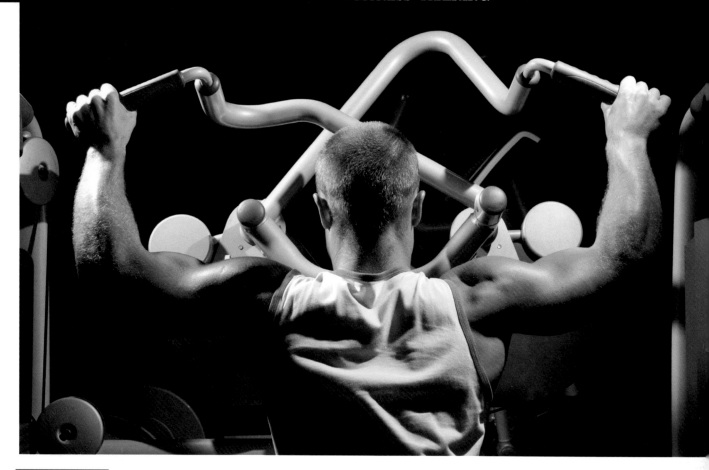

### Weight training

The two branches of weight training comprise weight lifting and weight training. Most people reading this book will not be interested in competitive weight lifting, which is concerned solely with the training of the body to lift heavier and heavier weights without any consideration of its appearance or functionality outside of this sport.

Weight training, by contrast, is concerned with the health and fitness gained from increased strength and stamina. The development of muscles purely for aesthetics is also a major aim of weight training, which is certainly not true of weight lifting. Furthermore, weight training is commonly used to support the development of performance in all major sports, whether rugby, martial arts, cricket or long-distance running. It is known that by developing power and strength and increasing the musculature certain gains can be achieved that may provide an edge over the opposition.

In weight training some form of weight – be it free weights or machine weights in a gym, or sandbags and rucksacks full of weight – is used as a form of 'resistance'. By increasing the weights used to perform certain specific exercises the muscles can be overloaded in a safe and productive manner over a sensible amount of time. Strength training programmes can be designed to help an individual train the strength needed for a specific sport, or can be designed to aid recovery from an injury. Whatever the reason, strength training is easy to tailor to the individual.

The acronym SPORT (specificity, progression, overload, reversibility, tedium) should always be kept at the forefront of your mind when designing a weight-training programme. It is easy to use someone else's programme, or to go on the Internet and download some special session that guarantees results, and you can certainly use these types of programme for ideas and inspiration; but you must also look at your own goals, your current fitness levels, and also whether or not these sessions are boring.

## Terminology

A 'set' is a number of exercises performed one after another. 'Reps' (or repetitions) are the number of exercises performed in that set. For example, I sometimes like to start or end my sessions with three sets of 50 press-ups. So I perform 50 'reps' three times, making three 'sets' of 50.

The '1RM' is the one repetition maximum, ie the maximum amount of weight someone can lift in a single repetition for a given exercise. For example, if an individual can lift 100kg on a bench press once and no more, his 1RM is 100kg. If in training he performs 87.5kg x 3 that is 87.5% of his 1RM. If the same individual bench pressed to failure using 66kg x 10, his training intensity would be 66% 1RM.

### The weights session

Ideally weight training should take place at least three times per week. It is not always necessary to ensure these days are preceded and followed by rest days, as if one body part is trained one day, a different one can be trained the next. However, for complete body recovery it can be more productive to train every other day.

It is imperative that a good warm-up takes place prior to a weights session. The muscles will be put under considerable stress, as will the ligaments, tendons and bones, and without a warm-up injuries will happen.

It is important to decide which muscles need developing for your chosen sport or goals and to choose exercises that will develop them. If your aim is to increase your pull-ups to join the Royal Marines then choosing exercises to strengthen the 'lats' of the back will be beneficial. However, doing very heavy squats three times a week will not help, although it will leave you with strong legs.

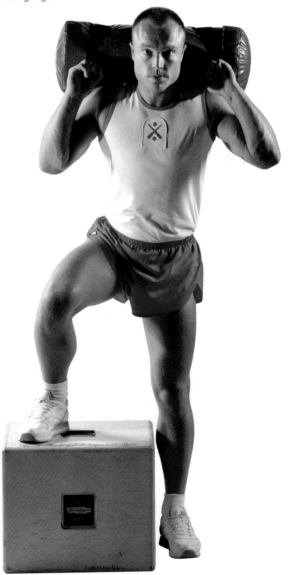

### ■ Strength training

For maximum strength gains it is necessary to do three sets of an exercise of four to eight reps (six being most beneficial) at near maximum weight.

### ■ Muscular endurance

For muscle endurance development at least three sets should be performed of 20–30 reps. the weight used should be around 40–60% of the 1RM.

### ■ Muscle power

To increase muscle power, at least three sets of 10–15 reps should be performed. These must be carried out at speed using weights around 60–80% of 1RM.

### Weight training tools

The following will be found useful in training many different areas of the body:

- **Barbells** – A weighted bar, between three and six feet long, usually with the major weighted portions at either end.
- **Dumbbells** – Resembling small barbells, these weights have small bars just big enough for a hand to grip (about 6in long). They come in pairs to allow similar exercises to those performed with a barbell, but with the hands working independently.
- **Kettlebells** – Weighted balls of iron (called bells) with an iron handle on top (called the horns). They work the core harder as the weight is 'easy' to manoeuvre.
- **Cable-weight stack machines** – A weighted stack or two weighted stacks with cables attached to which an array of handles can be attached to allow all sorts of exercises to take place. The advantage of cables is that resistance increases as the exercise reaches the finish position, as opposed to free weights where the resistance decreases.
- **Therabands, bungees, elastic or rubber surgical tubing** – Basically any specialist elastic for exercising. Being elastic, as it is pulled the resistance is increased.
- **Power-bags or sand-filled kitbags** – Sandbags have been used by the military for years to exercise. Power-bags are a mainstream, commercial version with handles attached.
- **Body weight exercises** – Press-ups, pull-ups, squats, sit-ups etc.

### Types of weight training exercises

Weight training exercises can be broadly classified anatomically into compound exercises and isolation exercises.

### Compound exercises

Compound exercises are multi-joint exercises that produce movement through two or more joints and involve many muscle groups in a co-ordinated effort. This not only develops all-round body strength but also inter-muscular teamwork (*eg* the deadlift, bench press and pull-up).

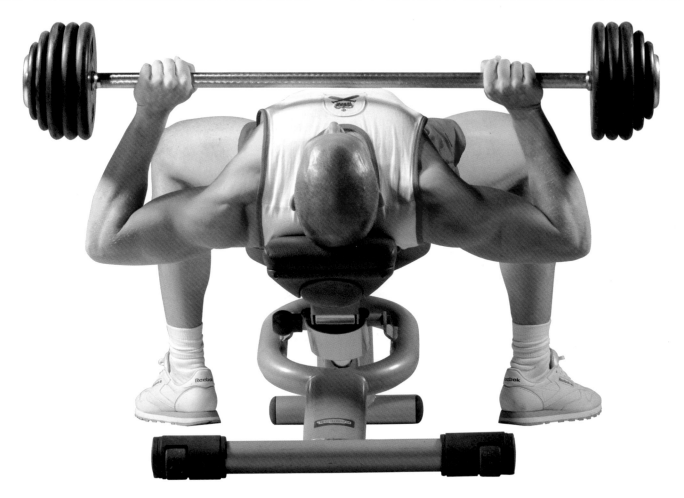

## Isolation exercises

Isolation (single-joint) exercises produce movement through just one joint (*eg* leg extension, bicep curl and triceps extension).

In general compound exercises are better for all-round fitness, as the muscles produce greater force (tension) when working as part of a group than when they contract alone. To put this into context, when in everyday life is the effort ever applied via a single muscle group? In reality, pushing a car, yomping or any sport uses many muscles at once. Furthermore, compound exercises will burn more calories than isolation exercises due to the larger number of muscles being used at one time.

### Injury avoidance

Although it often becomes too central in many young men's programmes, weight training is a very productive and rewarding method of physical training. However, if performed badly certain exercises can be at least painful and at worst crippling. Long-term poor exercise selection and/or poor technique can lead to chronic injuries that stop you training altogether and often decrease the quality of life in later years. Always be careful, and ensure correct technique and – perhaps even more importantly – sensible amounts of weight.

## Injury and Olympic weight lifts

Olympic weight lifts (the clean and jerk and the snatch) have not been included in this book for one specific reason: they should not be learned from a book. These exercises are technically very difficult to perform, but are extremely productive for developing power – hence their popularity amongst athletes, rugby players and rowers. However, they should be learned from a professional or a coach rather than a book. If these exercises interest you, seek a professional BWLA (British Weight Lifting Association) instructor.

### Weight training programme

The objective of any weight training programme is to develop all of the major muscle groups necessary with progressive overload.

Any beginner must develop technique-strength and conditioning (*ie* balance and flexibility) before building strength. The subsequent building of strength, skill and size will require a long-term outlook, which is to be measured in years not weeks. This long-term approach requires the consistent addition of weight via progressive overload.

It is important to have a period of 'breaking-in' training, which allows for the perfection of an exercise technique and the inducement of 'gaining momentum' when starting resistance training, implementing a new training system or returning to training after a lay-off or injury. This specifically gives the body (muscles, tendons, ligaments, bones and CV system) time to prepare and adjust for the gains to come.

## Weight training methods

### Training to beat failure
Training to beat failure is best described with an example. Using the bench press, during a six rep set the bar is lowered for repetition number six; it pauses at the chest, and although the weight would be threatening to defeat the trainee, he nevertheless pushes with every possible ounce of effort to complete the lift, thus beating failure.

For the next bench press session the trainee adds 5lb to the bar and the same amount of effort is repeated to complete six reps.

This may seem unlikely, but the positive mindset and psychological fitness discussed in earlier chapters is very important here.

### Training to failure
Using the example above, if this set was taken to failure, rep seven would be lowered to the chest but would not be possible to press back up, despite the lifter continuing to push as hard as possible. The 'spotter' would be required to complete the rep and rack the bar (hence the importance of always having a spotter).

This is a very hard way to train, but is necessary to stimulate muscle strength and growth, the advantage being that as long as rest and recovery are sufficient it will produce rapid gains over a short period of time. However, over time overtraining will eventually occur, due to the high intensity of this type of training. Furthermore, a decline in technique is often seen as it is very difficult to get the last rep.

### Progressive overload
The most effective way to train weight training for strength gains is to use 'progressive overload'. This basically means adding more weight on the bar or increasing the number of repetitions performed in each training session. This can be achieved by single progression or double progression.

#### Single progression
Single progression is the first choice for applying overload, and simply involves the addition of a small amounts of weight to the bar each training session.

It is important to ensure the percentage increase of weight is a sensible amount for the exercise – for example, increasing the weight from a 30kg to a 32.5kg dumbbell for a shoulder press represents a huge increase (2.5kg) for the relatively small muscles (deltoids and triceps), especially when compared to the same increase to a 100kg barbell for squats, which only represents a comparatively small increase for the far larger and stronger leg muscles.

#### Double progression
Double progression involves adding a repetition or two to each exercise until a selected target number is achieved. At this point a

small amount of weight – eg 2.5kg/5lb – is added to the bar, the reps are decreased, and the process starts again.

It is usually found that double progression is only successful when the target repetition range is small, eg 3–5, 6–8, 10–12 etc.

Double progression is especially useful for exercises using machines or fixed weights, where the addition of small increments of weight is impossible, as adding large weights will make the exercise too difficult.

### Exercise intensity cycling
Studies have shown that cycling exercise intensity produces the greatest strength and fitness gains of all weight-training systems. Supposedly, success comes from the variety of intensities stimulating the nervous system while also allowing the mind and body to rest at certain points and thus reducing the risk of overtraining. Furthermore, it is thought that technique-strength may even be improved during 'easy' training.

In simple terms, by reducing the amount of weight lifted to start with (by no more than 25% – ie a 100kg 1RM would be 75kg at it's lowest) a simple programme of 3 x10 reps can be started. By adding weight each session as described above for single overload progression, there will come a point where the number of sets or number of reps will have to decrease to cope with the weight. By doing this specifically in a set way you are 'cycling' the number of sets, number of reps and weight increases/decreases to see the biggest gains.

## Other training methods

### Eccentrics or 'negatives'
Lift the weight but accentuate the negative (eccentric) phase of the exercise by performing at four to six seconds lower. Ideally the weight used should be heavier than normally lifted. This means a spotter should be used to help lift the weight off the rack, but more importantly to help lift it back up following the eccentric lower.

Eccentric training causes more muscle growth and strength gains than regular training, according to studies. However, it also causes considerable DOMS (delayed onset muscle soreness) for one to two days. It is important to rest that muscle group following eccentric training or injury will occur. Eccentrics should not be performed more than once a week per muscle group. Ideally, perform only once or twice a month to avoid overtraining.

### Drop sets
Drop is a technique for continuing a specific exercise with a lower weight once the muscle has become too fatigued with the current weight and failed. This can be done with free weights or weights machines, but it is often the latter that is favoured as removing the weight quickly is thought by some to be extremely important.

As an example, while performing the bench press the lifter starts lifting a weight of 100kg and does as many repetitions as possible trying to maintain good form. When the muscles are fatigued and can no longer lift that weight, 5kg or 10kg is dropped, so 95kg or 90kg is pressed until muscular exhaustion is reached. Then the next drop is performed. These 'drops' could be done as many times as wanted. However, some research suggests that if performing very heavy drops no more than three distinct weights should be used.

### Tight drop/wide drop
Many variations of the drop set exist. The amount of weight shed is an obvious one to start with. The amount or percentage of weight dropped each time can be varied considerably. A wide drop set is one in where a large percentage (usually 30% or more) of the starting weight is dropped for each reduction. A tight drop set would only see 10% to 25% being dropped each time.

### Specific reps
Instead of taking the muscle to fatigue on each weight, a specified number of repetitions is performed at each weight (without necessarily reaching the point of muscle failure). As the weight is reduced, the number of reps increases.

### Overtraining
It is very easy to overtrain with drop sets. It is therefore necessary to curb the number of drop sets done per session. Ideally, no more than one to two drop sets per muscle group should be done in a workout. Furthermore, it is not recommended that drop sets be used as a recurring weekly session, due to the high intensity of the session.

### Supersets
Supersets involve doing two or three exercises one after the other. The exercises are usually for opposing muscles, but not always. For example, a simple superset might be 10 reps of bench press, 10 pull-ups and 20 press-ups, the lats and chest being the major muscles worked on these opposing exercises. The three exercises follow each other without rest. Biceps and triceps could also be exercised with a set of bicep barbell curls followed by a set of triceps 'skull crushers' with the same weight. Take two or three minutes' rest, and then repeat the two or three sets again.

### Twenty-ones
A favourite for many Royal Marines. The idea behind Twenty-ones is that it will exercise and therefore fatigue all ranges within a muscle. For most exercises there is a point in the range where the weight cannot be lifted, yet at other points it could. For example, on the bench press it is the portion close to the chest that is hardest and the range that usually fails first. Taking biceps as an example, Twenty-ones trains these ranges separately. The low range is from arms/elbow straight to a 60° lift, upper angle is from about 100° to the bar touching the chest/shoulders, and mid range is that in between. For Twenty-ones, perform seven reps in the low range, then seven in the mid range, then seven in the upper range.

To progress this, instead of doing your 21 then resting, then repeating for three to five sets, carry on performing sevens until the different ranges fail. For example, you may find that after 21 (7, 7, 7) you can still continue, so start the lower range again and do another 21. If the next time through the low range is fatigued go straight for the mid and upper, etc. Carry on until all three ranges are fatigued.

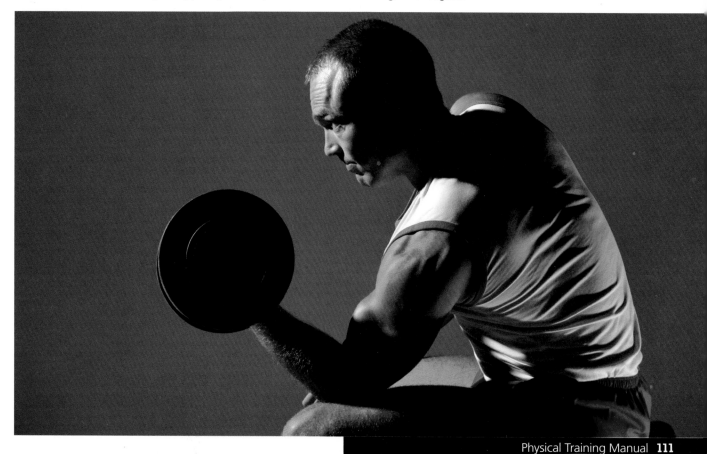

## Partial reps

These are usually used for muscle weaknesses/imbalances or areas that need rehab following injury. In a similar way to Twenty-ones, ranges are used, but only the perceived weak range will be exercised. For example, on the bench press most people can lift quite a lot more weight when only taking the bar halfway to the chest. By training this, they are only doing a partial rep.

## Gainers

Gainers (as I call them) are something I came up with for improving my ability to perform many of an exercise. The technique may already exist and be called something else by other people, and in fact it is basically a progressive overload of reps instead of weight. Nevertheless, I have included it specifically for anyone hoping to join the Royal Marines as a way of preparing for the RMFA.

I used gainers to improve the number of press-ups and pull-ups I could do prior to the RMFA on a specific course I was going on. It is very simple. All it requires you to do is choose the exercise you wish to train and the number of reps you wish to be able to perform with ease.

Let us take press-ups as an example. If you want to be able to perform 60 press-ups without a problem, perform a gainers press-up training session almost every day, if not then every other day. Start with a number of press-ups you can perform easily, for example 20 press-ups, which you perform three times with a minute's rest between each set, ie 20, one minute's rest, 20, one minute's rest, 20. Again, 20 is just the number you choose that you can do with ease – it could be 10 or 25.

The next session (or next day where possible) one rep is added, ie 21, one minute's rest, 20, one minute's rest, 20. The next day another is added, ie 21, 21, 20., etc, until eventually you are doing 50, 50, 50 with one minute's rest between each set.

This may sound easy, but it soon gets difficult. It may also sound like it takes a long time, and it does, but believe me, it works. Performing it nearly every day really builds up the muscular endurance. If you get to a point where the third set is nearly impossible, then stay at those reps for a week, ie for three or four sessions, to build strength and endurance and then increase.

If you have commitment and stick at this session, when it comes to the RMFA full marks are achievable.

## Detraining – losing all that you have worked for

The effects of 'detraining' can seem devastating to those of us that take our fitness seriously and have worked hard to achieve it. However, it is not a bad thing, it is just another motivation to continue training wherever and whenever possible.

It is suggested that losses in performance and efficiency occur when no training at all takes place for as little as two weeks. If several months pass by without training, the majority of the physical improvements previously achieved will be lost. Studies suggest that VO2 max can decrease by 25% over just 20 days of an almost sedentary lifestyle. Hence the reason why regular physical exercise is so important to Royal Marines. Not only could we be called upon at a moment's notice to deploy anywhere in the world, and therefore need to be physically and mentally

prepared to cope, but we have all worked hard to get where we are, and we don't want to lose it.

If, however, fitness improvements are lost, it is not the end of the world. Studies suggest that once a certain level of fitness is gained, even if it is lost again, it is easier to get back than if starting from scratch, ie than it was to achieve first time round.

## Overtraining

While writing this book, I noticed how many times I have mentioned overtraining. I have come to the conclusion that this is for two major reasons. Firstly, because it is a genuine problem that I see daily, be it among fellow Royal Marines, people I see in civilian gyms, or even my close friends and family. Secondly, it is something I have personally been guilty of, and have paid the consequences for. Consequently I cannot stress enough the importance of being aware of overtraining.

Overtraining can be defined as an emotional, behavioural and physical condition that occurs when the volume and intensity of exercise exceeds the recovery capacity of the body. In short, it is attempting to complete more exercise than the body can tolerate. The downside to overtraining is that is does not just halt progress, it also causes a loss of strength and fitness.

The most effective defence against overtraining is rest. A simple mnemonic (we love them in the Royal Marines, we have mnemonics for everything) can help you remember the importance of REST – Recovery Ensures Successful Training.

I have already spoken about the importance of 'knowing thyself'; it is imperative that we listen to our bodies. If you feel overtired and fatigued, you probably are, so combat this fatigue with a day's rest and appropriate nutritional intake. If you think of rest as a tool or a weapon to aid your training, you will use it effectively and appropriately.

It is so important to let the body recover from both general fatigue and local aches and pains, or DOMS (delayed onset muscle soreness). If training does take place too early, before effective recovery has taken place, it may well hinder the body's ability to recover, for body-builders this will mean that all the extra hard work will not go towards growing larger muscles, it will just lead to further fatigue and injuries. For endurance athletes, not allowing the body to recover adequately will lead to slower times, which leads to frustration and a feeling of needing to train harder; a vicious circle will ensue and possibly a downward spiral of continued fatigue. For a Royal Marine Recruit it could lead to poor results in physical tests, some of which may be criteria, and a fail results in a back-trooping. Worse still would be an injury that could see them put further back or even out of Royal Marines training. The overall consequence of fatigue and overtraining are too many to name. However, short- to long-term injuries are commonly caused by overtraining.

Again, I return to 'know thyself'. Obviously the fitter you get, the more intensely you will train. But it may be that your rate of recovery is also much increased, and therefore training can continue for longer or be more frequent without as much rest. This is not an excuse to start overtraining. Every person's individual rate of adaptation to exercise is different; however, they will all have

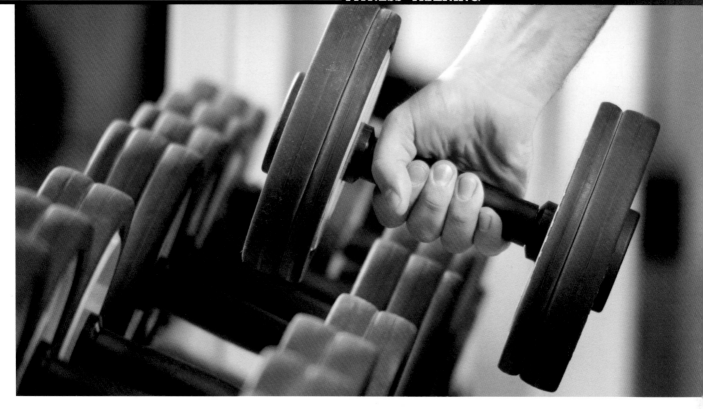

a limit at some point. No one can force their body to adapt and improve when there is no capacity left, and this is where training with a group or partner can backfire. If you partner is a little fitter, or their body is adapting and improving faster, it may be that they can cope with the excessive intensity and frequent sessions when your body cannot. Although it goes against all our competitive nature and may hurt our pride (well, a Royal Marine's anyway) it is important to take the rest *you* need, even if your training partner is raring to go.

Remember, only you have to cope with the consequences of overtraining. For many people, as the intensity of training increases the volume and frequency should decrease to allow for proportional rest and recovery. This is not the case for everyone, and it depends on the level of intensity increase too. As you get fitter, you can cope with much more intense sessions, but at the same frequency as you were doing previously.

**Overtraining symptoms**
Some or all of the following may be felt or seen if you are overtraining:

- Loss of performance.
- Inability to progress.
- Increased difficultly of easy sessions.
- Lack of enthusiasm.
- The need for increased recovery time.
- Muscular atrophy and associated weight loss.
- Heart rates (working and resting) become higher.
- Blood pressure becomes higher.
- Lowered immune system (leading to colds, infections and allergic reactions).

- Nausea.
- Loss of appetite.
- Emotional and psychological effects (lethargy, listlessness, procrastination, fear of failure, unrealistically high goals).
- Disturbed sleep patterns.
- Loss of libido.

## Conclusion

**The methods shown above, whether for weight training, continuous training, intervals training or whatever, are just examples of the many types that can be used. In training, Recruits will take part in all types of training including intervals, Parlauf, Fartlek, circuits and continuous. Although weight training is performed, it is infrequent and concentrates on functional strength rather than aesthetic muscle-building. The training sessions chosen from the examples above will, of course, depend on the goals of the individual. However, whether your goal is to add some size and strength or to lose weight and become aerobically fit, always remember the seven components of all-round fitness. If you are trying to lose weight, CV training is great, but increasing muscle tone will have a longer effect on burning calories throughout the day, as will interval sessions, so both should be trained. If trying to gain size and strength, performing some CV training will ensure a healthy and fit all-round system. It is important to ensure the heart grows with the body, which is why CV training is a must.**

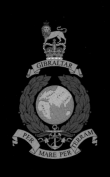

# CHAPTER 13
# THE EXERCISES

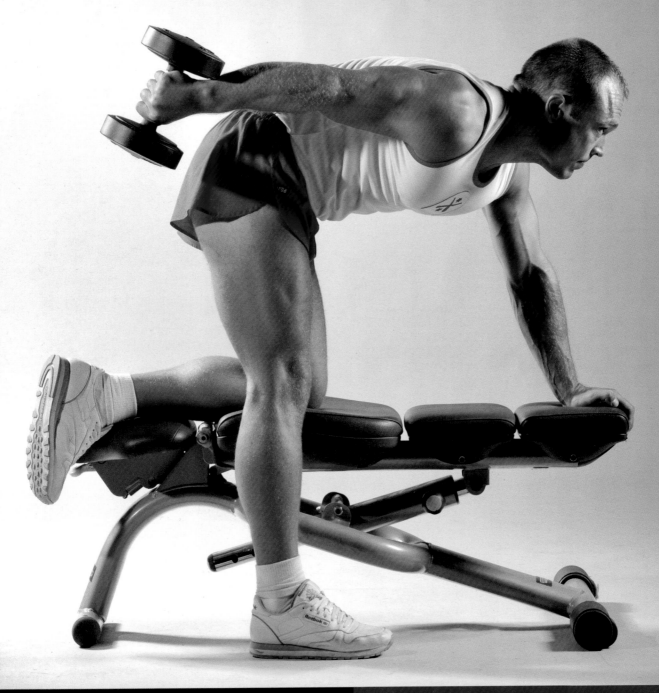

In order to achieve and then maintain a good level of fitness it is necessary to partake in a number of different kinds and types of exercise. As explained in Chapter 5, there are seven separate components to all-round fitness, and it is necessary to train in all of these areas. For Royal Marines certain areas are more important than others and this is likely to be true for most sportsman and casual gym-goers.

Where the training is to take place will have a large impact on the types of exercise that can be done. For example, in a gym nearly every exercise you can think of could be performed, as the kit and equipment are readily available. However, if exercising at home, in the park or, for Royal Marines, away on Operations in areas such as Afghanistan, only certain exercises will be possible. Having said that, it is the imagination that is the real barrier to overcome: with a good imagination exercises and sessions can be improvised anywhere. For the majority of Royal Marines pulling and pushing exercises involving your own body weight are those most commonly used, as they can be performed almost anywhere; they are also productive and provide a marker to work to. Furthermore, body weight exercises are cheap and simple to perform.

When you read and attempt the exercises below, please remember that this chapter is part of the book's 'fitness for all' section, meaning that the exercises outlined here are not those used by Royal Marine PTIs to train Recruits to be Commandos. Some of them are used, specifically press-ups, pull-ups and rope climbing, but in general a Recruit's training concentrates on functional strength and fitness revolving around specifics for the tests throughout Commando training, as explained in Chapter 9. However, as stated this chapter is about 'fitness for all', so Royal Marines around the Corps will undoubtedly have used some or all of these exercises at some point, whether during weight training sessions or during circuits organised by others.

Any good physical training session should be part of a training programme or at least some sort of general plan. The session should be planned beforehand and the areas to be exercised chosen and decided upon, which means that the exercises to be used can also be selected. Depending on the overall aim of training, the chosen exercises can be repeated over a set time period to see if strength gains are occurring, or a varied mixture can be used each time to simply improve general fitness and health. Remember, it is important to include variety, choose realistic goals and maintain motivation if you expect to see results.

### Concentric, eccentric and isotonic

It is important to understand these three terms, since they will be used throughout this chapter:

- **Concentric** – This is a contraction in which the muscle shortens as it contracts, meaning the ends of the muscles move closer together (*eg* the upwards movement of a pull-up).
- **Eccentric** – This is a contraction in which the muscle is put under tension as it lengthens, meaning the ends of the muscle move further apart (*eg* the downwards movement of a pull-up).

- **Isotonic** – This is a contraction that takes place when the muscle is working concentrically or eccentrically.

### The exercises

The exercises below can all be used in isolation or, in the majority of cases, incorporated into circuits and other forms of training. It is important to select the exercises that suit your aims and pursuit in terms of your fitness goals, as explained in Chapter 12.

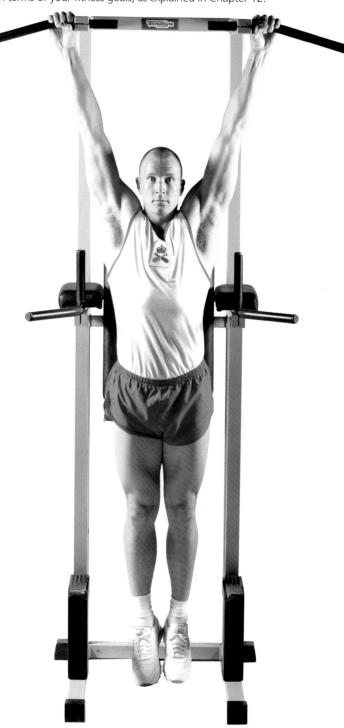

# PULL-UPS

A pull-up is an upper body pulling exercise in which the body is suspended by extended arms, gripping a fixed bar. (Such bars are available from High Street retailers and can be easily fitted in any doorway of your house, so no excuses!) The body is then pulled up until the elbows are bent and the head is higher than the hands and over the bar. For Royal Marines the overhand or pronated grip (ie with the palms facing away) is always used. In addition no swinging or 'kipping' (gyrating the body to obtain momentum) is allowed.

## Performing a pull-up

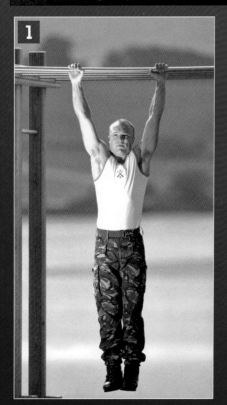

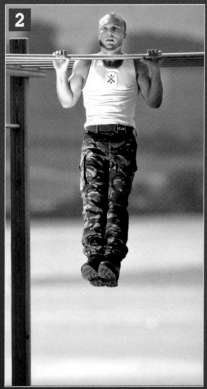

**1** Start with hands just a little more than shoulder-width apart. Hands should be pronated (with the palms turned away). Pull up, bending the elbows and bringing the upper chest up to the bar.

**2** At the top of the exercise, the chin should be over the bar, with the upper chest as close to the bar as possible, and the body should remain rigid throughout the whole range, up and down. The up and down movement should be controlled and steady.

The pull-up is an exercise that really separates the men from the boys. A large proportion of the population of this planet probably cannot perform even one pull-up, and there are very few who can easily do a pull-up if they have never attempted one before; even if they can they will not be able to perform many. Pull-ups are an exercise that requires training; they must be committed to and repeated often to see results. However, once they have been mastered, pull-ups are a great exercise to increase strength and muscular endurance.

A pull-up is a 'compound' exercise, meaning a multi-joint exercise that involves many muscles at one time. It works many muscles in the upper body as well as your overall core stability, as the body will naturally want to swing, which your core muscles will have to control.

Eight to ten reps is a good start. Sixteen to the bleep receives full marks on the new Royal Marines Fitness Assessment (RMFA) required on the PRMC and during the first weeks of training (eighteen in your own time gained full marks on the old RMFA). Anyone getting over 20 can consider themselves an accomplished pull-up performer.

# Regressions

## Assisted pull-ups

A friend or training partner can stand behind and place their hands on your hips and provide enough assistance for you to achieve the pull-up when working hard. Aim to reduce the level of assistance over time until pull-ups are achievable solo.

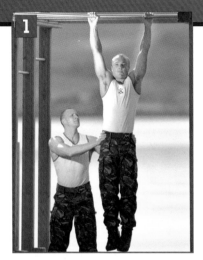
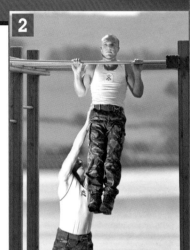

## Incline pull-ups

This exercise can be done with feet on the floor or on a bench. The idea is that the legs are rested on something so that the upper body does not have to pull up the whole of your body weight. Over time, raise the bar or stand up straighter, adding more weight to the pull-up until a standard pull-up is achievable.

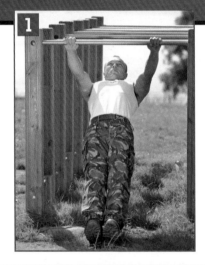
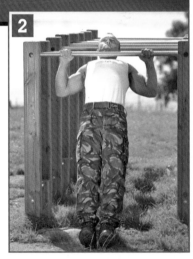

## Assisted elastic pull-ups

Specific elasticated supports for pull-up progression are now available with separate attachments to stay on the bar, and a piece of elastic with a knee cradle. Alternatively a piece of strong bungee/physio theraband can be tied to the bar just over shoulder-width apart. Rest the knees in the knee cradle or on the elastic theraband. The elastic should offer enough resistance to make it possible to perform the pull-up. Pull-ups can be practised in this fashion until enough strength is gained to perform standard unsupported pull-ups.

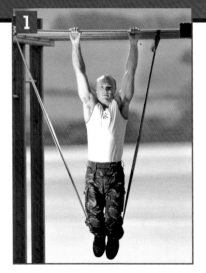
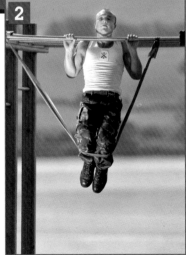

# Progressions

## Under-grasp pull-ups

As well as the upper back, this exercise also works other muscles such as the biceps. Hang from the bar with your palms facing towards you, still shoulder-width apart. Pull up so that your chin is over the bar and steadily return to the start position.

**Progression**

- **Close-arm chin-ups** – As above but with fists almost touching. Varying the distance between your hands when doing the pull-up is good for better all-round development of the muscles in the back.

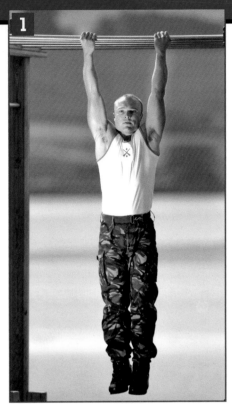
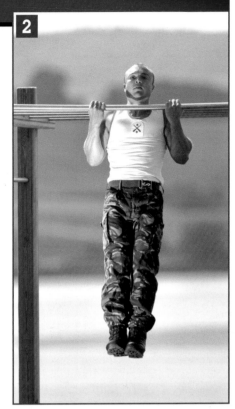

## Inward grasp pull-ups

Hang facing laterally, looking along the bar, with both palms facing inwards towards the bar. One hand should be in front of the other. Pull up and move your head to one side of the bar or the other. Lower to the start position and pull up again so that your head is to the other side of the bar. It is a good idea to vary the lead hand to ensure equal strength gains.

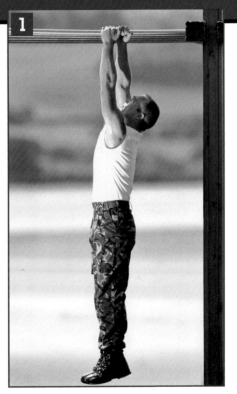
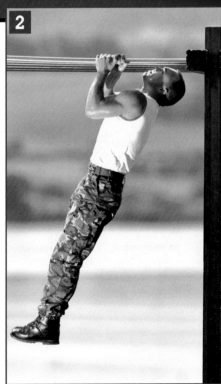

## L-shape pull-ups

This is an exercise that requires you to be very proficient in the pull-up, and also to have a strong core and strong hip flexors. The exercise involves performing a pull-up with your legs straight out in front of you at 90° to your body, forming an L shape. This is a very controlled exercise used extensively by gymnasts due to the wide variety of large muscle groups it works. To perform the exercise, hang from the bar and raise the legs to 90°, hold this position and pull up before returning to the start position. Due to your centre of balance changing considerably, it is necessary to lower with a huge amount of control to prevent the body swinging.

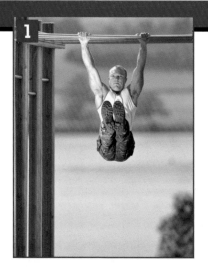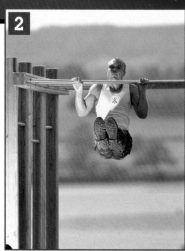

## Rope/kit pull-ups

This is a technique we use to work the grip, especially for Recruits when learning to rope climb; it involves performing pull-ups whilst hanging from a rope, ensuring the chest rises to the level of the hands. Not only does this work all the usual muscles associated with a pull-up, but it also requires a lot of grip strength and confidence in the grip. If training in a gym that doesn't have ropes (most don't these days) then use the 'triceps curl' rope by hanging the centre of it over the pull up bar and then taking hold of one side in each hand.

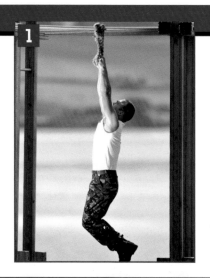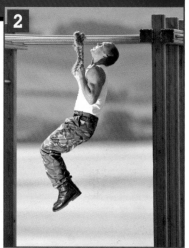

## Fingertips pull-ups

A very sports-specific exercise for climbers, but often a good test for those of us looking for a new pull-up challenge! Using a strong doorframe or an equivalent 'edge' (climbers purchase 'fingerboards' that hang on walls and bars for these pull-ups), try to perform pull-ups using your fingertips. The edge you use should be wide enough to just get the ends of your fingers over. Fingertip pull-ups are perfect for strengthening the fingers, especially if your chosen sport or activity requires strength in this area.

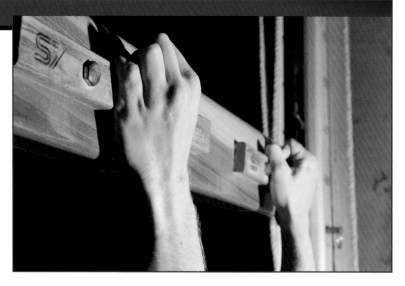

# Progressions

## Muscle-ups

Muscle-ups are a variation on the pull-up, that sort of combines the dip (described below) as well. The muscle-up is a gymnastic exercise that requires a lot of power (see explanation of power in Chapter 2). It requires hanging below the bar using an overgrasp grip and pulling up hard and fast, and then rotating the hands around the bar to allow the elbows to come up over it. At this point the chest can be almost rested on the bar. However, the exercise is not yet complete: the arms must now be straightened to completely raise the body over the bar. The hips will now be level with the bar and the arms straight. To repeat, allow the body to drop back below the bar and repeat the process.

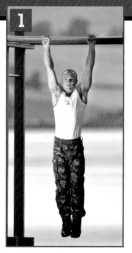 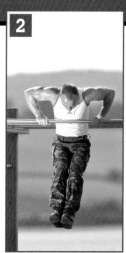 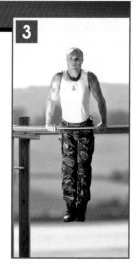

## Plyometric pull-ups

Unfortunately two bars are needed to perform this exercise, one above the other. The distance between the two bars can be varied as the exerciser becomes more proficient, so start at your minimum and work up. Again, a lot of power is needed to perform this exercise, especially over large gaps between the bars. To perform this exercise, hang on the lower bar in an overgrasp fashion, as if going to perform a normal pull-up. As with the muscle-up, pull up hard and fast, but as the chest reaches the lower bar release with the hands and reach up to take hold of the upper bar, and pull up on that as if completing a normal pull-up, chin over and chest to the bar. Drop to the lower bar, extend the arms and repeat.

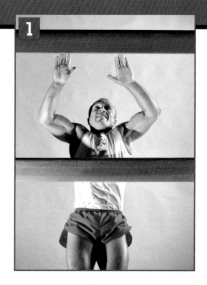 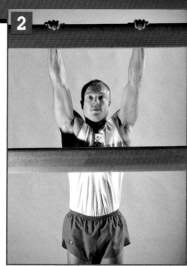

## Clap pull-ups

Similar to plyometric pull-ups, but instead of two bars only one bar is needed. Following an explosive overgrasp pull-up, allow the hands to release and clap them above the bar before catching the bar again, extending the arms and repeating. It is also possible to perform variations within a set, *eg* you could start with arms wide, perform one clap pull-up, then catch the bar in a close grip, perform a second clap pull-up and catch the bar in a regular grip, and so on.

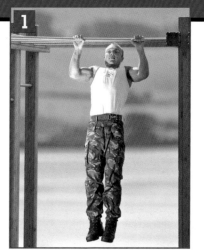 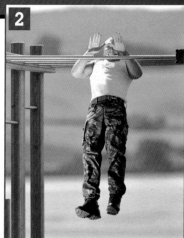

## Hand to chin pull-ups

A simple exercise from the regular overgrasp grip position, except that as you pull up allow your chin to travel left or right to touch and bypass the knuckles of one or other hand. Lower and repeat to the other side.

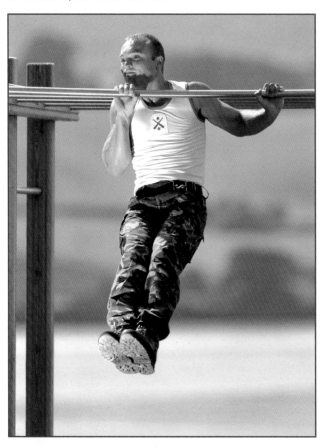

## Pull-ups with weight

Using a belt with weight added to it, or by gripping a dumbbell between the thighs, pull-ups can be completed with more than your simple body weight. A rucksack containing weight can also be used.

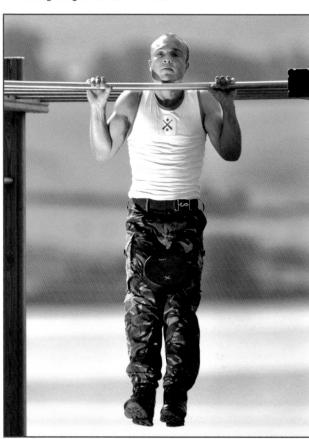

## Further pull-up variations

### ■ Static holds

Holding any exercise will improve static strength and aid in the development of muscular endurance. Holding the pull-up in a static position is no exception. However, hanging from the bar in the start position only really tests your grip strength, as the other muscles are not contracting, only using skeletal strength. But holding the pull-up halfway to the bar or with chin over the bar will certainly work your muscular endurance and strength. I guarantee it is not a position that can be held for long. Static holds can be performed from the over-grasp or under-grasp position. Try holding for a count of five or ten, or while a partner performs ten press-ups, then swap.

### ■ Eccentric pull-ups

A personal favourite of mine, especially when I am trying to improve someone's ability to perform regular pull-ups. Any pull-up can be performed eccentrically; it just requires that the return to the start position (ie the straightening of the arms following the pull) is done at a much slower rate than normal. A good way to do this is to count backwards from five, slowly.

# PRESS-UPS

Press-ups have taken their place as the cornerstone exercise of every military service across the world. This is probably because it can be executed pretty much anywhere, and unlike the pull-up can be managed by pretty much everyone. The press-up is an excellent exercise for working on muscular strength, and more importantly muscular endurance. The internet is also a great resource for seeing what progressions other people have come up with for the press-up – check out the 'planche' press-up.

## Performing a press-up

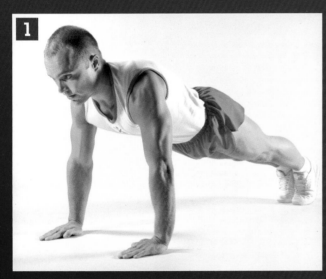

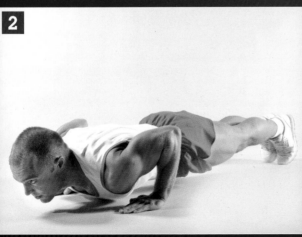

**1** To perform the press-up, locate a flat surface, clear of debris that might injure the palms of the hands. Start with the hands flat, shoulder-width or very slightly more than shoulder-width apart. The head should be up and looking forward (imagine you are looking out in case someone tries to kick you in the face). Most importantly, though often neglected, ensure that your back is straight and remains straight! The legs and feet should be together throughout, although variations exist which are described below.

**2** Bend the arms at the elbow so that the chest is about fist-height away from the floor. (When training I often use a couple of books or a few DVDs that equal fist-height below me, and ensure my chest touches them each time.) Once your chest is at fist-height, push down through your hands, thus straightening the arms until the elbows lock straight back at the start position.

This exercise is very easy to perform, but is equally easy to perform badly. Surprisingly, it is often performed badly even by Royal Marine Recruits, during their first few weeks of training. The most common mistake is dropping the hips. The back should remain straight at all times, and any movement should rotate through the toes as a pivot, not the hips. It is common to see the chest being lowered by rotating through the hips, but don't do this – it is not a press-up, and you are only cheating yourself. If done properly, the arms should be straight at the end of each rep, the back should be straight and the head should be up. Achieving 30 without rest is good to start with, but reaching 50 with ease is something to aim for.

# Regressions

## Incline press-ups

Put the hands on to a bench or perform the press-ups on a slope, so that the chest is higher than the legs. This will still exercise the muscles associated with the press-up, as well as some other areas, and is therefore a very useful regression. As stated, use a bench, table or wall to adopt the same start position as the regular press-up and perform the press-up in the same way. You should find that you can perform twice as many of incline press-ups as regular press-ups.

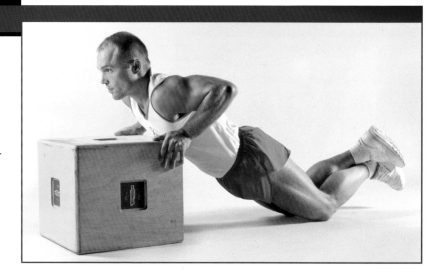

## Knees rested press-ups

Adopt a similar start position to the regular press-up, but with the knees rested. Your feet should be up in the air. The same press-up exercise is performed, but rotation is through the knees and not the feet. The chest is still lowered to the same point, and the back is still kept straight.

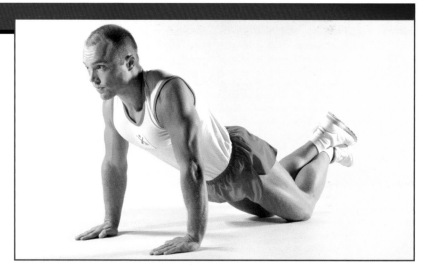

## Assisted press-ups

These are performed in the regular press-up position, but with a friend or partner beside or astride you. This person is positioned so that they can put their hands under your torso and on your abdominals/lower ribs. The exercise is performed in the same way, with a bend at the elbows, but on the upward portion of the exercise the assistor can lift gently at the abdominals/lower ribs area. It is important that there is not too much assistance and that the exercise is still challenging and will have the necessary effects.

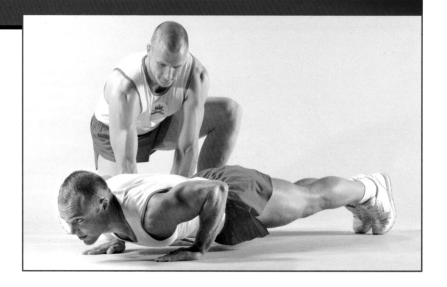

# Progressions

## Decline press-ups

To increase the weight needing to be pressed by the muscles used in the press-up (particularly the pectorals, deltoids and triceps), place the feet on to a higher surface. Aim to raise the feet only a small amount over a period of time until the body is at about 45° – any more than this and the focus of the exercise changes from the chest muscles to the shoulders. Remember to keep the back straight (this will be even more difficult in this raised feet position) and still lower the chest to the same point as with a regular press-up.

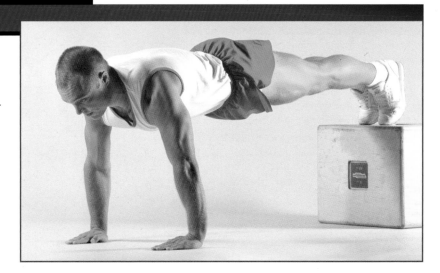

## Wide arm press-ups

Place the hands about one and a half shoulder-widths apart and perform the usual press-up exercise. By varying the distance between your hands, the exercise will focus on different muscles. The wider the hands, the more focus on the chest. Again, the 'form' of the exercise (straight back, chest down, head up) is the same.

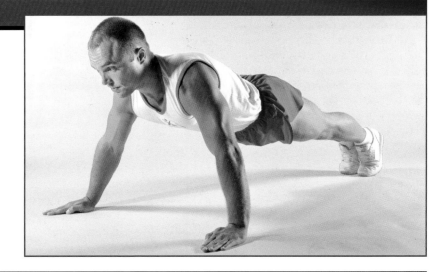

## Close arm press-ups

Similar to the above, but with the hands close together under the chest. A simple way of doing this is to form a diamond shape using the thumbs and index fingers of both hands and then perform the exercise. The closer the hands, the more the exercise focuses on the triceps. Form is the same.

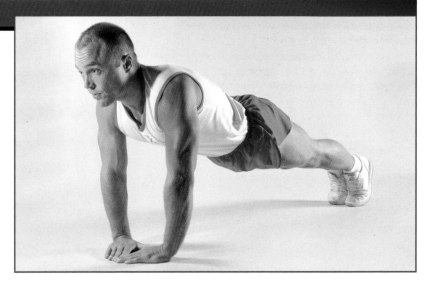

## Resisted press-ups

A friend or partner standing astride you presses down with their hands on your upper back/shoulders (between the shoulder blades) as you push up, thus resisting the press-up. The person pushing down needs to be relatively astute at judging the correct amount of resistance to use to ensure that you can still perform the press-up.

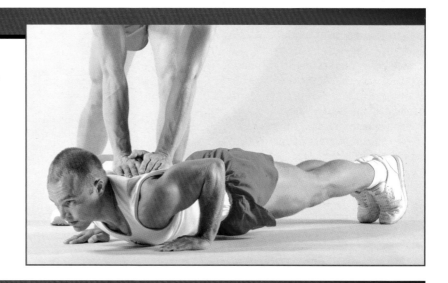

## Weighted press-ups

Weighted press-ups can be done either wearing a weighted vest, with a 'disc' weight from a gym placed on your back by a friend, or while wearing a medium-sized rucksack with weight added to it. The weight should always be through the upper/mid back, not the lower back/glutes, as this becomes more of a core exercise.

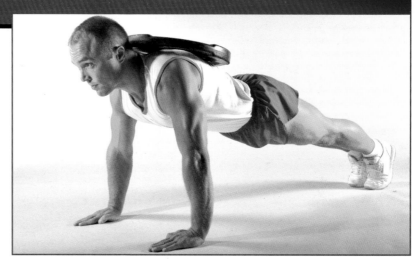

## Fist press-ups

Following an injury to my wrist I could not get much range of movement, so was forced to perform press-ups on my fists for about a year. Fist press-ups are not really any more difficult than ordinary press-ups, but varying the hand position adds subtle changes to the overall stability of the exercise. Be sure to lock your wrists to avoid them 'rolling' as the exercise gets tough, which can lead to sprains and strains.

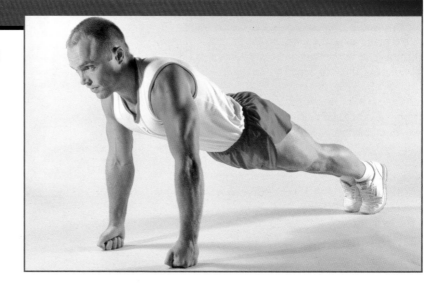

## Progressions

### Finger press-ups

Press-ups performed on the fingertips. Do not splay your hands too far or they may collapse. Ensure the fingers are kept locked and rigid for stability. As with pull-ups on the fingertips, this exercise is perfect for building finger strength, but more in the straight/rigid plane. It is therefore used extensively by martial artists.

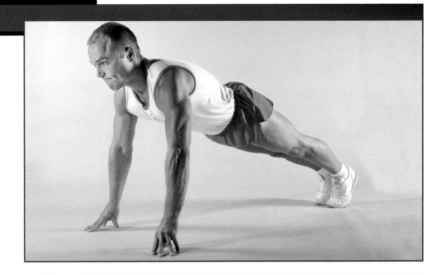

### Clap press-ups

Similar to clap pull-ups, in that the usual press-up exercise is performed but with a clap in the middle of it. Start in the normal press-up position. Lower to the ground in the usual way, but make the upward movement powerful and explosive, allowing the hands to come off the floor, clap, and then return to their original position. To avoid injury, enough force must be generated to have time to clap and return the hands to the ground.

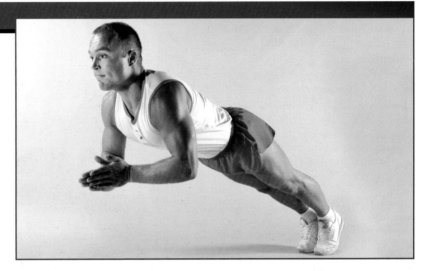

### Press-up stands

Available from any sports store, press-up stands are set on the floor at the width of the press-ups to be conducted. The hands grip them either laterally or longitudinally. The exercise is performed in exactly the same way as before, but the hand is now raised around 5cm from the floor, so the chest is lowered that much further, meaning the exercise is harder and the chest is exercised more fully. A set of these stands costs under £10 at the time of writing, and are an excellent addition to anybody's training kit.

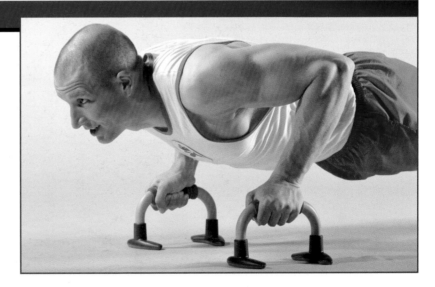

## Hand to chin press-ups

As with the pull-ups version, press-ups are performed in the same way as normal but the body weight is switched between the arms alternately by performing chin to alternate hand press-ups. The core is also worked to keep the body rigid as the centre of gravity is switched from side to side.

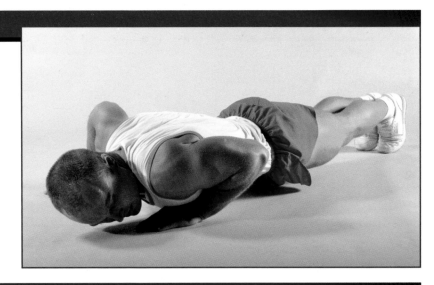

## Geckos

A gecko press-up is a press-up performed lifting one leg up off the floor and bending the knee up to the side until it is level with the waist. This movement causes the body to twist, lowering the shoulder towards the hand on the opposite side from the leg raised. The movement looks like that of a gecko.

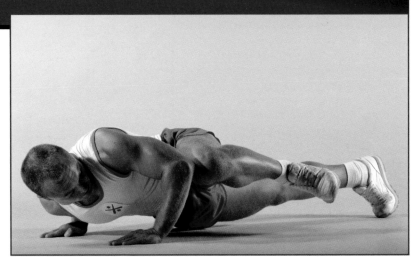

## Waist-level press-ups

As well as placing the hands closer or further apart, it is also possible to place them further down the body, still keeping them shoulder-width apart. If the hands are moved as far down as the waist, the exercise becomes considerably harder. When I have wanted to exercise, but had very little kit, I have often used this exercise and I find it reduces the number of repetitions I can do considerably.

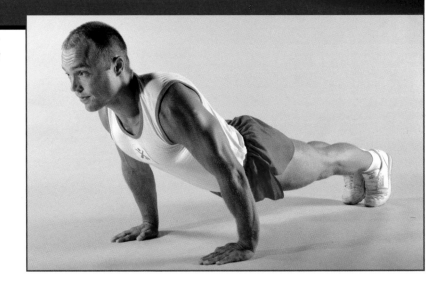

# Progressions

## One-armed press-ups

Not an easy exercise, but also not as difficult as it may seem. The important thing to remember when attempting the one-armed press-up is to open your legs to provide a wide base. Secondly, it is important to ensure that the hand being used to press is placed more centrally, *ie* directly under the centre of the chest. The hand not being worked should be placed behind the lower back to keep it out of the way. As the body is lowered, some people find it necessary to put in a slight rotation away from the arm doing the work, to maintain their balance. This exercise works the chest, shoulder and triceps to a high degree. Both arms should be worked equally.

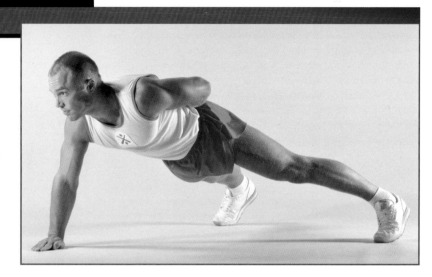

## One-hand raised press-ups

Using a step or a medicine ball (or even a small rucksack) one hand can be placed higher than the other, *ie* one hand is placed on the raised platform, the other on the floor but still in a normal press-up position. Press-ups are then performed as normal. Again, this will affect the core somewhat. It is imperative that both sides are worked equally to avoid a muscle imbalance.

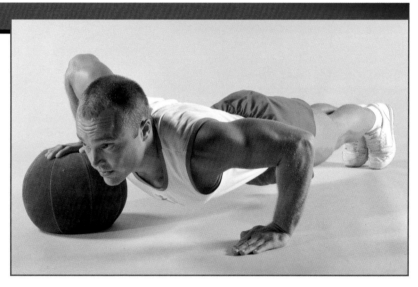

## Leg raise press-ups

From the normal press-up start position with arms extended, lower the body by bending the arms as normal. However, allow one leg to raise up off the floor by rotating through the hip. The leg raised should remain straight, and the back should remain flat. On the upwards press (arm extension) the leg is placed back down. On the next repetition the opposite leg is raised. This exercise is more demanding on the core and also works the glutes (backside).

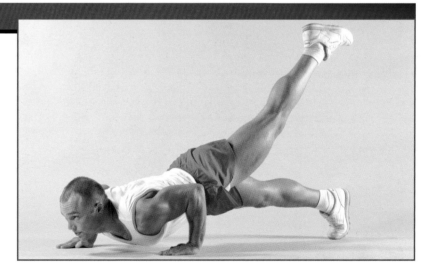

## Sniff the floor press-ups

This is one of the only press-up variations where it is acceptable to bend at the hips. This type of press-up is particularly difficult to perform and requires more work from the shoulders than regular press-ups. To perform this exercise, begin in the normal press-up start position with arms extended. Now raise your backside so that the body/back is no longer straight. Your body should now be an inverted V with hands and feet as the apexes.

To perform the exercise, lower your face towards the floor as if trying to sniff between your hands. Once lowered so that your nose is about a centimetre off the floor, lower your backside so that your body becomes straight again. This should move your head forwards away from your hands, running your nose along the floor. Straighten your arms when your back is straight, and repeat the exercise.

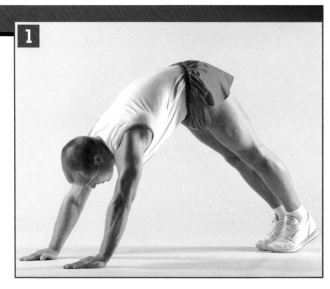

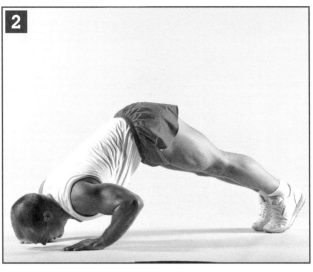

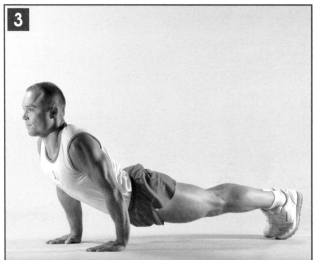

## Further press-up variations

### Static holds

In the same way as with pull-ups, static holds can increase strength and aid with muscular endurance. It is important, as always, to keep the back straight. Either hold in the arms fully extended position, which tends to use a lot of skeletal strength but is still very hard on the core and shoulders, or, for a more challenging exercise, hold at different points from the lowered position to the arms fully extended position.

### Eccentric press-ups

As with pull-ups, the lowering part of the exercise is performed slower than normal, but the upward part (as the arms are extended) is performed as normal. Again the use of a slow reverse count of five can be useful to ensure the slow eccentric lower is regulated.

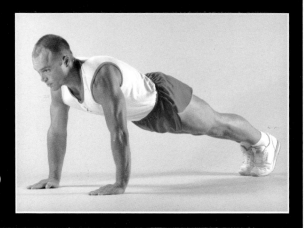

# DIPS

Dips are another great compound exercise for the upper body, and although not as easy to perform anywhere as the press-up, are still very user-friendly. Basic dips can be performed on the edge of any wall or chair, although full dips where the legs/feet are off the ground need certain facilities. The dips tends to work the chest, shoulders and triceps, and to some extent the core. The muscles worked depend on whereabouts the legs are and how the upper body is positioned.

## Performing a dip

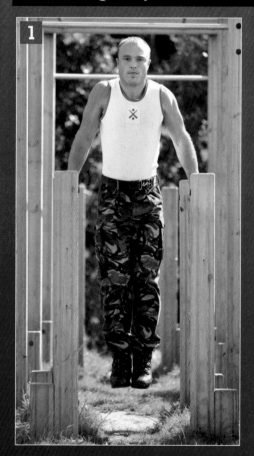 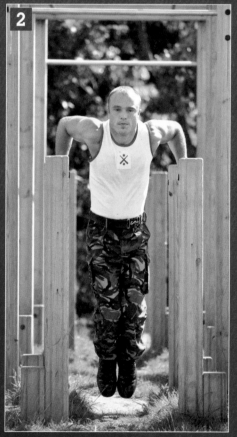

Although dips can be done with a bench behind the back and the feet rested, for some of us – certainly for Royal Marines – this is way too easy. Ideally you want the feet off the ground, so that the body is totally supported by the arms. To perform the exercise, start with two parallel bars, chairs or blocks, with the hands placed on these and the arms locked out. Keeping your head up and your back vertical, drop down under control so that your elbows are bent to an angle of 90°, hold, and push back to the top.

1 The best way to perform a dip is to have the feet hanging from a position where your hands are on parallel bars, which are shoulder-width apart.

2 Leaning slightly forward, drop down under control until your fists are a few inches from your shoulders. Anything over 20 repetitions is very good.

# Regressions

## Basic dip

As already stated, the basic, or regressed, exercise is to rest the feet, so that not of all the body weight is supported through the arms. Using a bench, wall or chair for the hands, and with the feet resting on the floor, the complete range of movement can still be performed, but is now focussed on the triceps.

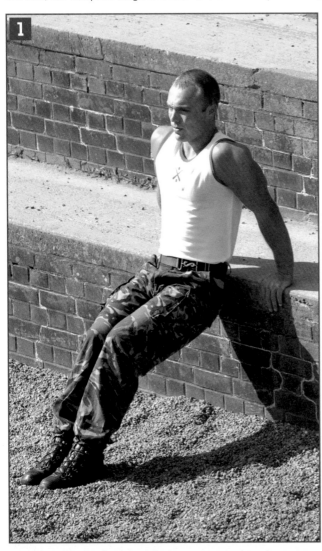

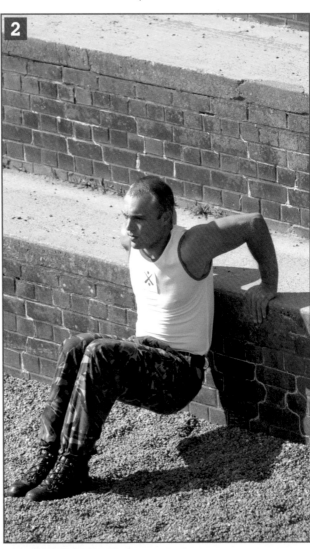

## Further dip variations

**■ Supported dip**
While performing the full dip, have a friend or training partner hold the feet so that not all of your body weight is going through the arms. The legs can also push against the support for extra leverage, thus making the exercise easier.

**■ Assisted elastic dip**
As for pull-ups, a specific elasticated support for dip progression is available. Alternatively a piece of strong bungee/physio theraband can be tied to the bars. This should be used to provide support through the knees until enough strength is gained to perform standard unsupported dips.

**■ Jump-up eccentric dip**
Adopt the normal dip position on the bar. Lower the body to the bent-arm position slowly to a reverse count of five, put the feet down, and 'jump' back to the start straight-arm position. Once the arms are fully stretched and the start position reached, repeat the eccentric lowering.

## Progressions

### Basic dip with weight

From the basic dip (*ie* with feet rested), a weight can be placed on the lap to add weight as the dip is performed. This exercise is often popular with body-builders for triceps work. However, I would rather see the full compound version performed than the easier version with an added weight.

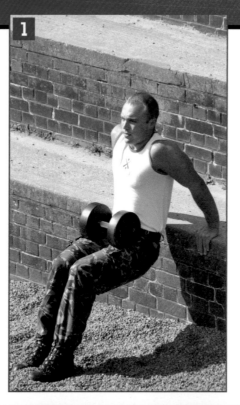
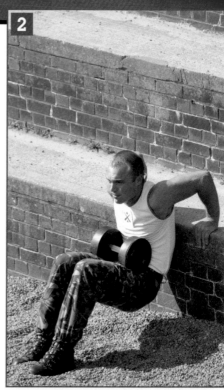

### Weighted dip

While performing the full dip, add weight by wearing a weights belt with a disc weight attached, holding a dumbbell between the thighs, or wearing a medium-sized rucksack containing around 10–15kg.

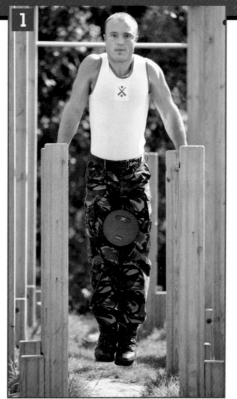
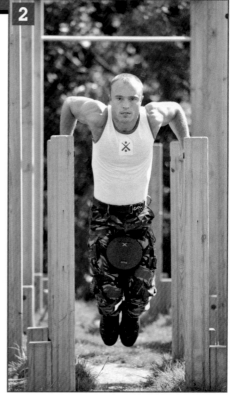

## L-shape dips

This is an exercise that requires you to have a strong core and strong hip flexors. The exercise involves performing the dip with your legs straight out at 90° to your body, as for L-shape pull-ups. To perform the exercise, raise the legs to 90°, hold this position and dip, before returning to the start position.

## Tucked dips

Used by gymnasts, this is similar to the above, but instead of an L shape the exercise is performed with the knees tucked into the chest. The abdominals will find this difficult to maintain for long.

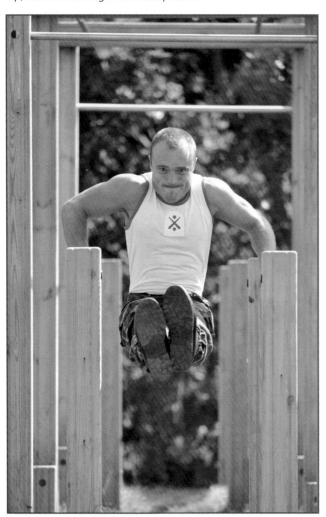

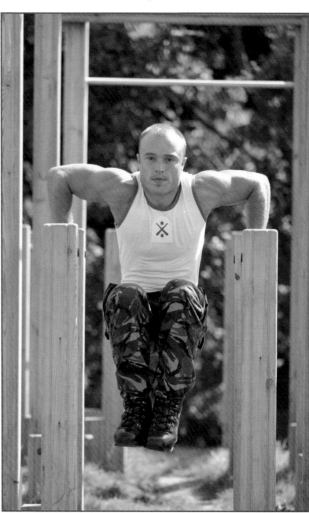

## Further dip variations

### Static holds

Holding the dip in a static position also improves muscular endurance and strength. If on bar in the start position the shoulders will still be worked but the majority will be skeletal strength; there is still some gain, but not as much as holding the dip halfway to the bar, which will certainly work the muscular endurance and strength. This is not a position that can be held for long.

### Eccentric dips

As with pull-ups and press-ups, eccentric work has been shown to lead to more strength gains than concentric. The lowering portion is done at a much slower rate than normal. A good way to do this is to count backwards from five, slowly. Then press up to the start position as normal.

# UPPER BODY EXERCISES

Upper body strength is imperative to a Royal Marine to allow him to perform all the tasks in his working day. The following exercises can be used to strengthen all the various muscles of the upper body. Royal Marine Recruits will use very few of these exercises through Royal Marines training, as their fitness is much more functional and specific. However, for the average trained Royal Marine or civilian training at home it is necessary to know a number of different exercises that can be put together in a training programme that will ensure increased strength, stamina and endurance of the upper body.

## Chest exercises

### Bench press

While laid back on a bench, a weighted barbell is taken from straight arms (above the chest) to bent arms, just touching the chest, before it is returned to the start position. Weights can vary from 5kg up to 200kg depending on the individual and the goals intended. It is a compound exercise that also involves the triceps and the front deltoids, and recruits the upper back muscles and traps. It is important not to 'bounce' the weight off the chest.

**Progressions**
- **Wide/close grip** – Vary the hand grip positions from shoulder-width (as regular) to wide and close grip derivatives. NB close grip will hit the triceps more, whereas wide grip and shoulder-width will concentrate on the chest.

- **Eccentric** – As for dips and pull-ups, the eccentric action involves lowering slowly, perhaps to a count of five. A friend (spotter) should be present to ensure the weight can be pushed back up following the eccentric lowering.

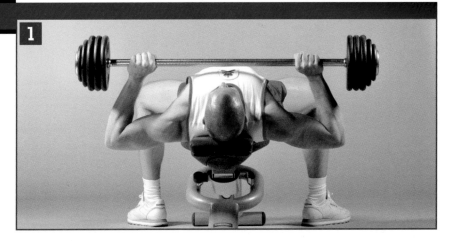

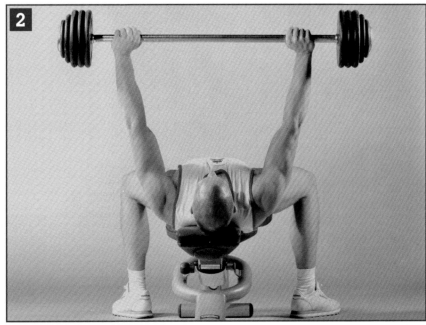

## Dumbbell press

Very similar to the bench press, but instead of a bar (barbell) two dumbbells constitute the weight to be moved. The individual weights could be 2kg each up to 60kg each depending on the individual and the gains being trained for. The exercise is performed in a very similar way to the bench press. Although a chest exercise, due to the instability of two dumbbells it is also good for the supporting muscles of the shoulders.

### Progressions
- **Rotated grip** – Instead of the dumbbell grip that is the same as the barbell, the grip is rotated 90° so that the weights are parallel with the body.

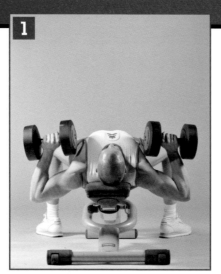
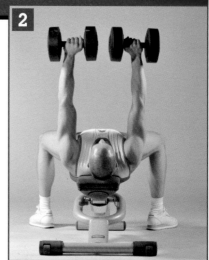

## Incline press

The bench press or the dumbbell press is done on a bench that is raised so that the body is no longer parallel with the floor, but is instead at anything from a 30° to a 60° angle, though most often 45°, head upwards.

**Progressions** As for the bench and dumbbell presses.

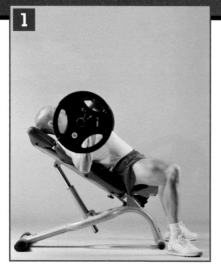
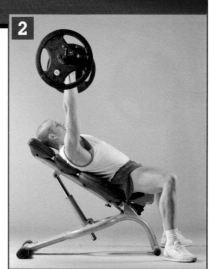

## Decline press

The bench press or the dumbbell press is done on a bench that is lowered so that the body is no longer parallel with the floor, but is instead at anything from a 30° to a 45° angle, head downwards. The chest is actually stronger at this angle for most people, so a larger weight can sometimes be lifted.

**Progressions** As for the bench and dumbbell presses.

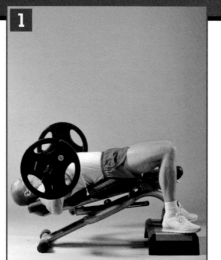
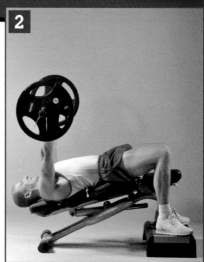

# Chest exercises

## Chest (pec) flies

Like the bench/dumbbell presses, this is performed while laid back on a bench, but with arms outspread holding weights. The arms are brought to the centre, together, above the chest. This is again a compound exercise for the pectorals, but also works the deltoids, triceps and forearms.

**Progressions** Similar to those above – incline, decline and eccentric variations.

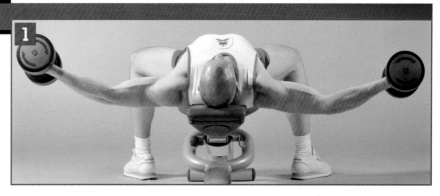

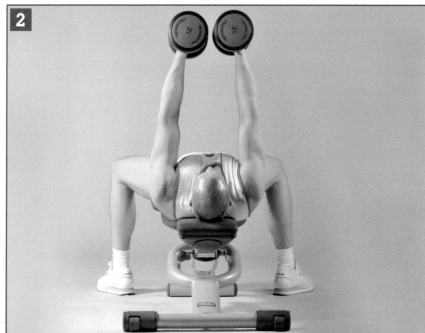

> ! Although I have described all of these exercises as if they are being done in a gym, they can actually be done anywhere by using sandbags, rucksacks, bottles of water, trees etc.

## Cable/elastic press

By tying pieces of elastic or theraband around a bar, or using a cable machine, a standing press/fly can be achieved that strengthens the chest, deltoid and triceps.

**Progressions** This can be performed eccentrically, or the height being pulled from can be altered, *ie* above head-height, below waist-height etc.

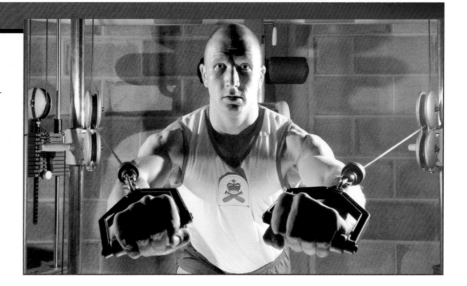

# Upper back exercises

## Lat pull-down

A specific machine is needed to complete this exercise. It is a compound exercise that also involves the biceps, forearms and the rear deltoids. Sit in the lat pull-down machine with knees securely fixed under the knee support. Grip the bar in a similar grip to that used for pull-ups (just wider than shoulder-width, with palms turned away) and pull the bar down to the top of the chest. Hold for a split second and then return to the starting position under control. Try to keep the body upright and rigid so that it is the lats performing the exercise. Try not to swing or lean back and involve the lower back muscles to initiate the movement. **NB:** This exercise is very good at improving the muscles associated with performing a pull-up if this is an area of weakness.

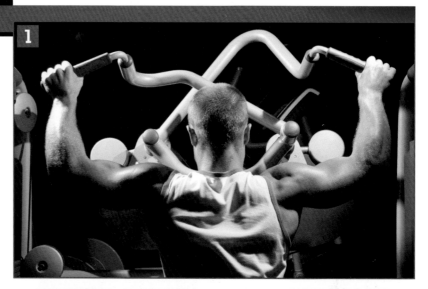

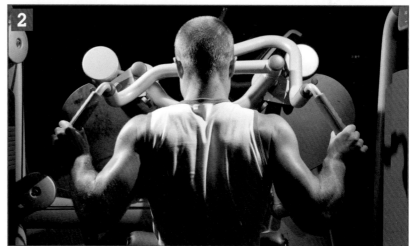

### Progressions
- **Eccentric** – Perform the release back to the start position eccentrically.

- **Vary grip** – Wide grip is usually harder, close grip can be taxing if the weight is increased. Palms inward grip can be used as well. This will target the biceps more.

## Bent-over barbell row

This exercise is performed while leaning over, holding a barbell in both hands. The bar is then pulled up into the lower chest/abdomen. It is a compound exercise that also involves the biceps, forearms, traps and the rear deltoids. It is very important to fix the back and keep the core tight. The back should be straight, and not curved. Some people find this position difficult to maintain, so you should be very careful as it is easy to injure the back if you have bad posture. For this reason some heavy lifters wear lifting belts to help support the lower back.

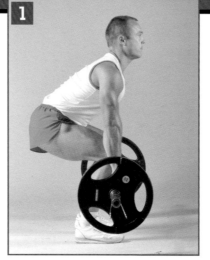

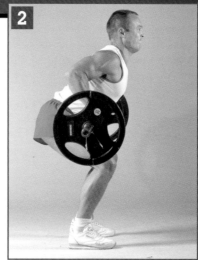

# Upper back exercises

## Bent-over dumbbell row

As barbell row on previous page, but holding dumbbells in both hands. It is again important to protect the lower back.

### Progressions

■ **Single-arm dumbbell row** – As above, but performed while leaning over a bench holding a dumbbell in one hand. The opposite hand is rested on the bench, and the leg on the same side is knelt on the bench. The back must be fixed in a safe position, ensuring it is straight and not curved. The weight is then pulled up into the abdomen/upper chest. The same muscles as above are exercised. It is again important to protect the lower back.

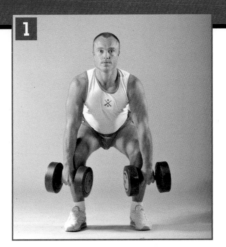

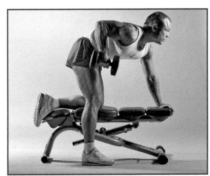

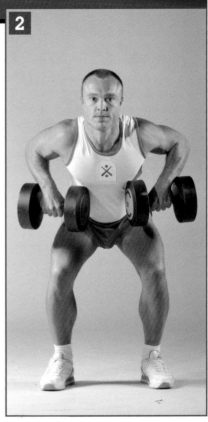

# Central back exercises

## Barbell shrug

Hold a relatively heavy barbell with your palms facing in, about shoulder-width apart, with your feet about shoulder-width apart as well. Ensure the arms are fully extended. It is easy to injure the back if this exercise is performed badly, so ensure the core and lower back are controlled. Shrug the shoulders as high as possible towards the ears, thus lifting the weight up, pause briefly, and then lower the bar back into the starting position. This exercises the traps, deltoids and upper back.

### Variation

■ **Dumbbell shrugs** – As above but performed with two dumbbells. They should hang naturally at the sides of the body and the exercise should be performed as above.

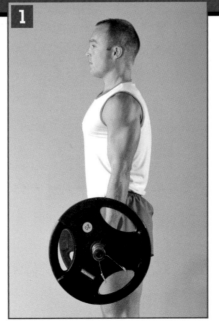

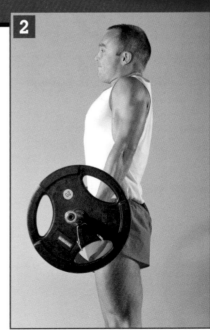

# Lower back exercises

## Deadlift

The deadlift is a compound exercise that works the lower back, the glutes (backside), adductors (inside of the legs), hamstrings, quads, lats, traps and grip strength. To perform a deadlift, place a (light to start with!) barbell on the ground in front of you with the bar touching your shins. Take hold of the bar with your hands a little wider than shoulder-width apart, ensuring the hands/arms are placed outside your legs. Many people prefer a 'split grip' (*ie* one hand overgrasping, one hand undergrasping), but it is personal preference. Ensure thumbs are around the bar. Arms should be straight, head should be up with chest up and out. It is important to look straight ahead with shoulders back in order to keep the back straight. Take a big breath and hold it to make to body/core/back solid and tight. Lift the bar in a slow controlled manner, exhaling as you complete the lift. Pulling is done by extending the legs and hips and pushing your feet into the floor. Arms and back remain straight and the bar is kept close to the body. At the top there should be a slight pause before holding your breath and returning the bar to the floor under control, pushing the hips back.

**NB:** Ensure the back is kept straight at all times! Always return the weight to a 'stop' on the floor before repeating – do not bounce the weight.

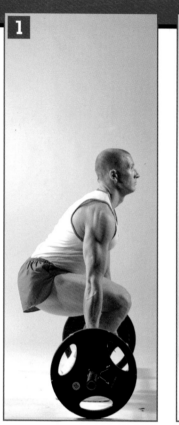
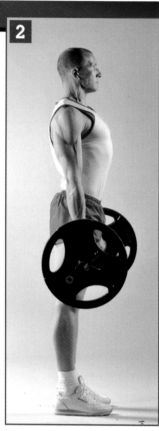

## Good morning

This involves placing a bar/barbell across the shoulders behind the neck. Stand with feet shoulder-width apart, ensuring legs are kept straight and back is straight and not rounded at all. While keeping the head/eyes looking forward, bend forward until the upper body is parallel to the ground. Hold for a split second, then return to the start position.

**Progression** – The same exercise but holding dumbbells instead of a barbell across the shoulders. Dumbbells have to be held, not rested. This is a harder exercise as the shoulder/arms must also work.

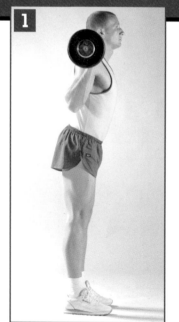
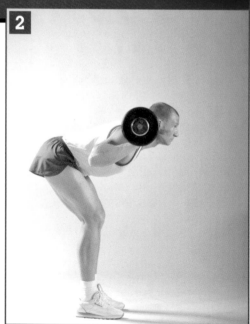

# Lower back exercises

## Superman dorsals

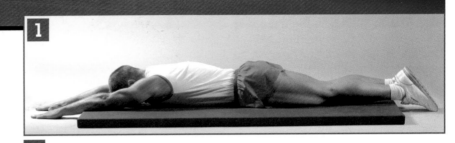

To perform this exercise, lie on your front with legs straight and arms extended above your head. Lift one arm and the opposite leg a few inches off the floor and hold for a few seconds. Once complete, slowly lower back to the floor. Repeat for the opposite arm and leg.

### Progression

■ **Superman on all fours** – The same exercise as above with alternate arms and legs raised, but this time from the all fours (hands and knees) position.

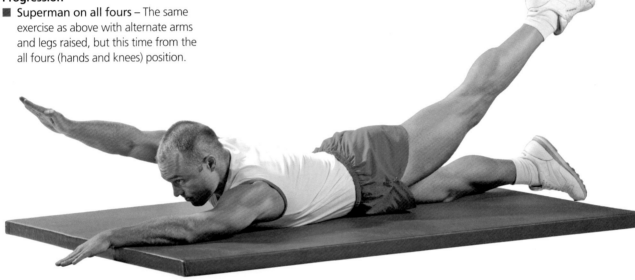

## Pelvic lifts/bridging

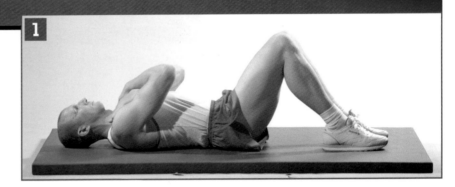

To perform this exercise, lie on your back with your knees bent and arms at your sides. Raise the pelvis up towards the ceiling so that the shoulders, hips and knees are in line. Hold this position for a few seconds, ensuring the glutes (buttocks) are squeezed while holding. Release the position and lower back to the floor. This exercises the lower back, abdominals, glutes and hamstrings.

### Progression

■ **Fitball bridge** – As above, but with feet on fitball. The core is exercised more in this variation.

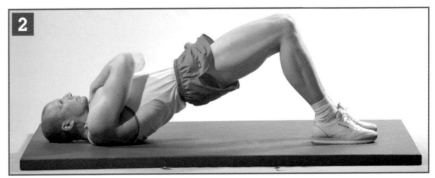

## Dorsal raise

Perform the dorsal raise by lying face down on the floor with fingertips on temples and shoulders relaxed. Lift your chest off the floor while keeping the lower body on it. Hold briefly, then gently lower to the floor, breathing out. This exercise trains the muscles of the erector spinae of the lower back.

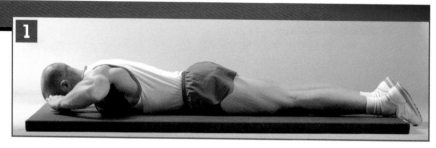

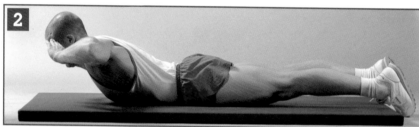

## Leg lift bridge

As for pelvic lifts, but once in the upper position extend one leg from the knee until it is straight. Lower this leg and repeat with the other leg. There is a lot of control in this exercise. It is important to try to keep the hips steady and level – do not allow them to 'dip' or drop to one side. The core is exercised more in this variation.

**Progression**
- **Fitball bridge** – As above, but with feet on fitball.

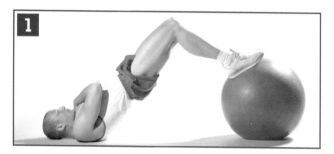

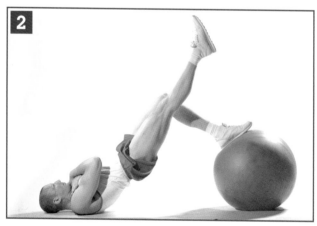

## Dorsal raise on fitball

As above, but with hips/lower abs resting on a fitball and the upper body curled over it. Toes should be in contact with the ground, with feet wider than shoulder-width apart for stability. Lift up and hold for a second before curling the upper body back around the ball.

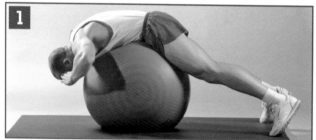

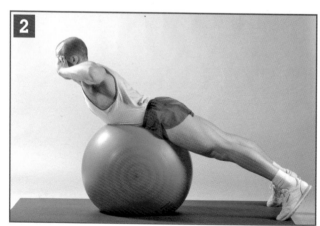

# Shoulder exercises

## Shoulder press

The shoulder press can be performed while seated or standing with a barbell (or two dumbbells – see below). The weight is held above the head and then lowered to just above the shoulders/the top of the shoulders, and then raised again. It is a compound exercise that also involves the trapezius and the triceps.

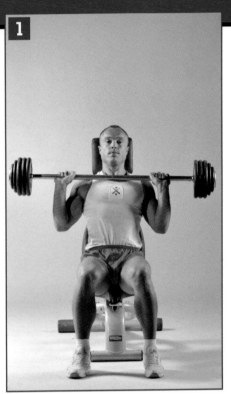

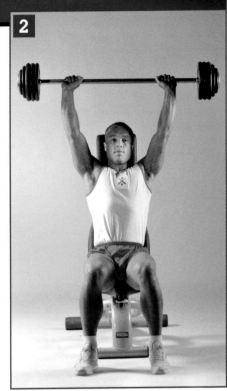

## Military press

This is similar to the shoulder press but is always performed while standing and with the feet together (not shoulder-width apart). It is named the military press because of its similarity in appearance to the 'at attention' position used in most armed forces. As it is performed in this position as opposed to the seated/feet apart shoulder press, the military press exercises the core stabilisers to keep the body rigid and upright. It is therefore a more effective compound exercise.

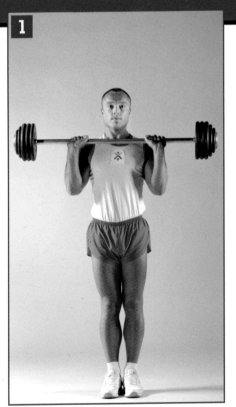

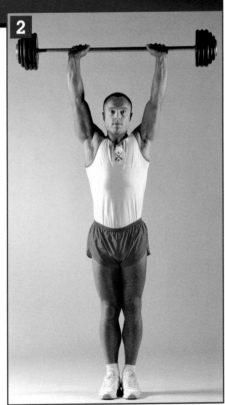

## Arnold press

As for the shoulder press with dumbbells, but the start position (weights rested on the tops of the shoulders) has the palms facing the body. As the weights are pressed they are rotated so that the palms face outwards when the weights are overhead.

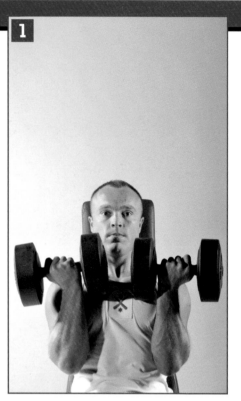
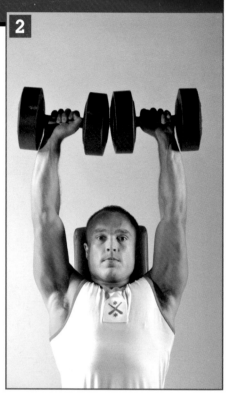

## Upright barbell row

This exercise is performed while standing. It involves holding a barbell at the centre with thumbs touching. The weight is then lifted straight up to the collarbone/chin, with the elbows of both arms leading and reaching a height around the top of the head. It is a compound exercise that also involves the trapezius, upper back, forearms, triceps and biceps.

**Progression**
The narrower the grip the more the trapezius muscles are exercised, the wider the grip the more the deltoids are worked.

**Variation**
■ Upright dumbbell row – As above, but instead of holding a barbell in the centre, two dumbbells are held.

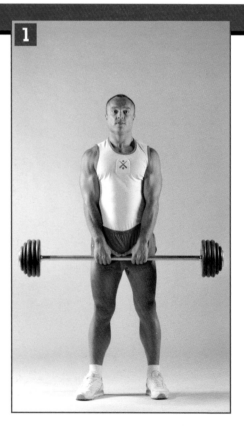
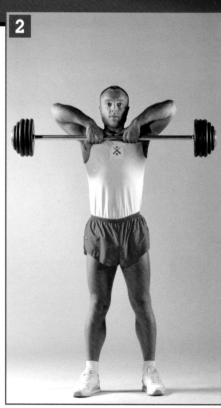

# Shoulder exercises

## Lateral raise

This exercise can be performed seated or standing. A dumbbell should be held in each hand and the arms should hang naturally down at the sides of the body. Both weights should be lifted out to the sides at the same time until at the same level as the shoulders. The lateral raise is an isolation exercise for the deltoids, but also works the forearms and traps.

### Progressions

- **Little finger high** – While lifting the weights upwards, turn the hands so that the thumb points downwards and the little finger is highest. This hits the deltoid that little bit more.

- **Full raise** – As above, but with a smaller weight. Instead of stopping when in line with the shoulders continue all the way up until the weights touch overhead. Again, this will work the deltoids that little bit more.

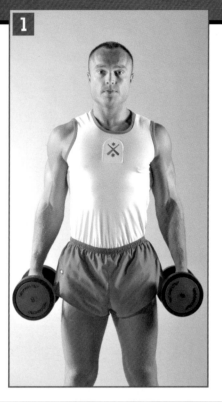

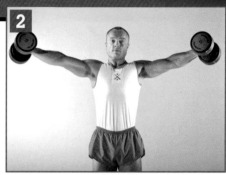

OR

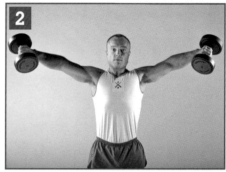

## Front raise

This exercise can be performed seated or standing. A dumbbell should be held in each hand and the arms allowed to hang down at the sides of the body. Together or separately, they should be lifted up to the front of the body until at the same level as the shoulders (just below eye-level). It is again an isolation exercise for the deltoids, but also works the forearms and the core due to the changing centre of gravity.

### Progressions

- **Single weight** – Instead of two dumbbells, use a sandbag or a single disc weight (like those put on an Olympic bar). Perform the same exercise, but obviously both arms are lifting at the same time and working together. This works the core and tends to hit the deltoid that little bit more.

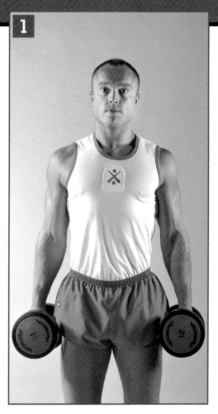

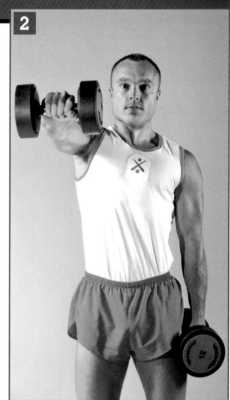

## Bent-over raise

Performed in a similar position as for the bent-over row. With the back straight and fixed, dumbbells are held in each hand and allowed to hang naturally down the sides towards the ground. The weights are lifted with straight arms almost like a reverse pec (chest) fly until they are parallel with the ground (*ie* at shoulder height). This exercises the rear of the deltoid and the traps.

### Progressions

- **Lying rear deltoid raise** – This is the same basic exercise but performed lying face down on a bench, allowing the weights to hang at the sides. However, a very high bench or very short arms are necessary if the weights are not to hit the floor.

- **Seated rear deltoid raise** – The same exercise, this time performed sitting on the end of a bench, leaning forward. Again, the back must be kept solid.

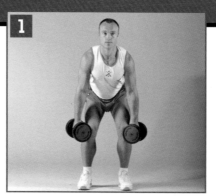
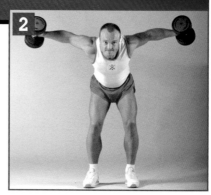
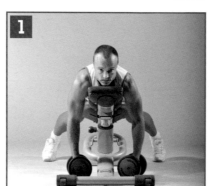
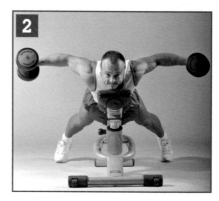

## Cable/elastic raise

The front and side raise exercises explained above can be replicated using a cable machine or a piece of elastic/theraband tied to a post/bend or even trapped under the foot. The same muscles are worked and the same techniques apply.

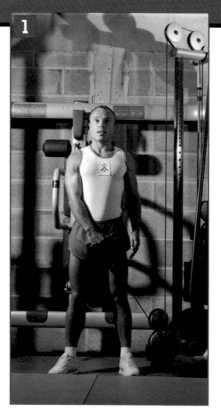
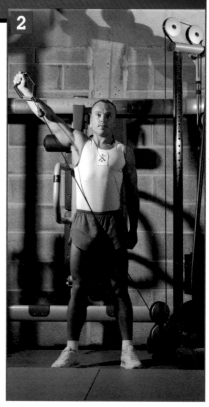

# ARM EXERCISES

Strong arms make a Royal Marines life much easier, whether carrying his SA80, loading stores for an Operation or just impressing the girls on the beach during his post Operational leave. The following pages show a number exercises that can be used to strengthen the bicep and triceps. By incorporating some or all of the exercises shown into your circuits and training programmes both endurance and stamina in the arms can be increased, not to mention strength and power as well. As before, these exercises will seldom be used by Recruits in training, although trained Royal Marines may well use them in their own time or in organised circuits.

## Barbell curls

This exercise is performed while standing with the hands holding a barbell (palms facing away from body), which hangs down to rest on the thighs. The weight is then curled up to the shoulders. It is important to try to keep the rest of the body, especially the back, still, and to keep the elbows in at the hips.

**Progression**
- **EZ bar curls** – More of a variation than a progression. The EZ bar allows a slightly different hand position for curling that some people prefer.

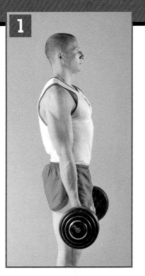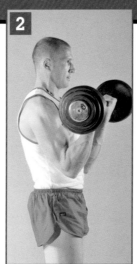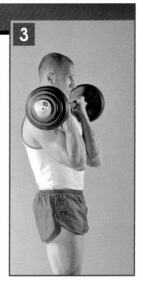

## Dumbbell curls

As above, but two dumbbells are held, hanging naturally at the sides of the body. This can be performed standing up or sitting down. As the weights are curled up towards the shoulders they are twisted so that the palms are facing the shoulders.

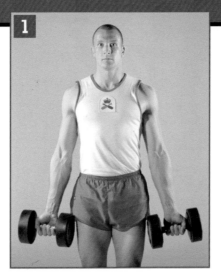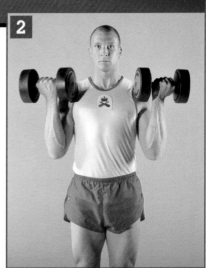

## Hammer curls

As above, sitting down or standing up, but the weights are not curled to face the shoulders – instead, the palms stay facing inwards towards the body so that the weights stay like 'hammers'.

### Progression

■ **Alt curls** – As for dumbbell curls or hammer curls, but instead of curling both weights at the same time the weights are curled one at a time.

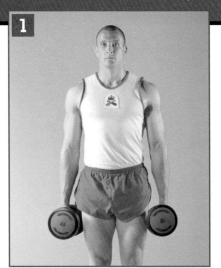
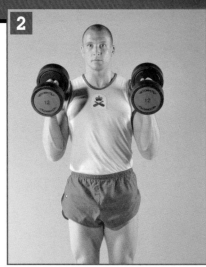

## Concentration curl

Usually performed sitting on the end of a bench. Each arm is exercised independently with a dumbbell. Sit with the legs apart and the exercising arm in between them, with the elbow against the inside of the thigh and the dumbbell in the hand. Curl the dumbbell up to the shoulder and return, repeat, then change arms and repeat the same number on the opposite side. This is an isolation exercise for the biceps.

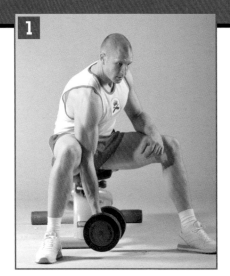
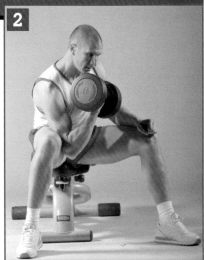

## Incline curl

Similar to the seated dumbbell curl, but with the seat at an incline of 45° (or thereabouts). As the body is at an incline and the arms are hanging naturally at the sides, the biceps are again isolated.

### Progression

■ **Arms turned out** – By performing the same exercise, but turning each arm slightly outwards, the biceps can be hit that little bit more.

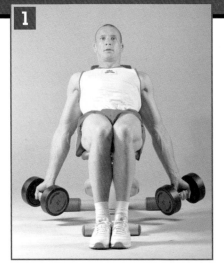
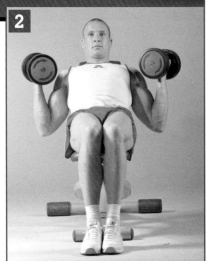

## Close grip bench press

Hold the weight with the normal bench press grip but with your hands about six inches apart. Lower the weight to the chest, ensuring the elbows remain at the sides. Press back to the top. Although the chest and shoulders are also used, the triceps are exercised above all.

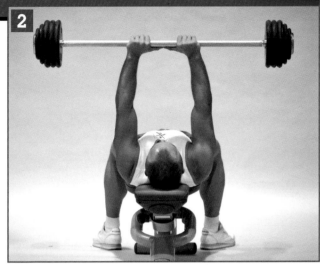

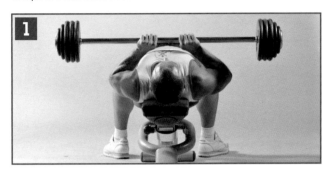

## Lying triceps barbell extension

Performed lying on the back holding a barbell in both hands directly above the eyes, with hands about six inches apart. Keeping the upper arms still (elbows pointing directly up), allow the lower arms to lower the weight down towards the top of the head/forehead. Pause at the bottom and then straighten the arms back to the start position.

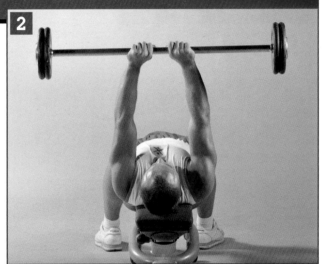

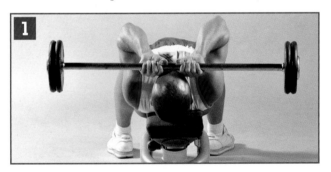

## Dumbbell kickback

Performed leaning over a bench in the same way as for the single-arm dumbbell row but with a much smaller weight and the arm holding the weight raised so that the elbow is about shoulder-height. The lower arm and weight point towards the floor, hanging naturally. Keeping the upper arm still, the lower arm is brought up to the same level, raising the weight by extending at the elbow. Pause slightly at the top before lowering to the start position.

### Progression
- Both arms kickback – By either bending forward or kneeling on a bench with both legs and bending forwards, both arms can be put in the position above and exercised at the same time. It is again important to have a straight back in a good position.

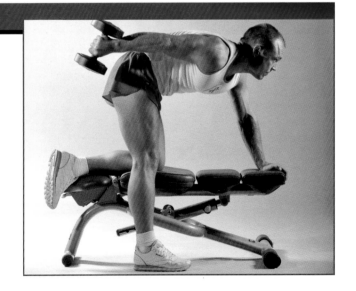

## Dumbbell extension

This exercise can be performed sitting down or standing up. A dumbbell is held in one hand behind the head, with the elbow pointed straight up in the air. The arm is extended so that it is fully straight, with the upper arm kept stationary with the elbow pointing upwards. It is then lowered to the start point. Ensure both arms are exercised equally.

### Progression
■ **Two-arm dumbbell extension** – As above but with both hands on the weight. It is held behind the head, and then extended in the same way as before.

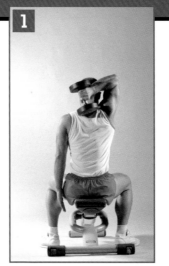
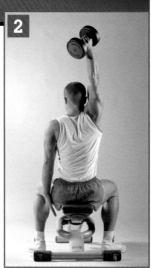

## Triceps pushdown

Usually performed on a cable machine using a straight or inverted 'V' bar. Take hold of the bar with both hands (no more than ten inches apart) and ensure the back is straight – if anything lean slightly forward so that the shoulders are over the hands, but ensure the back does not curve. Fix the elbows into the sides so that the upper arms are parallel with the body. Cock the wrists by rolling the hands away (opposite to revving a motor bike) so that the wrists are strong. Bending from the elbow, straighten the arms, keeping the upper arm locked into the sides. Pause, and return to the top. The arms should be completely straight at extension.

### Progressions
■ **Rope pushdowns** – The same exercise, but a rope is used instead of a bar. Where possible the hands should be kept apart and not allowed to come together. Everything else is exactly the same.

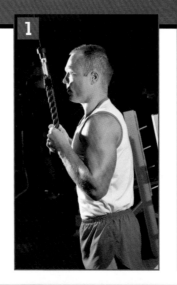
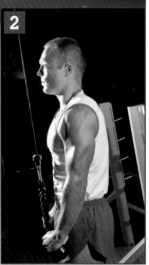

## Triceps overhead extension

Using the same cable machine and bar as the pushdown, but held overhead, with the cable stretching back to its origin behind the body. Step forward so that one foot is in front of the other, as if performing a calf stretch. The upper arms should be parallel to the ground with elbows pointing towards the opposite side of the room. The upper arms should be fixed, and the lower arms extended until straight. A slight pause, then return under control to the start point.

### Progressions
■ **Rope overhead extension** – The same exercise but using the rope attachment. Again, the hands must be kept apart and not allowed to touch. Try to keep the elbows in and not allow them to skewer out to the sides.

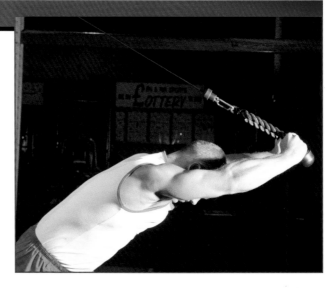

# LEG EXERCISES

During his time in training a Royal Marines Recruit will develop such strong legs he is able to achieve feats he would have assumed impossible before joining. Recruits' bodies, particularly their legs increase considerably in their ability to 'yomp' very large distances carrying considerably heavy weights. Many Royal Marines will use some of the exercises outlined in the following pages to increase and maintain this strength. Recruits also touch on a few of these exercises, just to ensure some real muscular strength and size develops in their legs. Again, these exercises can be included in specific sessions or as stations in circuits.

## Step-ups

This exercise can again be done with or without weight. The basic premise is to have a step (around a foot high) in front of you. You then step up with the right foot, then the left foot, down with the right foot, then down with the left foot. This can be repeated for a certain number of reps, or repeated over and over for a set period of time. Always ensure the whole foot, not just half, is placed on to the step. It is important to change the lead foot so that they equally share the initial (harder) step-up. For example, perform ten right foot first, then ten left foot first, then back to right etc. This works the quads, hamstrings and glutes.

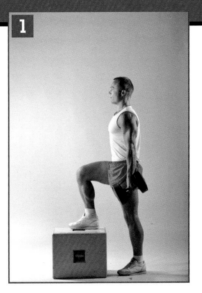
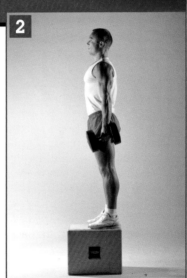

**Progressions**

- **Barbell** – As for squats/lunges. The exercise is performed with a bar across the shoulders or a rucksack containing weight.

- **Dumbbells** – As for squats/lunges. The exercise is performed with dumbbells in the hands.

- **Higher step** – The higher the step, the more difficult the exercise.

- **Side step-ups** – The same exercise, but performed standing side on. The lead foot must step on far enough to allow the other foot to fit on as well. Remember to change sides. Any weighted variations could be used.

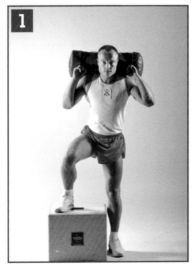
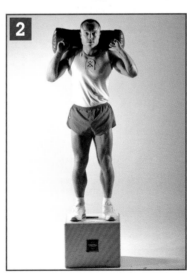

# Squats

Squats can be performed as a body-weight only exercise, or with weight added. The technique for either is basically the same. Without weight, stand with the feet parallel to each other, pointing forwards, shoulder-width apart. Ensure the arms are out of the way, so that they do not start pushing on the tops of the thighs if the exercise becomes difficult. For Recruits we teach them to cross their arms across their chest (right over left – military order!), holding the tops of their shoulders.

To perform the squat, bend at the knee until the upper leg is parallel with the ground, *ie* the knee is at a 90° angle. While squatting down it is imperative to keep the back straight and upright, and not to bend forward. Furthermore it is important that as the knees bend they go forwards over the big and second toes of the foot, and that the heels remain on the floor at all times. On the way up, the back should remain tight and upright, the heels flat and the buttocks (glutes) should be squeezed. Once completely upright, repeat. This will work the quads, hamstrings and glutes.

## Progressions

- **With weight** – The basic exercise is the same, but a barbell is placed across the back of the shoulders behind the neck, the hands gripping the bar either side of the head. Once you have mastered it, the weight should nestle on the traps and will not cause discomfort, though at first a lot of people use padding or find they bruise slightly. It is even more important when using weight to ensure that the back is kept upright, as if any forward leaning is allowed the balance can be lost. Again, ensure the heels remain on the ground. A rucksack with weight can, of course, be used instead.

- **Front squat** – Similar to the normal squat but with the bar across the front of the shoulders. More emphasis is placed on the quads. The arms are crossed and the bar gripped with palms down and knuckles into the collarbone. It is important to keep the elbows up high, at shoulder height or higher. Keep the head up and looking forward. Squat as normal so the knee is about 90° before returning to the start position.

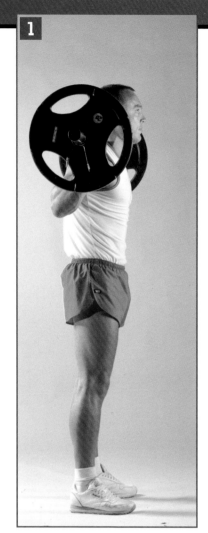

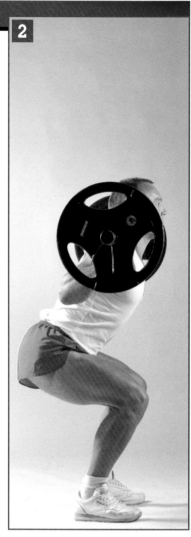

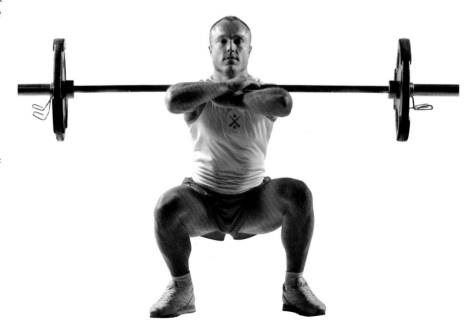

## Lunges

Like the squat, the lunge can be performed with or without weight. Again, it is basically the same in either case. To perform the lunge stand with feet parallel to each other pointing forwards just under shoulder-width apart. As with the squat it is important to keep the hands from supporting the legs, so the arms are crossed in front of the body as before. With one foot, say the right, take a large step forward, around a shoulder's width and a half. Ensure both feet remain pointing forwards as if on train tracks.

With the right foot planted, the right leg should be bent until the upper part is parallel with the ground and the knee is just under an inch off the floor (it should not touch the floor). The right knee should not go further forward than the right foot. If it does, then a longer step must be taken next time. It is important to keep the back straight and upright – do not lean forward. The right leg then 'powers' the body upright by pushing off the floor and the right foot is retuned to its starting point next to the left. Repeat for the left leg. This will work the quads, hamstrings and glutes.

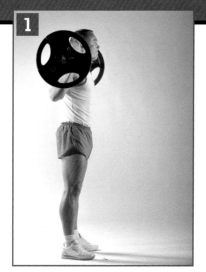
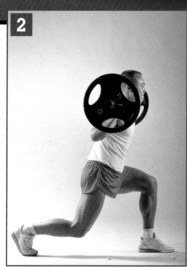
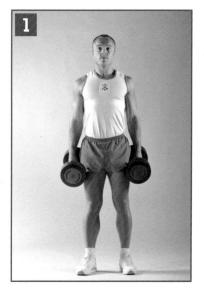
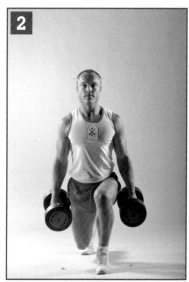

### Progressions

- **Barbell lunges** – With the barbell in the same position as it was for the squats, the same exercise is performed, paying particular attention to staying upright and taking a long enough stride forward each time. Again, a rucksack with weight in could be used instead.

- **Dumbbell lunges** – As per normal lunges but a dumbbell is held in each hand (equal weight) and allowed to hang naturally at the sides of the body. It is important to stop the dumbbells swinging wildly. This exercise therefore has some effect on the grip (forearms) and shoulders.

- **Walking lunges** – This exercise can be performed with or without weight and for either of the weighted variations. The exercise starts in the same way, but instead of 'powering' back to the start position off the right foot, the left foot steps forward to meet the right foot. The exercise is then performed on the left leg. In this manner, a predetermined amount of ground can be covered using 'walking lunges'.

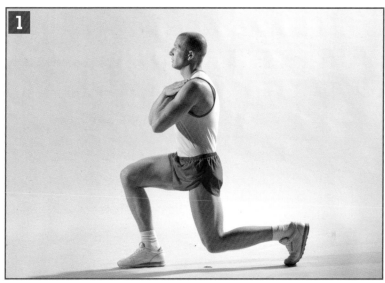

## Single Leg squat

Similar to the normal squat but performed with one leg only. The opposite leg is raised forward for balance. Squat down to 90° or just beyond raising the opposite leg and both arms to the front for balance. Push down through the foot from the lowest point to return to the top. This exercise requires considerable balance and core stability beyond the obvious leg strength.

### Progressions
- **Weighted Single Leg squat** – Same exercise with weight held either across the chest, or in outstretched arms.

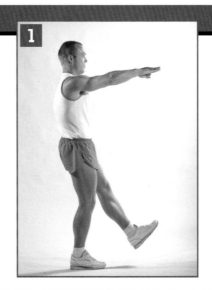
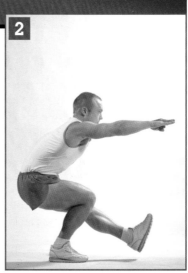

## Leg press

A simple weights machine that mimics the squat action. Although it is effective, it is not as good as the real squat exercise. However, it is good for inclusion in a general muscular programme, and especially good for building strength following an injury or long period of inactivity, as it requires less stabilising muscles than the squat. Sit in the machine, ensuring the knees are at around 90°, select a sensible weight and press the weight through the heels. Control the weight and never just 'drop' it.

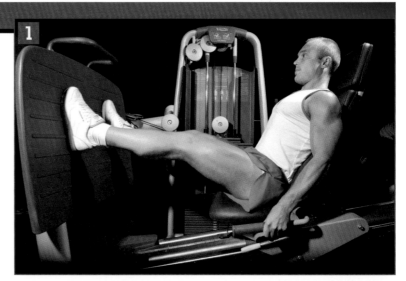
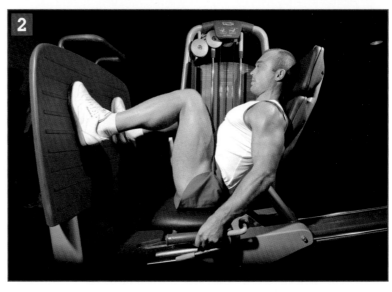

## Leg extension

An isolation exercise for the quads using a specific machine. Especially good following injury or to correct a muscle imbalance, but not as good as the more functional leg exercises mentioned above. Sit in the machine, ensuring the cushioned supports are in the correct place for your body. The padding you push against should be in the ankle/lower shin area, not the foot as this will cause injuries to the ankle ligaments.

### Progression

A similar exercise can be improvised by sitting in a seat that allows the legs to dangle above the floor, and gripping a dumbbell or a small rucksack with weight in it between the feet. The legs are then straightened, lifting the weight, and lowered again.

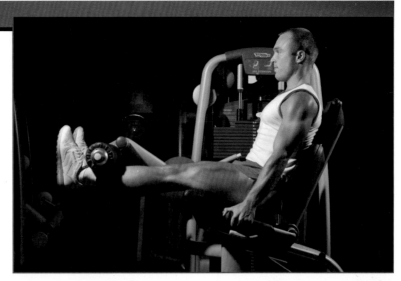

## Leg curl

An isolation exercise for the hamstrings using a specific machine. Especially good following injury or to correct a muscle imbalance, which many people have in their hamstrings when compared to their quads. However, in general this exercise is not as good as the more functional leg exercises mentioned above. Lie in the machine, ensuring the supports are in the correct place for your body. The padding you push against should be at the bottom of the calf. A common mistake is to lift too much weight, so be careful – the hamstrings are easy to pull. Ensure you do a thorough warm-up prior to this exercise.

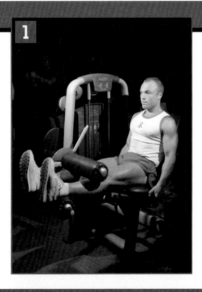
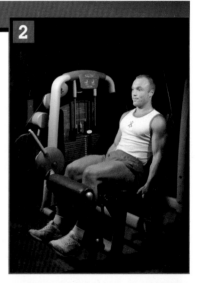

## Calf raise on leg press machine

It is possible to exercise the calf muscles using a leg press machine. By fully extending the leg, ie pressing the weight, the feet can be adjusted to the bottom of the plate so that the weight can be pressed by the toes by rotating through the ankle. Again, a pause is paramount for good technique. Be aware that the ankles/Achilles area can be at risk if the feet are positioned too low and the weight is dropped by slipping. For this reason some gyms do not allow this exercise on a leg press machine.

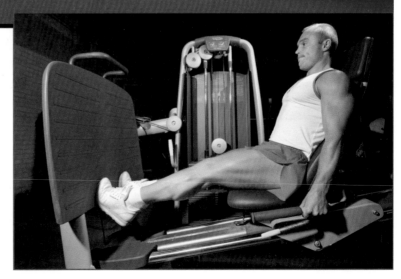

## Leg curl with partner

Kneel on the floor in an upright position, crossing the arms across the chest. A partner then sits on and supports the lower portion of the leg/calf muscle. Lean forward in a gentle and controlled manner, contracting the hamstrings to prevent the body from crashing to the mat. Prior to a point of no return, contract the hamstring fully and return back to starting position.

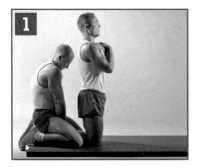

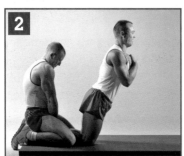

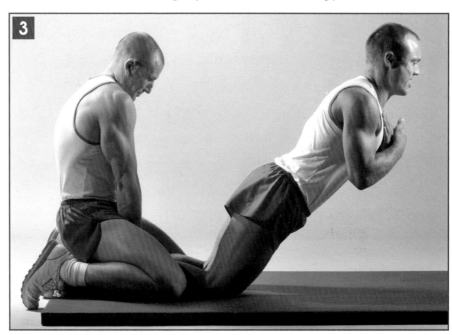

## Standing calf raise

Either from the floor, or on the edge of a step, the calf raise involves going up on to tiptoe from a position with the feet pointing forwards just under shoulder-width apart. A momentary pause at the top should be followed by a slow return to the start point. Some balance is required for this exercise.

### Progressions

■ **Barbell calf raise** – As above, but performed with a barbell on the shoulders as for the squat. Control must be maintained to ensure the weight does no cause the body to 'fall' forward. Therefore the core must be kept tight and the back upright. A rucksack with weight in can again be used instead.

■ **Dumbbell calf raises** – As per lunges, raises can be performed with dumbbells held in either hand. Balance is again key, and the heavy dumbbells also work the grip/forearm.

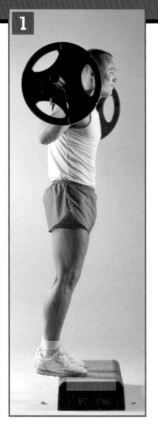

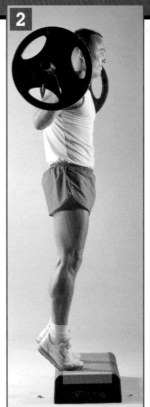

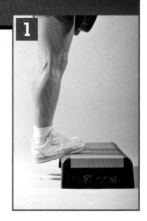

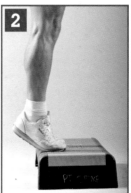

# ABDOMINAL EXERCISES

Abdominal exercises are some of the most important exercises to be performed. From their first days in Recruit training to the day they leave the Corps, every Royal Marine will perform some form of abdominal exercise every week. The abdominal muscles protect the internal organs, aid in good posture and prevent injuries to the back. The following shows some of the exercises that Royal Marines will perform in circuits and in their own individual sessions. Many other abdominal exercises exist, so don't just stick to the ones you like. Vary your exercises, include them in circuits and remember variation prevents boredom and the plateau effect.

## The sit-up

While lying down on the back with the legs bent, feet together and knees together and fingertips on the temples, sit up under control to a near vertical position so that the elbows can touch the tops of the knees. Ideally the feet should remain flat on the floor and the fingertips in touch with the temples. Do not be tempted to put the hands behind the head and pull up through the arms, as this will injure the neck. Once vertical, lay back under control, so that the head, shoulders and elbows are back in contact with the ground. Repeat the exercise, ensuring your form is correct. Achieving 30+ is good. However, in their RMFA most Royal Marines will achieve the maximum score of 85, so this is something to aim for.

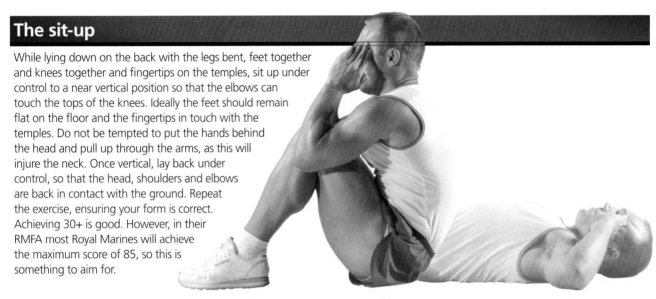

## The half-sit

If you are finding the regular sit-up extremely difficult, try putting your hands on the tops of your thighs and sliding them up the thighs to touch the tops of the knees. This should gently lift the torso off the floor and start exercising the correct muscles to improve regular sit-ups. However, do not allow the body to 'flop' back down to the ground, as this will injure the back. Lower under control, almost eccentrically.

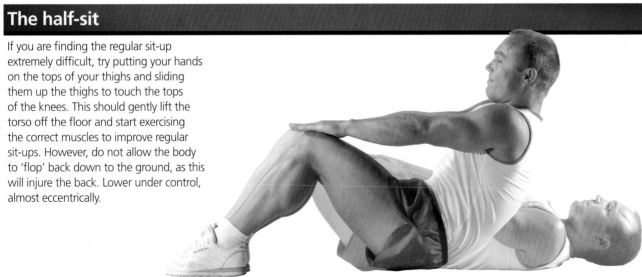

## Sit-up progressions

- **Alternate sit-up** – Similar to the regular sit-up, but more effective for exercising the obliques. Instead of sitting up completely straight and placing the elbows on top of the knees, as you sit-up twist the torso from the waist to touch the elbow on the top of the opposite knee. Return to the start position and do the same on the opposite side.

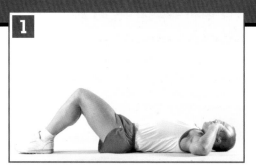
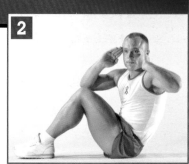

- **Weight across chest** – As for the regular sit-up, but instead of placing the fingers on the temples, cross the arms across the chest (as done for squats without weight). By placing some form of weight on the chest under the crossed arms, the abs have to work harder when sitting up.

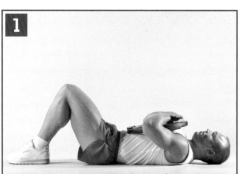
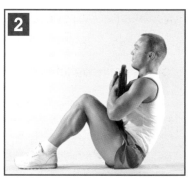

- **Weight outstretched** – As above, but instead of holding the weight across the chest it is held up in the air, directly above the head. As the sit-up is performed the weight stays above the head, on the way up and on the way down. It is important to keep it directly above the head and not allow it to come forward over the chest (which makes the exercise easier). This exercise has some effect on the shoulders depending on the weight held.

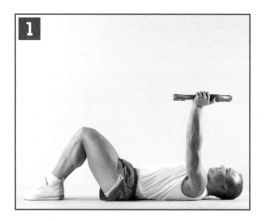
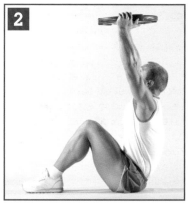

## Sit-up feet fixed

As for the regular sit-up, but instead of trying to keep the feet on the floor they are trapped under a bar (these can be purchased from sports shops to attach to door frames), under furniture, or held down by a friend or training partner. This makes the exercise much easier by recruiting the hip flexor muscles (13 different muscles make up the hip flexors). This is not so good for exercising the abdominals, but is excellent for improving rope climbing or other techniques that require a lot of hip flexor strength.

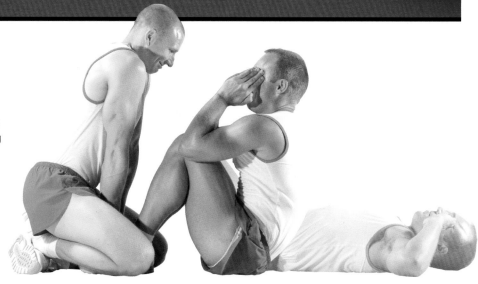

## Crunchies

Laying flat with your fingers on your temples, raise your feet off the ground about six inches, but keep the knees at 90°. Sit up and bring the knees to your chest simultaneously. Return to the start position without allowing your feet to come into contact with the ground. Repeat.

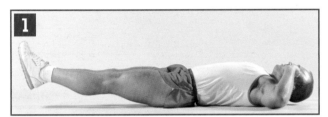

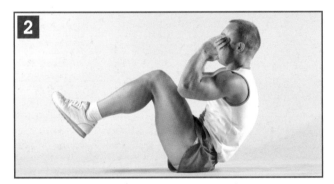

## Reverse crunch/rock backs

Lie on your back with your hands on the ground to your side or just under your buttocks/lower back. Keeping your upper and middle back on the floor and your legs in the same position, rock the knees towards the face, ensuring the hips/lower back are curled off the floor, and feel the abdominals contract.

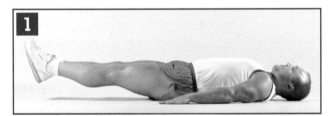

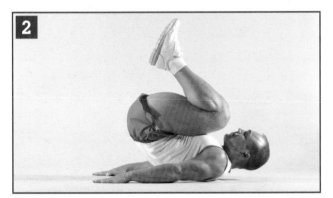

## Bicycle crunchie

This exercise is very similar to the crunchie, but performed in a continuous peddling motion with the legs and with a twisting rotation through the hips so that alternate elbows touch alternate knees. It is said to resemble a fly dying on its back!

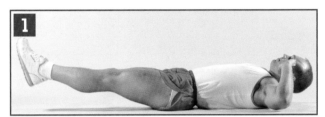

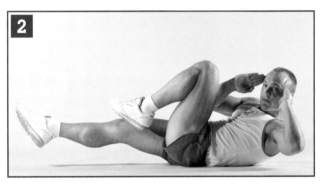

## Flutter kicks

Lie on your back with your hands on the ground to your side or just under your buttocks/lower back. Raise your legs about six inches off the ground and perform 'flutter' kicks in the air as if you were laying on your back in water and trying to propel yourself along (kick from the hip). Keep the legs as straight as possible at all times.

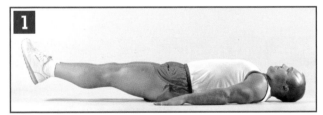

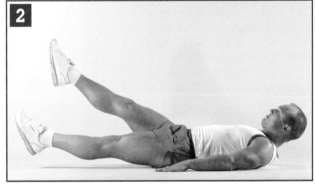

## Straight leg hip extension

Lie on your back with your legs straight up above you at 90° to your body. Place the hands next to the body, or just under the buttocks/lower back. Push up from the abdominals with your legs pointing straight up. Aim to force the toes as high as possible. Lower under control (don't flop!) and repeat.

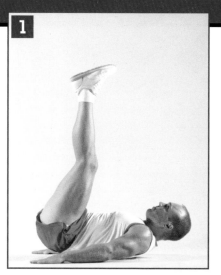
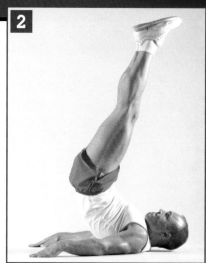

## Heel push/hamstring contracted sit-up

In complete contrast to the above, instead of fixing the feet the heels are used to pull against something. Anything put between the heels and the buttocks under the bent legs can be pulled against by the heels – a small rucksack, a 20kg disc weight or even a football could be used. By using the heels to pull in against the object, the hamstring muscles are contracted. Using the agonist/antagonist model discussed in Chapter 5, this means that the hip flexors must relax. By relaxing the hip flexors, this exercise becomes very abdominal specific/isolationary and is thus surprisingly difficult at first.

## Ab crunch

The ab crunch is a relatively simple and easy exercise. In the position used for the original sit-up, curl up from the abs, raising the upper back off the floor. The pivot is more at the centre of the abs than the lower back and hence a crunch is performed rather than a full sit-up.

**Progressions**
- **Leg raised crunch** – As above, but instead of performing the crunch with the feet flat on the floor they are raised so that the lower legs are parallel with the ground. The crunch is then performed.

- **Vertical leg crunch** – As above, but the legs are this time pointed straight up in the air.

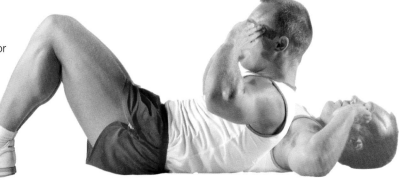

## Oblique crunch

This exercise is performed on one side for a certain number of reps and then the other side. Lie on your back in the regular sit-up position, but while leaving one foot on the floor pick the other foot up and place the side of it on the top of the thigh of the bent leg. The oblique crunch is now performed by crunching up to touch the opposite elbow to the knee that is raised. Control back down and repeat. Make sure both sides are exercised equally.

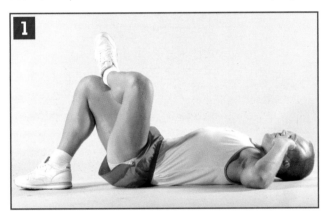

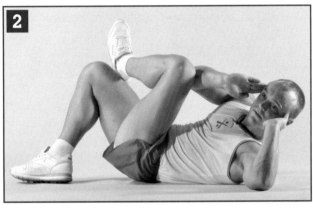

## Heel taps

While lying on the back in the regular sit-up position, a sort of 'half-crunch' is performed and held at the top. The torso is then dipped to one side and then to the other to allow the hand on either side to tap the heel on that side. This is repeated.

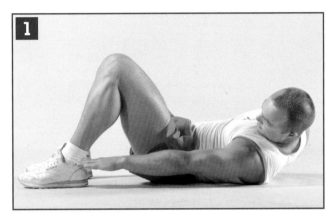

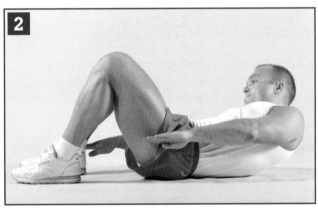

## Scissor kicks

Lying on the back with the hands under the lower back or backside, the legs are raised out in front about six inches off the floor. They are then opened as far as possible and brought back into the centre, and one foot passes over the top of the other. The legs are opened again and then closed again to allow the opposite foot to pass over the top of the other. This is repeated a set number of times.

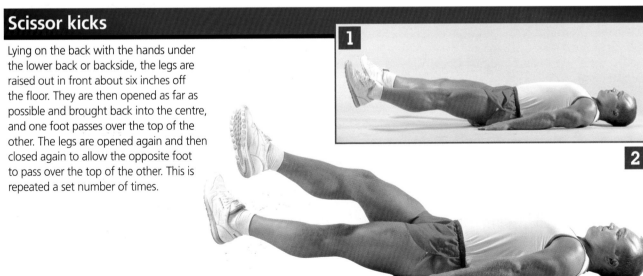

## The plank

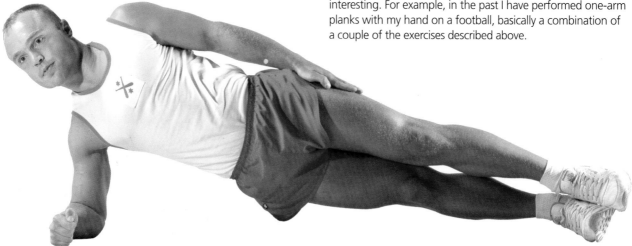

The plank is one of the most underused and underrated core exercises around. It is so simple and has so many variations that a whole workout can be designed around it. Yet despite its apparent simplicity it is actually a relatively hard exercise and commonly performed badly.

To perform the plank lie face down on the floor, keeping the feet and legs together, and raise the upper body up by leaning on the forearms and elbows. The head should be kept up and not allowed to hang down. The shoulders, hips, knees and ankles should be in line at all times – the waist/lower back in particular should not be allowed to sag to the ground or be raised into the air. Once the correct position has been achieved it should be maintained for a set period of time. Try 30 seconds to begin with, then increase to a minute at a time. A five-minute plank is particularly impressive.

### Progressions

■ **On hands** – The same exercise, but instead of resting the weight on the elbows the hands are used. Basically the fully extended press-up position is held.

■ **Feet raised** – The normal plank is held, but a box or bench is used to raise the feet. Again, the straight body position is imperative.

■ **One arm** – Either on the forearm/elbow or on the hand, the same plank position (with the front of the body facing the floor) is performed but with only one arm in contact with the ground. The other arm should be placed out of the way behind the back.

■ **Leg lift** – The normal plank is performed, but once the position is achieved the legs are raised alternately off the ground, completely straight, rotating from the hips. This works the glutes (buttocks) but also unbalances the plank and causes the core to work harder to readjust. This can be performed for a set time, or a certain number of raises.

■ **Arm lift** – As above, but instead of raising the legs the arms are raised alternately. The feet are kept together and on the floor. Again, when raising the arms imbalance makes the core work harder.

■ **On fitball** – By placing either the feet or the arms on a fitball when performing the plank the exercise difficulty is greatly increased. The instability of the ball means that the core really has to work hard to maintain the plank position.

■ **Side plank** – The body is turned to face one side or the other and the plank is performed on the one arm (forearm in contact with the ground) that is directly under the shoulder on that side. It is important to again keep shoulder, hip and knee in line and not allow the hips to sink to the floor.

### Combinations

The different planks exercises outlined above are just some of possibly hundreds of variations, and it is only your imagination that will limit you changing your exercises and keeping things interesting. For example, in the past I have performed one-arm planks with my hand on a football, basically a combination of a couple of the exercises described above.

## Hanging knee raises

Hang from your pull-up bar and with straight legs. Bend the legs and raise the knees up to the chest, curling the hips up by contracting the abdominals. It is important to keep control of the exercise and work hard to stop yourself swinging. Lower and repeat.

### Variation

- **Captain's chair knee raise** – As above, but instead of hanging by the arms, which requires a certain amount of forearm/grip strength, the arm rests on the captain's chair are used to enable the forearms to support the body weight.

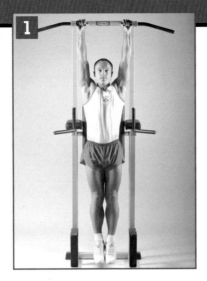
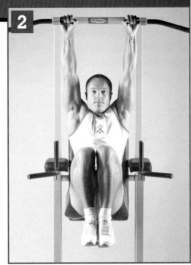

## Hanging leg raise

As above, but keep the legs straight at all times during the exercise. The legs should be raised to a horizontal position so that they are parallel with the ground, followed by a slight pause before controlling them to the dead hang again. As above, it is important to stop the body swinging.

### Variation

- **Captain's chair leg raise** – As above, but instead of hanging by the arms, which requires a certain amount of forearm/grip strength, the arm rests on the captain's chair are used to enable the forearms to support the body weight.

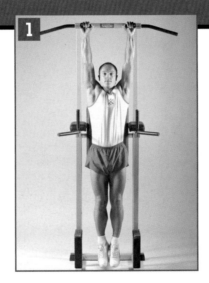
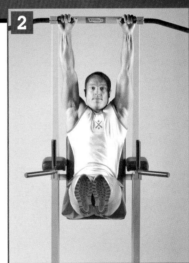

## Hanging leg raise, toes to bar

As for the normal hanging leg raise, but the legs are raised past 90° so that the toes can touch the bar in between the hands. The legs are then lowered, under control, to the start position.

### Progression

- **Eccentric toes to bar** – As above, but once toes have touched the bar the legs are lowered to a reverse count of five.

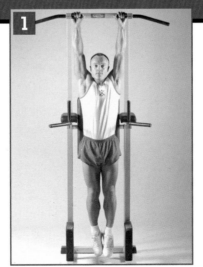
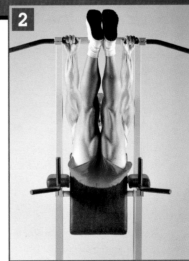

## Side bends

This is an oblique specific exercise that involves standing up straight with feet shoulder-width apart, holding a dumbbell or other form of weight in one hand. Imagine that the body is in between two panes of glass, so that it cannot bend forwards or backwards. Bend sideways to lower the hand holding the weight until it is in line with the knee, then lean all the way over to the opposite side to touch your free hand on the opposite knee. Repeat a certain number of times. Ensure you perform the same number on the other side as well. Depending on the weight held, some grip/forearm strength can be improved.

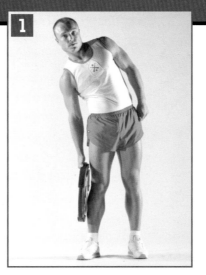
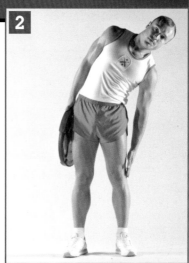

## Saxon side bends

Still imagining yourself between two panes of glass, a weight is held above the head with straight arms. A bit like a tree swaying in the wind, the body pivots at the waist to one side and back to the centre, then to the other side and back to the centre. It is best to start with a small weight first, as this is quite a challenge.

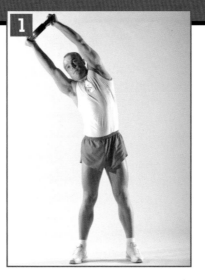
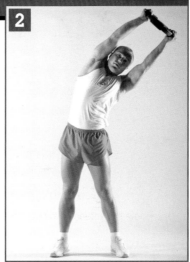

## Oblique twists

This is another oblique exercise and an excellent ab builder. To perform it, take an Olympic bar with a weight disc (not too heavy to start with) on one end. Wedge the non-weight end into the corner of a wall. Hold the bar at the end above the weight disc, as if holding a baseball bat. Keep the head up, looking forward. Twist the torso and bring the hands (and therefore the weight) down to one hip. Pause, then powerfully rotate the hips back to the start position and lift the weight back to the start. Repeat for the other side.

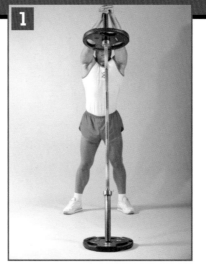
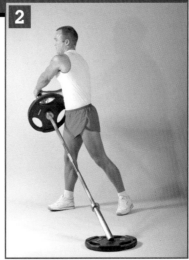

## V-sits

This is a relatively difficult and advanced exercise. While lying flat on the back, with your hands stretched out above the head, a sit-up and leg raise is performed so that the hands and feet meet in the middle above the waist, with the body and legs forming a 'V'. It is important to keep the arms and legs as straight as possible, and also to control the exercise to avoid injuring the lower back.

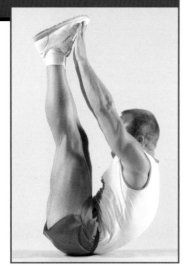

### Progression

- **Alternate V-sits** – As above, but the legs are raised alternately while the arms are still raised together to meet the single leg in the centre. Ensure you exercise both legs equally. Again, control is paramount.

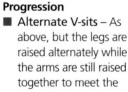

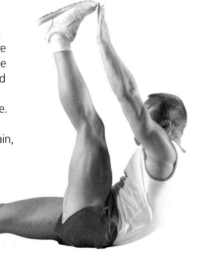

## Gymnast crunch

Performed from the same start position as the V-sit, but instead of raising the legs and arms to meet straight, a 'tuck' is performed as if a front somersault is being performed on the ground. To tuck, bring the knees to the chest and hands down towards the knees as if about to grab them. This will raise the shoulders as if crunching. It is important to hold for a slight pause once 'tucked' before returning to the outstretched start position. A certain amount of control and co-ordination is required.

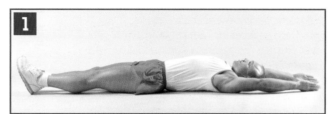

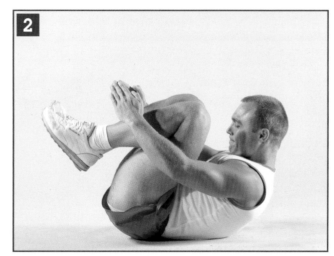

## Russian twist

Sitting on the floor with the knees bent and feet flat on the floor, some form of weight is held in the hands (a dumbbell, a medicine ball or a bottle of water). The upper body is then moved to an angle of 45° by leaning back. This also means the feet come off the floor by about an inch. The arms then lift the weight to one side of the body, so that it is in line with the hips or behind the back. It is then lifted to the same point on the other side of the body. This is repeated a set number of times.

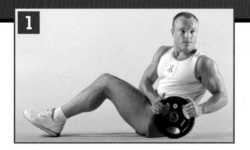

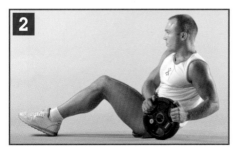

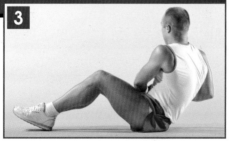

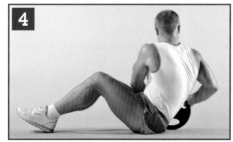

## Rollouts

Perform using a rollout wheel or a small barbell. This is not an easy exercise and should be built up to by performing a variety of sit-up and plank exercises. To perform the rollout, choose an area free of obstructions. A six-foot mat is perfect. Starting on the knees, with the arms straight down from the shoulders holding the handles on the wheel, allow the wheel to roll forward and in doing so stretch the whole body so that the face, chest and hips are about an inch off the floor. Only the knees and wheel should be in contact with the ground. Return to the start position, leading with the backside, by contracting the abdominals, *ie* pull the wheel back as you return to the start position. Repeat. It is very important to make the core/back tight when performing this exercise, as it is quite tough on the lower back at full extension.

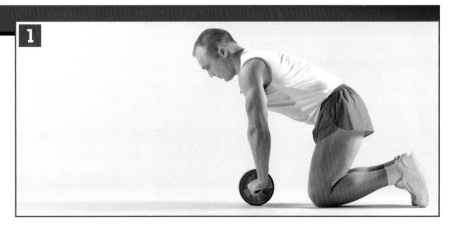

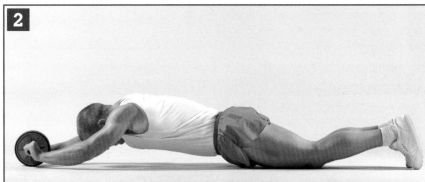

## Standing rollout

As above, but instead of starting on the knees start from standing with the wheel between the feet, held by the hands. On rolling out, only the feet and wheel should be in contact the ground. At first it may be necessary to do this facing a wall that will restrict how far you can roll out, until you have the strength to do a full standing repetition. This can be progressed further by performing it wearing a weighted vest/rucksack with weight.

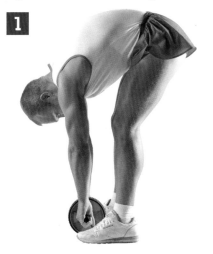

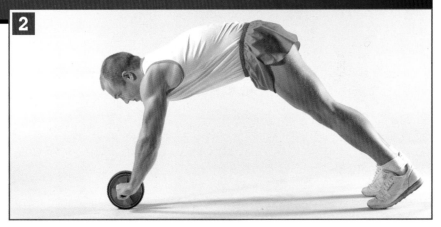

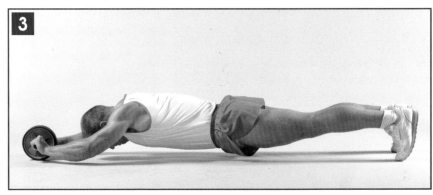

## Shovel pick-ups

The same set-up of bar and weight as for the Russian twist is laid out on the floor. Approach the non-weight end of the bar and stand with feet shoulder-width apart. Bend down and grip the bar with a split grip as if deadlifting it (the hand nearer the weight end should use an undergrasp). Stand up as if deadlifting the bar. The arms should now be extended with the bar on the hips and the weighted end stuck out at one end. Holding the core tight, rotate the hips and arms to bring the weight in towards the direction the body is facing in an arc. Once the weight is in line with the direction the feet are pointed in, return to the side position and repeat. Ensure both sides are exercised equally.

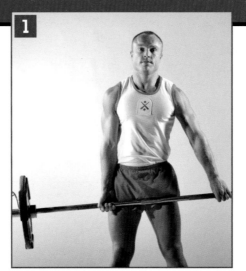
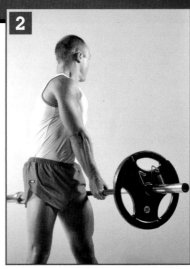

## Dragon raises

This is a very advanced and tough exercise. It is easy to hurt the lower back and hence a good progressive programme should be undertaken before attempting this exercise. Using a weights bench or similar that is fixed to the ground, lie on it face upwards. Take hold of the end of the bench over the head with a tight grip. Raise the legs to 90° by performing a normal leg raise, and by contracting the abs and pulling on the arms push the feet as high as possible directly upwards. You should now be fully extended up in the air, with only the shoulders and neck in contact with the bench. The arms holding the bench are keeping your balance. By tensing the core, abs and lower back the body tension should be kept completely rigid, keeping the ankles, knees, hips and shoulders in line. Pivoting from the shoulders, the body is now lowered back to the bench, but completely straight and rigid. The waist should not be bent. Once back on the bench, repeat.

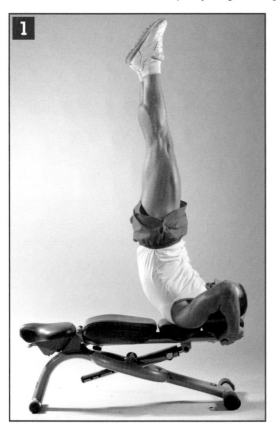
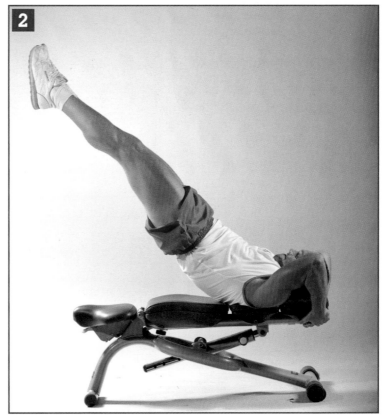

## Fitball Kneeling

Kneel onto the fitball but do not sit back on the heels. Kneel completely upright so that the kness, hips and shoulders are all inline. To regress this perform in front of a bar or wall and hold on with both hands, 1 hand, 1 finger etc until it is not needed. Ensure the core (abdominal) muscles are contracted during the exercise. Perform timed periods in the position.

> **!** **Many of the exercises explained in this book can also be performed on a fitball for added instability and therefore increased abdominal workout. There is not enough space to explain all the various fitball exercises, however, many books or websites exist on the subject.**

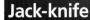

## Jack-knife

Get into the press-up position but with hands on the floor and feet on a fitball. From here, bring the knees into the chest by contracting the abs, allowing the backside to go up in the air and rolling the toes along the fitball. Return to the extended press-up position and then repeat.

**Progression**
- **Jack-knife with press-up** – As above, but every time you return to the start position perform one press-up.

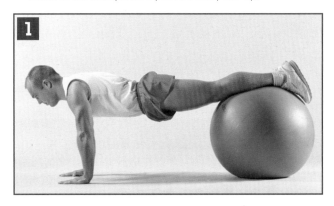

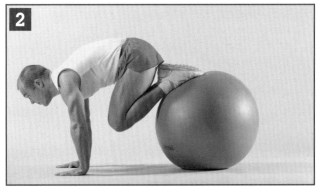

## Fitball Squats

From the kneeling position put both hands onto the ball as well. Now move 1 foot up so the sole of the foot is on the ball, then the other foot so both feet and hands are on the ball. Keeping the back straight and core tight, stand straight up to stand on the ball. Perform timed periods in the position, ie 30 second, 1 minute etc. Or perform squats in the normal fashion but on the ball.

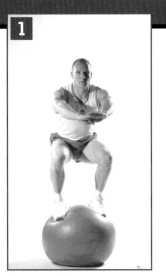

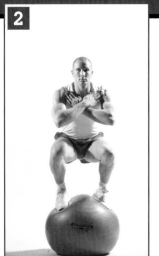

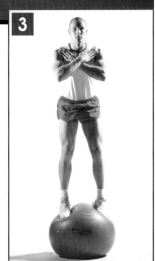

# CV/ALL OVER EXERCISES

These exercises are excellent for getting the pulse rate up and the CV system working hard, to complement running, cycling and swimming training. Some of them may seem very leg specific, but this is because, as the largest muscles in the body, the legs require more oxygen when working and hence get the CV system working quickly. These types of exercise can be performed as separate exercises or as parts of a circuit, mixed in with other types of exercises. When performing these types of CV exercises you should aim to do high reps or do the exercise for set amounts of time, working as hard as possible throughout. Setting a stop watch and performing burpees for 1 or even 2 minutes will soon have your heart pumping and your breathing rate increased.

## Burpees

Start in the standing position with your legs shoulder-width apart. Drop to your haunches with your palms on the floor shoulder-width apart. Keep your head up, back straight and backside almost resting on the back of your heels. From here shoot both legs to the rear so that you are in the press-up start position, then reverse the manoeuvre to the standing position. Repeat as quickly as possible for a certain number of reps or for a certain amount of time.

### Progressions

■ **Jump burpee** – As above, but once back in the start position jump up as high as possible into the air. On landing, go immediately into a burpee.

■ **Long-jump burpee** – As above, but jump forwards, not upwards.

■ **Tuck jump burpee** – As per jump burpee but with knees to the chest while jumping.

■ **Jump-over burpee** – As per jump burpee, but jump over an obstacle or hurdle between burpees.

■ **One-armed burpee** – Use only one arm for the whole exercise. Alternate arms either every time or every ten or so reps.

■ **Dumbbell burpee** – As per regular burpee but holding light dumbbells in the hands throughout. Any of the variations could be used.

■ **Press-up burpee** – A press-up is performed prior to returning to the start point.

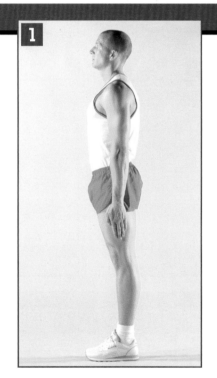
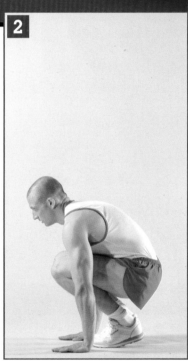
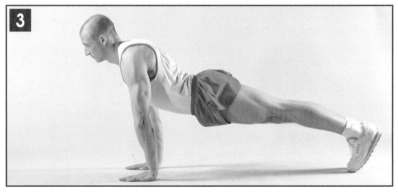

## Squat thrusts

Very similar to the burpee but without standing. The squat thrust starts in the press-up position and the knees are brought into the chest (feet as close to between the hands as possible) and then forced back to the rear as quickly as possible. It is important to concentrate on technique, as it is easy to neglect this. Try not to slide the feet on the ground and do not shorten the step throughout the session.

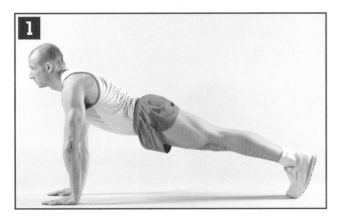

## Alternate squat thrusts

As above, but instead of bringing both legs forward and back alternate the movement of the legs. Bring one leg up while leaving the other out straight and then swap, so that as one moves forward the other moves back at the same time.

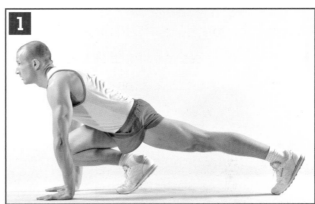

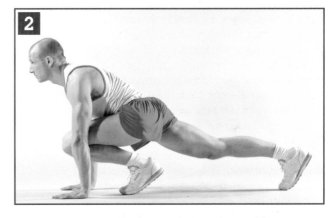

## Squat jumps

Just like the squat without weight mentioned above, but once the downward portion has been completed, instead of simply standing up to return to the start position you should jump up into the air as high as you can. Land and repeat as quickly as possible. A good way of ensuring you go down to the right level is to have your arms hanging at the side of the body and allow your hands to touch the bone on the outside of each ankle. Once these are felt, jump up in the air as high as possible as stated above.

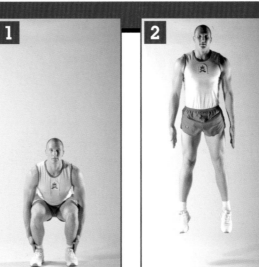

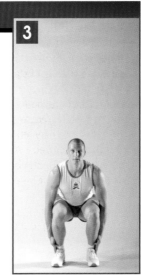

## Star jumps

Starting from a crouch position on your haunches with back straight and head up, push down through the legs and jump up as high as possible. When in the air throw the arms and legs out into a 'star' position. On landing, adopt the same start position and repeat as fast as possible.

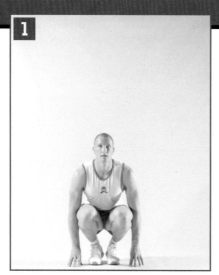
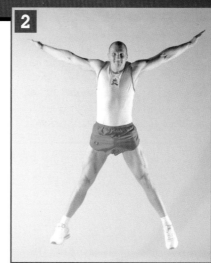

## Stride jumps

Standing in a normal start position, feet shoulder-width apart, hands by the sides, jump up in the air and open the legs and raise the arms into a 'star' position. Return to the normal start position prior to landing and immediately repeat.

■ **Regression** – Sometimes this exercise is done landing in the 'astride' star position and then jumping up again and landing back in the start position. This version is very easy.

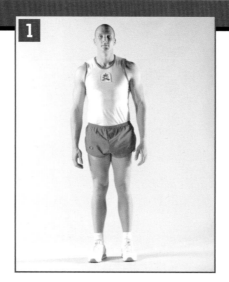
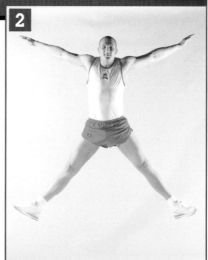

## Tuck jumps

From a normal standing position, jump up as high as possible and bring the knees to the chest at the top of the jump. On landing try to repeat immediately, although a small pre-jump is acceptable. Repeat as quickly as possible.

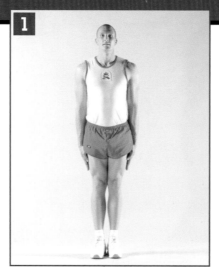
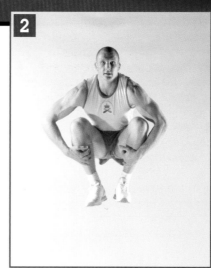

## Bench jumps

Find a bench or box that is approximately a foot high and around the same width. Stand astride the box, *ie* one leg on one side and one on the other, and sit down on it. Then jump up and land with both feet on top of the box. On landing, immediately return to the start position with legs either side of the box and repeat as quickly as possible.

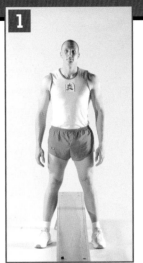
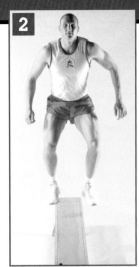
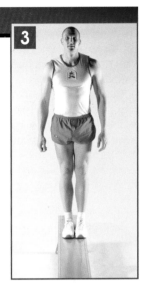

## Ski jumps

Starting in a 'lunge' position (see lunges above), *ie* with one leg forward and one to the rear, with the rear knee almost touching the floor, jump up high and while in the air bring the rear foot forward and take the forward foot to the rear. On landing in the same position as the start but with legs reversed, repeat as quickly as possible.

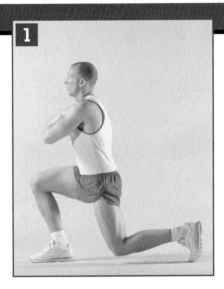
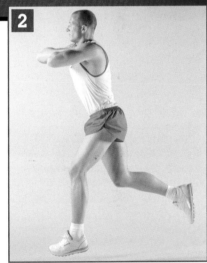

## Box jumps

With a box between one and two feet high in front of you, stand facing it with feet shoulder-width apart. Jump up on to the box from a standing start. Step/jump down carefully and repeat a set number of times as quickly (but controlled) as possible.

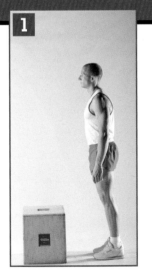
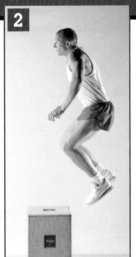
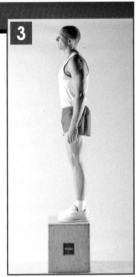

## Wood chops

Usually performed holding a light weight, though it can be performed without, this exercise works the core as well as the legs. Holding the weight/arms out in front at about eye/chest level, bend the legs and rotate the torso to one side and lower the weight to the floor beyond the foot on that side. In a fast explosive movement, rotate the torso back and bring the weight back to the centre and beyond to the highest point of the opposite side (as if diagonally from the floor/foot on the opposite side). Once the weight/arms are at the high point, repeat the exercise as quickly, but still as controlled, as possible. In this manner it looks like chopping wood. Ensure both sides are exercised equally (the above describes the procedure for one side only).

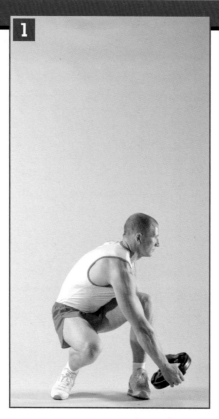
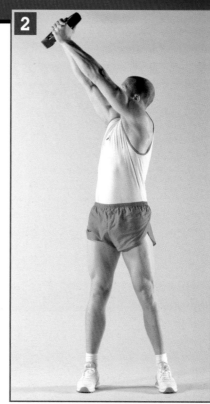

## Step-ups

Although step-ups has been included previously in this book as a leg strengthener, it can also be used as a CV exercise. In the case of step-ups as a CV exercise, a smaller weight, or no weight is used to perform the exercise in exactly the same way, however, instead of low repetitions to build strength, the exercise is performed for set periods of time (say 1 - 2 minutes) or for high repetitions, i.e. 20 - 50 reps each leg.

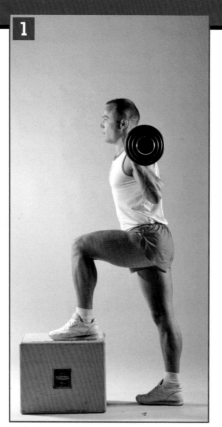
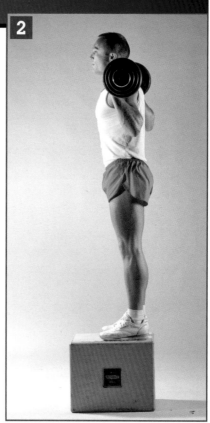

## Skipping

Normal skipping with a skipping rope for a set time or for a set number of jumps. If you have never skipped before it may at first seem difficult to skip without making mistakes and having to constantly restart, but with a bit of perseverance it will soon become second nature. The great thing about skipping is that a skipping rope does not take up much room and skipping can be completed almost anywhere.

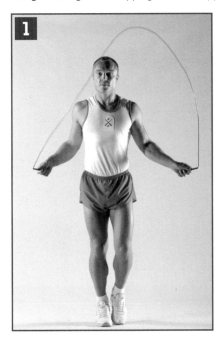
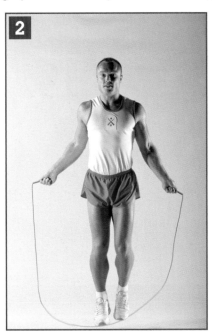
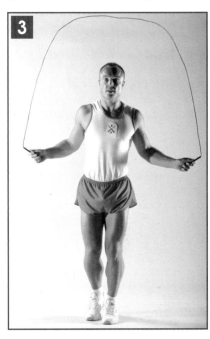

## Bench-hops

Using a bench about a foot high and the same width, stand with both legs to one side and place the hands on the bench, taking hold of one side in each hand. Using the arms like a pivot, jump the legs over the bench to the other side. On landing, immediately repeat back to the starting side. Repeat for a set number of repetitions or set amount of time.

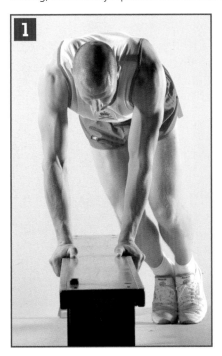
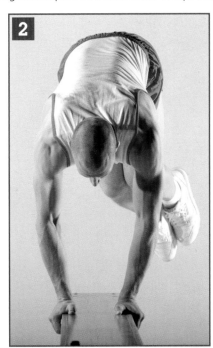
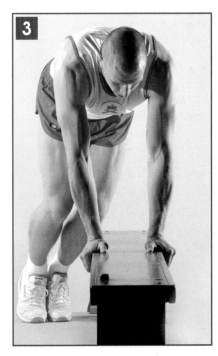

## Farmer's walk

Relatively heavy objects (usually dumbbells) of equal weight are held in each hand and then carried as quickly as possible to a specific point, or round a point and back. Grip, core, upper back and a whole host of muscles are tested, making this a real burner of an exercise. The weights cannot be dragged.

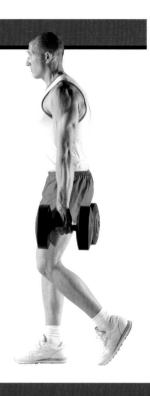

## Tyre/object drag

Using a climbing harness, chest harness or simply by tying a piece of rope around the waist, attach an object such as a tyre to the other end. Select a certain distance or certain time and pull the object for that time or distance as quickly as possible. This exercise is best performed on grass or sand, but can be performed on concrete if necessary.

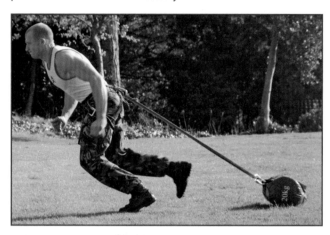

## The Turkish get-up

Lying flat on your back, the kettlebell (or a dumbbell or even a small rucksack) is held straight arm above the head (pic 1). Keeping the arm straight and weight above the head at all times throw the leg on the side of the raised arm over the opposite leg and post up onto your elbow (pic 2). Stand-up on the foot of the same leg thrown over the other leg and post up onto the hand, ensure the bell remains straight above the head (pic 3) and lastly stand-up straight standing on both feet with kettlebell above the head with a straight arm (pic 4). Ensure the weight is always above the head and NEVER take the eyes off the weight. This will ensure balance is maintained. Once standing up straight, lie back down using the reverse technique, then repeat a set number of times equally on each arm.

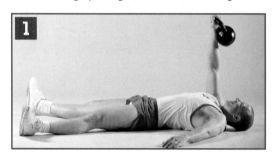

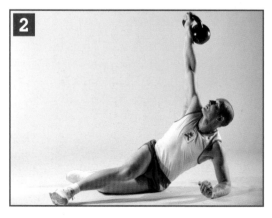

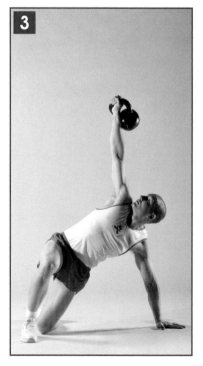

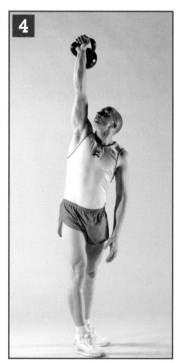

# Kettlebell swing

Place the bell in between the legs with handle parallel to the shoulders. Squat down and take hold of the handle, keeping the back straight and head up. Perform a powerful squat, paying particular attention to driving the hips forward (a hip thrust) and squeezing the glutes together. In doing this, momentum allows the bell to come up to around eye level by rotating through the shoulders. As the bell starts to drop (gravity), bend the legs into the squat position again; as the bell comes in between the legs, drive up again and thrust the hips forward. Repeat for a certain number of reps or for a set time.

## Progressions

■ **One-hand swing** – As above but instead of two hands only one hand holds the bell. The other arm is kept out of the way. Ensure the shoulders remain square and parallel with the feet. Do not allow the bell to drag the body away. This works the core more. Repeat equally for both sides.

■ **Two-hand swing on to step** – Perform the regular kettlebell swing but in front of a step. As the bell is thrust forward and swinging to its peak, step up on to the step and down again leading with one leg. On the next swing do the same but leading with the other leg.

■ **Walking two-hand swing** – Perform the normal two-hand swing, but take a step with alternate feet each swing, *ie* first swing the right foot, then swing the left foot etc. Do so for a certain distance or number of swings.

> ❗ **The kettlebell is a great fitness tool that has seen a revival in the last few years. It allows CV and strength training to take place using a single piece of apparatus. Unfortunately this book is not big enough to allow all the kettlebell exercises available to be described.**

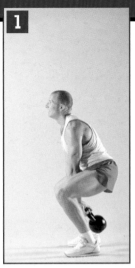
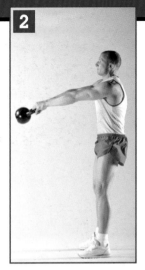
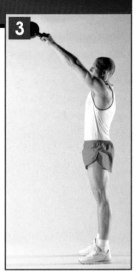
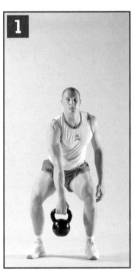
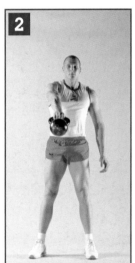
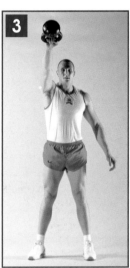
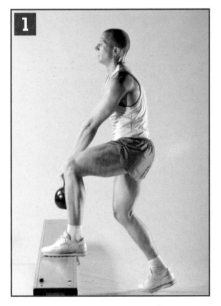
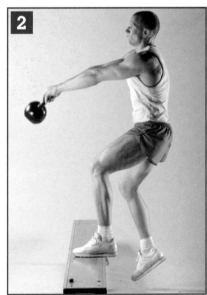

## Fireman's carry

A dead weight is carried in a similar way to the previous exercises, but this time it is a human being across the shoulders. For Royal Marine Recruits the test involves picking the partner up on to the shoulders and then carrying him 200m in 90 seconds or less over grassy and muddy terrain, with both men wearing their 21lb of webbing and carry their 10lb rifle.

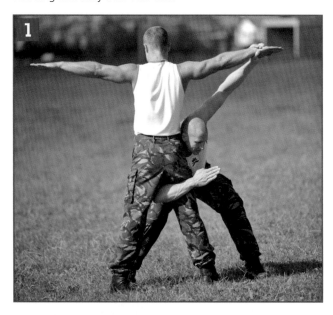

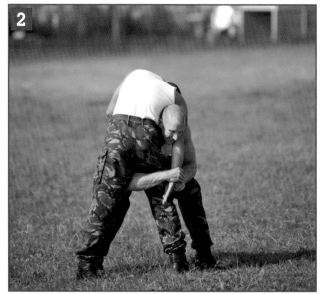

■ Person to be carried adopts the 'star' position. Carrier puts right arm between legs and takes partner's right wrist with left hand

■ Person to be carried leans over carriers shoulders. Carrier passes partner's right hand from his left hand to right hand so his own head is now in gap between partner's right leg and right arm

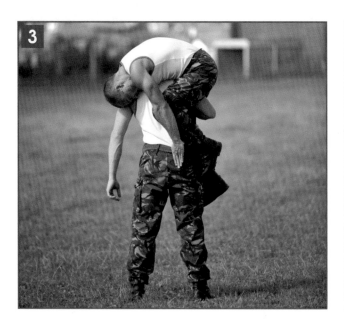

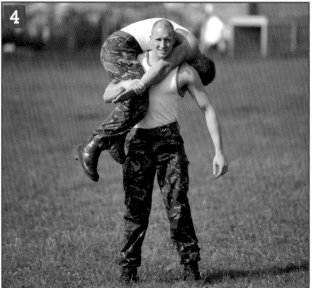

■ Carrier (or instructor if as a group) says 'prepare to lift (pause) LIFT'. Carrier squats up as partner jumps onto back fully. Carried person takes hold of the back of the carrier's belt/trousers and curls himself into a tight ball

# Combat Conditioning

For many Royal Marines this type of training will make up a vast majority of their training. However, this is largely because they have the base level of strength and fitness to cope with it. For most people starting out on a fitness plan or most casual gym-goers, this type of training would be too intensive and lead to injuries and possibly even put them off exercising altogether. Hence why I have decided to only include a small paragraph on the subject. It must be stated that strength and conditioning are quite different. Weights training will make your muscles strong, conditioning exercises will make your muscles anaerobically fitter for a specific sport/role. In general the conditioning exercise should mimic the intensity of the role being trained for.

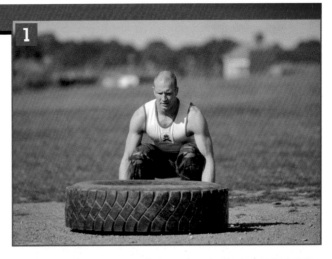

Combat conditioning actually has a large crossover with plyometrics and improvisation, as many exercises build/require power and often the kit and equipment used is not the normal kind of thing you would associate with exercise training. Combat conditioning has become very popular in recent years with the growth and publicity of 'Mixed Martial Arts' as it has become 'the' training of that sport. The exercises not only provide strength gains to the athletes but also the robustness and power that they need when fighting, something which obviously crosses over nicely with the aims of Royal Marines.

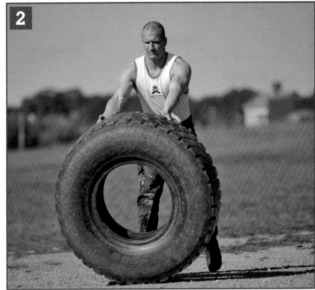

**Exercise examples are:**

- Farmers walk (as shown on page 174)
- Tyre flips (as shown on the right)
- Object drags (as shown on page 174)
- Sledgehammer tyre strikes – striking a large tyre with a sledgehammer repeatedly for time or reps
- Axe training – simply chopping wood with an axe for time/finish
- Med ball slams – throwing a medicine ball into the ground or at a wall as hard as possible catching and repeating for time or reps
- Wheel barrow training – heavy weight in wheel barrow for time or distance reps
- Car/vehicle pushing – pushing a vehicle for distance or time
- Sandbag running/sprints – performing CV exercise carrying a sandbag
- Kit loading – lifting object from floor to a higher platform for time/reps
- Sandbag/tyre throwing for time/reps

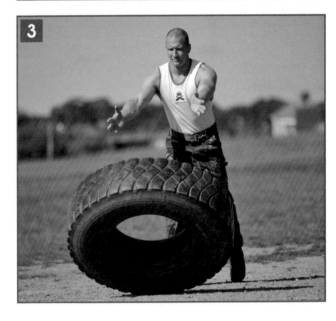

There are many different sessions to be found on the internet for Combat Conditioning. Just remember these sessions are hard, and require a considerable amount of strength and aerobic fitness, therefore they should not been performed without some physical preparation as laid out in this book.

# ROPE CLIMBING

I have left this exercise until last for two reasons. Firstly, it is hardly ever seen in gyms these days – very few gyms or parks have 15–40ft ropes that people can use for strength and fitness gains. And secondly, it is probably the exercise that is ingrained into every Royal Marine for life. Even if a Recruit leaves Royal Marines training after only one month, he will still leave being able to climb a 30-foot rope easily and with confidence. For Royal Marine PTIs, rope climbing becomes second nature. They not only develop a near-perfect technique, but they learn tricks (like the 'reverse' – yes, upside down on the rope) to improve strength and confidence.

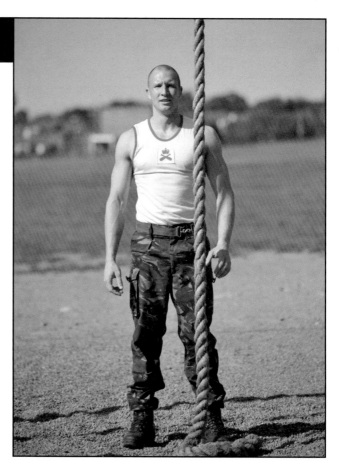

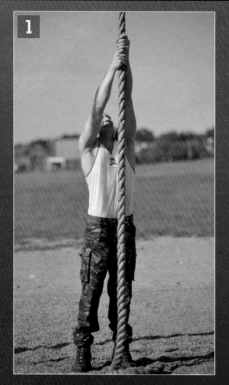

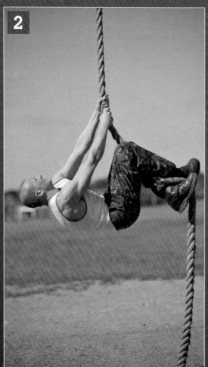

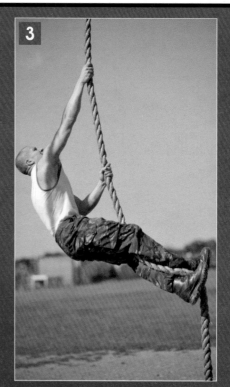

# Rope Climbing technique

Climbing a rope seems near impossible. Unless you are quite strong it can indeed be very difficult, and even if you can climb a 30-foot rope with arms only, I would be surprised if you can do it twice! As explained earlier in this book, rope climbing is fundamental to the development of Recruits in Commando training, as it combines all the elements we expect of Royal Marines: strength, cardiovascular fitness, the ability to perform a technique or skill under pressure, and performing while outside of their comfort zone (in this instance at height). Again as already explained, Recruits are tested in rope climbing, eventually having to climb 30-foot (9.14m) ropes outside, wearing boots and carrying 31lb (13.6kg) of kit.

To climb a rope with ease and grace a specific technique must be mastered. Although this technique has seen little changes over the years, and despite there being some variations, used particularly by the Army when they come on the All Arms Commando course, the technique explained below is that taught today at the Commando Training Centre.

- Ensure you have the correct kit on – a pair of trousers (shorts will cause abrasions to the legs; most PTIs, including myself, have the scars to prove it), a pair of *old* trainers (they will get abrasions) and a T-shirt.
- Stand in front of the rope, with the rope running down the centre of the body a few inches in front of you.
- Reach up on tiptoes and take hold of the rope as high as possible so that the arms are completely straight.

- Taking a big bounce or jump, pull on the rope to bring the knees up to the hands. It is imperative to throw the head backwards (take your eyes of the rope to do this) to allow the knees to come up to the hands. If you don't throw the head back, it is impossible to get your knees to your hands.
- It is now necessary to grip the rope between your knees and feet. This is usually the difficult part at first, but once mastered seems simple. The rope should run down from the hands and straight between the knees, and should be gripped by the bony part of the inside of the knees (yes, this hurts a little when done right). The lower parts of the legs are then crossed so that the rope runs at the front of one shin and the rear of the opposite calf. It then goes between the feet on the inside of both shoes. Note that the feet are parallel, the rope is *not* stood on.
- To really grip the rope with the legs it is necessary to straighten the legs out towards the wall, *ie* once straight they will be almost parallel with the ground (the body and legs are now an L shape). Use the big muscles of the legs to squeeze hard on the rope so that it locks between the bony points on the knees, *not* the soft area of the thighs.
- Once the legs have locked, reach up as high as possible and re-grip the rope with both hands.
- Release the legs and repeat: throw the head back and bring the knees up as high as possible to the hands to re-grip the rope with the legs.
- Remember: perfect practice makes permanent.

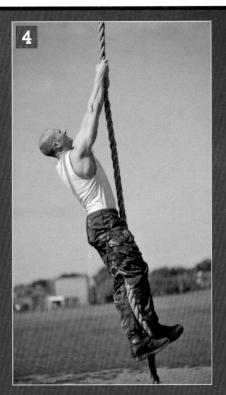
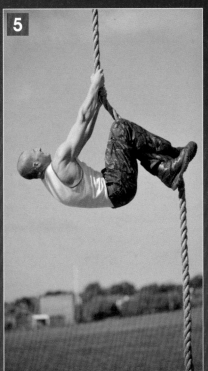
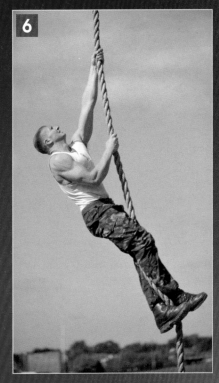

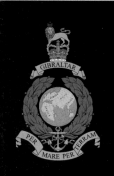

# CHAPTER 14
# CIRCUIT TRAINING

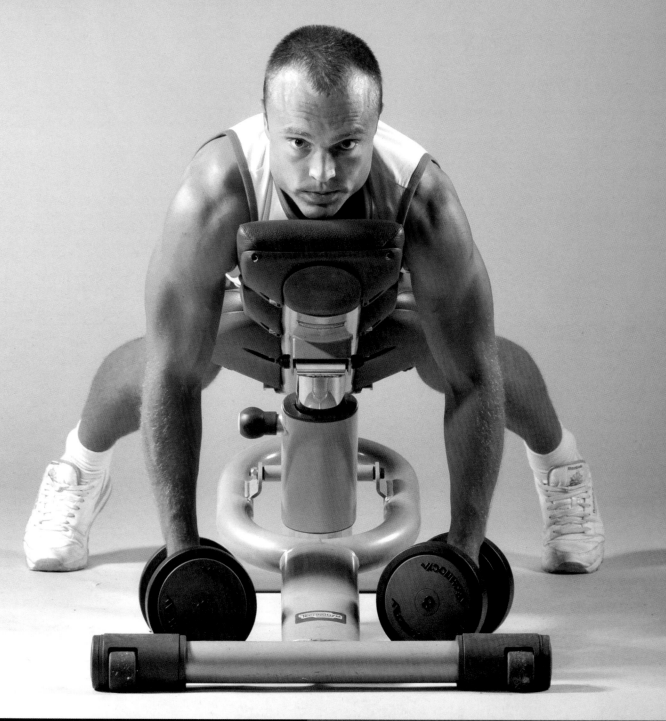

For general, non-specific fitness, circuit training is probably the best one-off method available to develop endurance, stamina and strength. Due to this, circuit training has become an integral part of physical training throughout the Royal Marines. For Royal Marines, circuit training is both highly effective and time-efficient. Furthermore, it allows just one instructor to exercise a large group of individuals almost anywhere. All PTIs are taught on their course that the variations in circuits are limited only by the instructor's imagination, ingenuity and the application of his knowledge. All RM PTIs have to pass a circuit training practical exam in order to pass their course. The real crux of this exam is ensuring that the PTI delivers the benefits of a circuit through meticulous planning, inspirational and enthusiastic supervision and continuous coaching throughout.

## Using circuit training

The physiological aim of circuit training is said to be the progressive development of musculo-circulo-respiratory fitness. However, although circuit training is a superb fitness tool, it is just that – a tool. It should not be used in isolation for increases in fitness. Circuit training is a supplement to the other training modalities, and should always be used as such. Consequently only one or two circuit training periods per week should be undertaken, and these should be combined with goal or sport specific sessions.

## Fitness improvements from circuit training

- Improves both the aerobic and anaerobic energy systems.
- Assists in improving the creatine phosphate energy system.
- Improves the lactate threshold.
- Boosts the body's ability to deliver and use oxygen.
- Increases the body's VO2 max score.
- Increases stamina/muscular endurance.
- Provides some improvement in strength (more for the untrained than the trained).
- Increases lean muscle mass.
- Reduces body fat levels.
- Burns more calories than most other activities of the same duration.

## Circuit exercises

### ■ Muscular

During any circuit fatigue will build up and it is because of this that exercise technique may suffer. Therefore it is best to avoid complex, difficult exercises that require specific technique. Any exercises that require the lifter's safety or need a 'flat-back' (eg a weighted squat or weighted bent-over row) should be avoided. For best results, circuit training should combine body-weight exercises with resistance exercises (free weight and/or machine). Any torso exercises should include both abdominals and lower back exercises. Basic core stability is also a very good inclusion and often a good rest station.

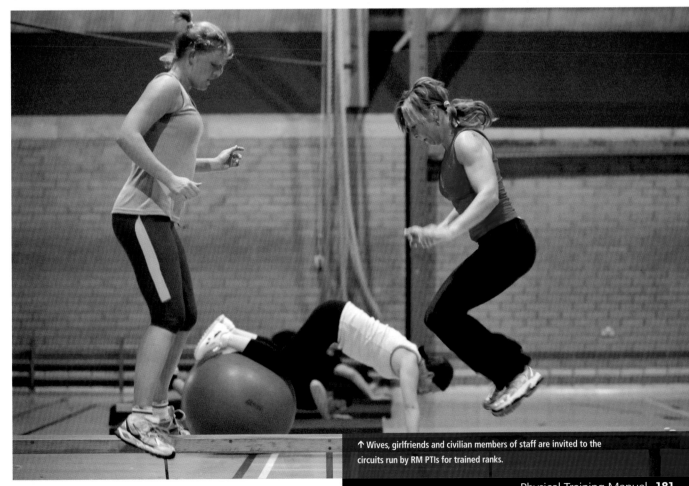

↑ Wives, girlfriends and civilian members of staff are invited to the circuits run by RM PTIs for trained ranks.

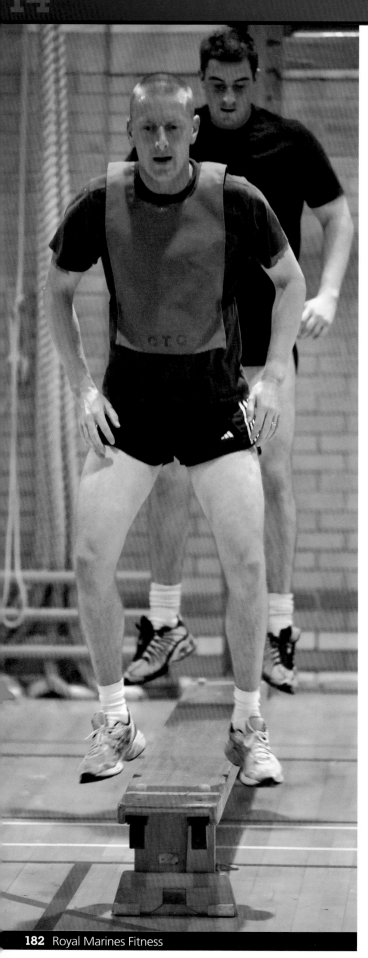

### Aerobic

CV exercises can also, of course, be included in circuits. Where possible, resistance exercises should be compound exercises as these induce the greatest demands on the CV system. The inclusion of isolation exercises is fine but they are often better as abdominal exercises or placed as 'easy' stations within the circuit, as they allow the CV systems to recover somewhat.

In general, aerobic exercises are excellent stations to include in the circuit. Examples such as running (shuttle or laps), cycling or rowing improve the benefits of the circuit on the CV system and thus VO2 max. Aerobic stations can be part of the circuit, or can be placed between exercises or circuits as a separate part for added benefit. For maximum effect the aerobic exercises should be more than one minute in duration.

### Plyometric

Exercises from the simpler end of the plyometric spectrum can be included, such as squat jumps. As these exercises are so dynamic they will raise the heart rate more than their static counterparts. They will also provide some power training to the circuit.

### Types of circuit training

- General circuit training.
- Individual circuit training.
- Colour circuit training.
- Sports-specific circuit training.

### General circuit

Consists of 3, 6, 9, 12 or 15 (or more, in multiples of three, if required) stations that alternate arm, trunk and leg exercises. The exercises are performed for a set amount of time, and generally three circuits are performed. It is common practice to vary the length of the exercise duration from one revolution to the next (often longest for the second rotation and shortest for the last) – for example, 30 seconds first time through on each exercise, 45 seconds the second time and 20 seconds the last. Strengtheners (like press-ups or pull-ups, or even an aerobic exercise) may be included in between each circuit.

#### Advantages of the general circuit

Performed indoors or outdoors.
Performed in limited space.
Requires no equipment or equipment can be improvised.
Varied abilities catered for and can work concurrently.
Progress can be measured if required.
Large numbers can work simultaneously.
Adapted for all components of physical fitness.
Adapted for specific sport training.
Unlimited circuit variations.

#### Disadvantages of the general circuit

Easy to cheat on exercises when in large groups.
Exercise technique can deteriorate with speed.

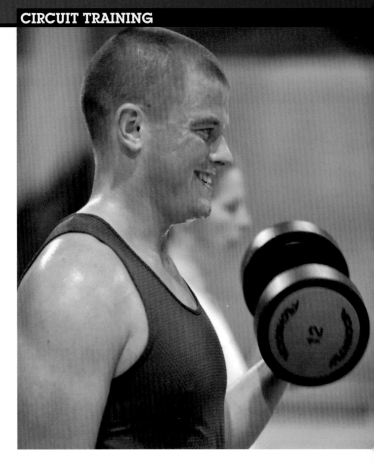

### ■ Individual circuit

There are various examples of individual circuits, some of which are outlined at the end of this chapter. However, the following is actually called 'the individual circuit'.

The individual circuit is a specific circuit for an individual to monitor their own fitness progression. It involves two major phases, a test phase and a timing phase. For the test phase a number of exercises are chosen (any exercises could be selected) and each exercise is performed for a maximum number of repetitions within a set amount of time, up to a maximum of 60 seconds (so could be 15 seconds, could be 30 seconds, could be 60 seconds etc). Rest should be taken between the tests, but no more than 60 seconds.

For the timing phase, the maximum number of repetitions performed in the test phase should then be halved and performed for three laps of the circuit against the clock. The time in which to achieve the exercises is 70–85% of the test time. This will give a realistic, yet challenging, target.

The circuit should be performed for 8–12 weeks or until the target time or number of reps is achieved.

### ■ Colour circuit

These comprise a circuit with varying exercises where each colour denotes a predetermined number of repetitions to be performed on each exercise station. This works well when a group has very varied abilities; it means that everyone does the same exercises, but simply do more or less reps.

The same can be done for timings, with a longer or shorter time being spent on each exercise instead. The most common example of a colour circuit can be found on 'trim-racks', where a route around a field to and from exercises and each actual exercise has a number of reps specified 'beginner', 'intermediate' and 'advanced', which are often colour-coded for ease.

### ■ Sports-specific circuit

A sports specific circuit should have a clear objective and ultimately improve the performance of an individual at their chosen sport. Sportspersons often enjoy their sport but not the associated fitness training, and should not have to rely solely on

circuit training to improve their conditioning. A good sports-specific circuit can really break up the rigmarole of a hard weight-training programme associated with their sport. If used correctly such a circuit can be useful in improving motivation towards fitness training by involving aspects of and techniques used in the individual's sport.

### Circuit training station timings for specific goals

The following table gives an idea of the timings that should be used for a circuit to train the various different energy systems and muscular areas.

| Component | Load/resistance | Rest between stations | Min–max work | Remarks |
|---|---|---|---|---|
| Aerobic endurance. | Light–moderate. Not to induce muscular failure. | Less than 30 seconds. | 30–60 minutes. | Include aerobic stations of 60 seconds or more. |
| Muscular endurance. | Moderate–high. Induce muscular failure at 15–25 repetitions. | Work = rest time. | 20–45 minutes. | Repeat high levels of work. Pre-exhaust and overload muscle groups on subsequent stations. |
| Strength. | High. Induce muscular failure at 1–8 repetitions. | One minute plus. | 20–60 minutes. | Repeat heavy work. Alternate muscle groups with compound exercises. |

# Typical 'Bootneck' circuits

## Down and ups, 'whatever' down to one

A simple circuit used by Royal Marines wherever they are, this can be done with one specific exercise or combining two or three. The basic idea is to choose an exercise – the most commonly chosen is press-ups, so that will be our example – and a start number, let's say ten for ease (ten down to one). This circuit is best done in pairs or in a group, but it can be done alone.

To perform the circuit, one person does ten press-ups, then the other person (or everyone else if in a group) does ten. The first person then does nine, and everyone else does nine, then the first person does eight, and everyone else does eight etc, all the way down to four. For three, two and one, six reps are performed, as three, two and one individually are too easy. Once everyone else has done six, then the original exerciser starts going back up: so six are performed for one, two and three, then four, then five etc, all the way back up to ten, and everyone else follows him.

If on your own, just use a stopwatch to give yourself rest in between your exercises. I usually rest for 10 seconds, 20 seconds or 30 seconds depending on the number of the exercise I am doing, ie the rest decreases and increases as the exercise numbers do.

Down and ups can be performed for pull-ups, sit-ups, squats, bicep curls etc, almost any exercise – just ensure good quality repetitions are performed at all times.

Combinations are possible, in which you do two different exercises, for example sit-ups and leg raises. You do ten sit-ups, then nine leg raises, then eight sit-ups, then seven leg raises etc.

For press-ups, 25 to one and back up to 25 is very impressive. For pull-ups, ten to one and back up to ten is not easy and is a good effort to achieve.

To regress such circuits, just do ten down to one but don't go back up again.

## Overload endurance circuits

### ■ Upper body

The overload circuit is something I have seen Royal Marines do all over the world. It is straightforward because it simply requires a barbell or two. A number of different variations are in use, but in general any overload circuit can be constructed with a barbell or two dumbbells. The following is an example to try, but try to add to it subsequently, or come up with your own variations.

A relatively light barbell is chosen, let's say 15kg. Four (or five) exercises are performed one after the other: shoulder press, upright row, bent-over row, biceps curl and possibly press-ups. With the four/five exercises completed (a total of 80 or 100 reps in all), the bar is handed to the partner to do the same, or if working alone two minutes' rest is timed. The 80 reps (or 100 if doing press-ups as well) should be done three to five times through.

The barbell is now increased by 5kg, for this example, to 20kg and the same circuit is performed, again three to five times through, but only ten reps of each exercise are performed. Press-ups can again be included, either in regular sets of ten or with the feet raised. I have also done this with ten pull-ups instead of ten press-ups.

| Exercise | Reps 1st circuit | Reps 2nd circuit | Remarks |
|---|---|---|---|
| Shoulder press. | 20 | 10 | First time circuit 3–5 times through with weight performing 20 reps. Second time circuit 3–5 times through performing 10 reps with 5kg heavier barbell. |
| Upright row. | 20 | 10 | |
| Bent-over row. | 20 | 10 | |
| Bicep curl. | 20 | 10 | |
| Press-up/pull-up. | 20 | 10 | |

At first this circuit is not easy and requires considerable muscular endurance. The biceps and the grip strength are particularly challenging. However, once mastered it can be advanced so that the two barbells increase in weight, but still 5kg apart, or a third set can be added in the middle using a barbells 2.5kg lighter than the heavy bar and 2.5kg heavier than the light bar, of which 15 reps are performed. Also try it with dumbbells equalling the same weight.

### ■ Lower body

Using either a barbell or a sandbag/powerbag over the shoulders, or a rucksack with sandbag/powerbag inside (my preference), perform the following circuit. The weight should be between 10kg and 30kg, but start low! Exercises should be performed without a rest between:

- 20 step-ups each foot (40 in total).
- 20 side step-ups each foot (40 in total).
- 30 squats.
- 20 walking lunges each leg (40 in total).
- 20 step-overs each leg (40 in total).
- Two minutes' rest, then repeat.

The circuit should be done two or three times through at first, then four and finally five. Once five times is achieved a few times, up the weight and return to two or three. This circuit is excellent for building up the legs and CV ready for 'yomping'-style exercises.

## Playing card circuits

Playing card circuits are one of my favourite types of session. Whether training alone or in a group, using a deck of cards keeps the circuit fresh, fun and interesting. When in a group it can also add some humour, especially if you are not the first to go!

Using a deck of cards for the circuit is easy. Basically, four exercises are chosen – for example, press-ups, pull-ups, dips and shoulder presses, or if for an abs workout, sit-ups, leg raises, Saxon side bends and rollouts. Each suit in the deck is assigned an exercise. I also always find it helps to invent some sort of association between suit and exercise to help remember them, rather than having to refer to notes: so press-ups is always hearts, as the heart (chest) is lowered to the floor, etc.

The deck is shuffled and placed face down. All the necessary kit for the circuit is gathered in the area (barbells, dumbbells, rollout wheels etc) and an order of march (order of who exercises when) is agreed. The first card is then turned over and everyone does the exercise of that suit the number of times on the card, ie a two of hearts would be two press-ups, a four would be four press-ups. Picture cards and aces are ten. Some exercises (like press-ups) are always doubled, as they are otherwise too easy. The whole deck is done in this fashion.

If using barbells/dumbbells, unless you have more than one set of kit there is an order of march, if press-ups, sit-ups etc requiring no kit, then either everyone goes together or the same order is kept to. The next card is never turned over until the last person has finished.

For added fun the jokers can be shuffled in and either be ten of each exercise or a special exercise, like a 500m running or rowing interval etc.

## 'Cube' (dice) circuits

Using a set of dice (or cubes – or mice, as they are known to Royal Marine PTIs), a similar circuit can be done to that above. A certain number of exercises can be chosen – six works well as the dice has six sides (however, three exercises can be done with each having two numbers, or 12 exercises with two dice being used). Each exercise is given a number. The dice is rolled, and the number shown is the exercise to be performed. The dice is then rolled again and that number of the exercise is performed. The exercises can be the same as above (sit-ups, press-ups etc), but dice can also be used for running or cycling, with the second dice-roll denoting the number of times round

a track or course etc. If used for exercises, then a total number of that exercise could be agreed beforehand and then crossed off every time some are done until none are left. Or a set time for the circuit could be set, and the dice keep rolling and the exercises keep coming until the time is up.

The downside of the cube circuit compared to the card circuit is that the same number of each exercise at the end cannot be guaranteed, whereas with the cards it can.

## Rolling or roaring circuit

For this, some paper and a pen – or, if a large number of people are doing, it a whiteboard and markers – will be needed, since a table with the exercise names and people doing the circuit must be drawn up.

All the repetitions have to be achieved, but not in one go. Individuals mark how many repetitions of each exercise they have achieved on the board. For example, someone may start with 15 press-ups, which they then mark off. They then perform 20 sit-ups and 20 dorsals, which they mark off, followed by a chase circuit. They return from the chase circuit, rest for a minute and perform ten pull-ups before marking and moving to the next exercise. Like the cards circuit, it is possible to perform this circuit on your own, but doing it as a group is far more rewarding.

All of the above have been deliberate, specific circuits that I have done, or seen used in the Corps. For each, if done in a group, the atmosphere and enthusiasm of combined effort usually makes the circuit more enjoyable and makes you work harder. Where possible it is always worth getting a stereo and some good music to train to; if on your own, headphones and an MP3 player are fine.

| Exercise | Repetitions | Remarks | Names | | | |
|---|---|---|---|---|---|---|
| | | | Al | Baz | Caz | Deb |
| Pull-up. | 30 | This circuit works best with an 'oppo' or as a team. Exercises can be performed in any order. Move from one exercise to another in your own time and aim for quality exercises and not speed. Perform the chase circuit at a good pace, working to at least 80–90% effort. | | 10 | | |
| Sit-up. | 60 | | | 20 | | |
| Burpee. | 40 | | | | | |
| Dip. | 50 | | | | | |
| Dorsal. | 70 | | | 20 | | |
| Bench jump. | 20 | | | | | |
| Press-up. | 60 | | | 15 | | |
| Rock-back. | 50 | | | | | |
| Squat thrust. | 40 | | | | | |
| Shoulder press. | 50 | | | | | |
| Half-sit. | 40 | | | | | |
| 300m chase course. | x 4–6 | | | 1 | | |

# General circuits

### Arm, trunk, legs basic circuit

| Exercise | 1st lap | 2nd lap | 3rd lap |
|---|---|---|---|
| Press-up. | 30sec | 45sec | 20sec |
| Sit-up. | 30sec | 45sec | 20sec |
| Squat. | 30sec | 45sec | 20sec |
| Shoulder press. | 30sec | 45sec | 20sec |
| Leg raise. | 30sec | 45sec | 20sec |
| Lunge. | 30sec | 45sec | 20sec |
| Strengthener – 400m run lap. | x 1 | x 3 | 0 |

This could have been 6, 9, 12 etc exercises. Equally it could have been done on reps instead of time, as long as adequate and realistic weights/exercises are provided:

| Exercise | 1st lap | 2nd lap | 3rd lap |
|---|---|---|---|
| Press-up. | 20 reps | 25 reps | 15 reps |
| Sit-up. | 20 reps | 25 reps | 15 reps |
| Squat. | 20 reps | 25 reps | 15 reps |
| Shoulder press. | 20 reps | 25 reps | 15 reps |
| Leg raise. | 20 reps | 25 reps | 15 reps |
| Lunge. | 20 reps | 25 reps | 15 reps |
| Strengthener – 500m row. | x 1 | x 1 | x 1 |

### Arm, trunk, legs aerobic endurance circuit ('rolling')

Basically a variation on the theme above, but making things more interesting.

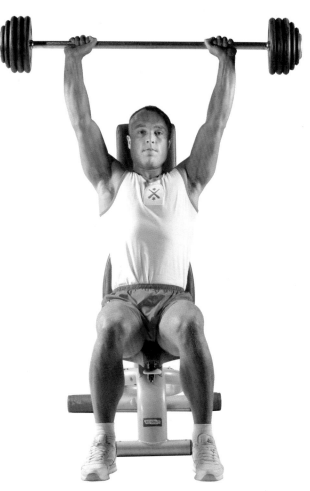

| Exercise | Circuit/reps/timings |
|---|---|
| 1. Press-up.<br>2. Crunch.<br>3. Alternate squat thrust. | Circuit 1:<br>Perform exercises 1–3 for 8 reps, then exercise 10 for 1 lap.<br>Perform exercises 1–6 for 12 reps, then exercise 10 for 2 laps. |
| 4. Bench dip.<br>5. Leg dorsal raise.<br>6. Squat. | Perform exercises 1–9 for 15 reps, then exercise 10 for 3 laps. |
| 7. Bench press-up.<br>8. Bench crunch.<br>9. Step-up. | Circuit 2:<br>Perform exercises 1–9 for 15 reps, then exercise 10 for 3 laps.<br>Perform exercises 1–6 for 12 reps, then exercise 10 for 2 laps. |
| 10. Steeple chase course (indoor). | Perform exercises 1–3 for 8 reps, then exercise 10 for 1 lap. |

The same set-up and exercises can be used for two separate circuits.

### Muscular endurance circuit ('rolling' or 'roaring')

| Exercise | Reps | Explanation |
| --- | --- | --- |
| Station 1:<br>Squat jump.<br>Full dip. | 30/25/20/15<br>25/20/15/10 | Station 1: 30 reps squat jump, jog across to dips do 25, return to squat jump – continue until all set-reps are completed. |
| Station 2:<br>Step-up.<br>Bench dip. | 30/25/20/15<br>25/20/15/10 | Station 2: As above, step-ups, then bench dips, then back to step-ups until all sets done. |
| Station 3:<br>20m grid sprint.<br>Press-up. | 10/8/5/5<br>25/20/15/10 | Station 3: As above but sprints and press-ups. |

### Strength circuit

Whereas the circuits above are completed with exercises immediately following each other, this strength circuit gives 60 seconds of rest between exercises to ensure sufficient recovery to let the low reps/high weight exercises remain achievable.

| Exercise | Reps | Remarks |
| --- | --- | --- |
| Station 1:<br>20m farmer's walk.<br>Crunch.<br>Full dip.<br>Side-bend right side. | 1 x failure<br>1 x 10<br>1 x 5–8<br>1 x 5–8 | Perform each exercise within the station for the prescribed repetitions with 60sec rest between exercises.<br><br>Perform stations 1 and 2 three times through. |
| Station 2:<br>Pull-up (under grasp).<br>Side-bend left side.<br>Military press.<br>Step-up. | 1 x 5–8<br>1 x 5–8<br>1 x 5–8<br>1 x 5–8 | Perform station 3 just one time through. |
| Station 3:<br>Object drag (heavy). | 3–5 | |

The exercises may be chosen for a specific goal that an individual has or to cater for weaknesses that they want to improve. Again, these are just examples – substitute the exercises you want to train, or design your own circuits using the examples and guidelines given.

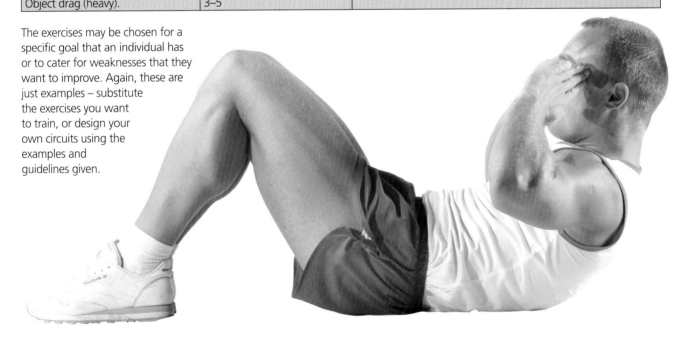

# Further examples of circuit training

## Specific circuit: stamina

| | Circuit 1 | Circuit 2 | Circuit 3 |
|---|---|---|---|
| 1a | Static cycle | Shuttle sprint | Ergo rower |
| 1b | Trunk exercise | Upper body exercise | Lower body exercise |
| | 20 reps: | 20 reps: | 20 reps: |
| 1 | Twisting crunch | Press-up | Lunge |
| 2 | Ab crunch | Incline pull-up | Weighted step-up |
| 3 | Dorsal raise | Military press | Hamstring bridge |

Perform 'a' for three minutes and then 'b' for 20 reps per exercise but continue for a further three minutes. Then move on to the next station and do three minutes and three minutes again. Obviously, if three minutes for 'b' is too hard for you take this down to one or two, but try to increase over time.

## Overload circuit: leg overload

1   20m object drag
2   Weighted step-up
3   20m shuttle sprint
4   Walking lunge
5   Bench dip
6   Crunch
7   Press-up
8   V-sit
9   Incline pull-up
10  Dorsal raise

Between circuits, two minutes of step-ups without weight as quick as possible.

## Countdown circuit

| | Circuit 1 | Circuit 2 | Circuit 3 |
|---|---|---|---|
| 1 | Lunge | Weighted step-up | Deadlift |
| 2 | Press-up | Incline pull-up | Bench dip |

Each exercise is performed for 20, 18, 16, 14, 12 repetitions – *eg* 20 reverse lunges, 20 press-ups, 18 reverse lunges, 18 press-ups, 16 reverse lunges etc. Any exercises can be chosen that are specifically appropriate to you and your training.

## Competitive circuit: ergo row

1   Press-up
2   Sit-up
3   20m shuttle sprint
4   Bench dip
5   Leg raise
6   Lunge walk
7   Incline pull-up
8   Superman dorsal
9   Squat thrust
10  Ergo row

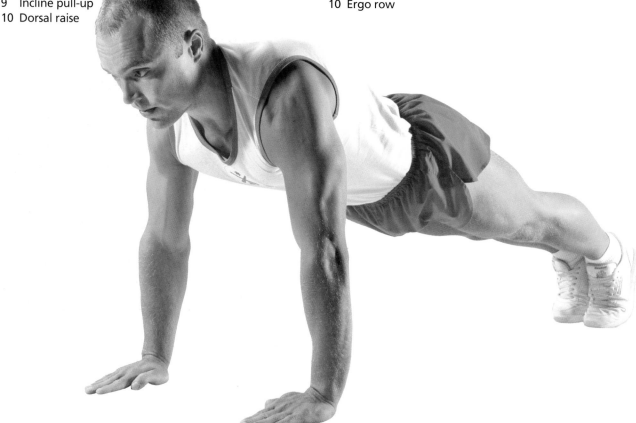

Perform exercises for 45 seconds and row as far as possible in 45 seconds. If more than one person is doing the circuit, see who rowed the furthest in 45 seconds.

## Competitive circuit: cross training

1 500m on ergo rower
2 Full dip x 30
3 Feet fixed sit-up x 50
4 1km run
5 Dumbbell squat jump x 40 (10kg each hand)
6 Overgrasp pull-up x 20
7 Burpee x 30
8 Press-up x 50

These are performed against the clock as a team relay or as individuals. Any number of different exercises can be chosen for a cross-training circuit to test true all-round fitness.

## Sports-specific circuit: rugby league

### ■ Circuit 1
60 seconds per station in pairs (swap with partner after 30 seconds).

1 Ground pass to partner sprinting along puddings
2 Scrummage (against each other, therefore work for whole 60 seconds)
3 Dive for try, past opposition
4 Upper body strength:
   Shoulder press
   Pull-up
   Weighted press-up

### ■ Circuit 2
60 seconds per station (swap with partner after 30 seconds). Between circuits, ball-pass in lines.

1 5m resisted sprint (like object drag but partner is object and resists)
2 Side-step partner to score a try
3 Sprint 10m, tackle bag and hold. Partner attempts to pull bag from tackler for three seconds. Tackler retreats 10m and repeats
4 Lower body strength:
   Weighted step-up
   Ski-jump
   Hamstring bridge

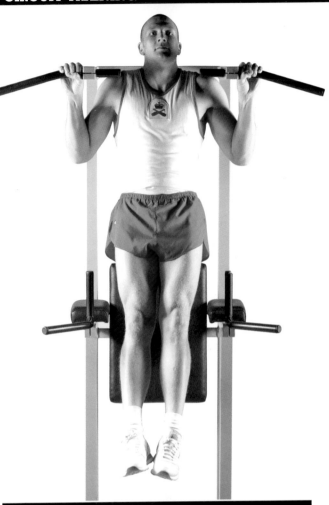

# Conclusion

Circuit training is almost unbeatable for developing general, non-specific fitness. Depending on the type and structure of the circuit, endurance, stamina and strength can be worked separately or all at once. It is for this reason that circuit training plays such a big part in the general physical training of Royal Marines in the UK and throughout the world. This chapter has highlighted the numerous pros of circuit training for both Royal Marines and casual gym-goers, as well as sportsmen and women training for excellence in their given sports.

Despite its evident success at delivering fitness improvements, it must again be emphasised that circuit training should not be used in isolation for fitness training, but should be seen as a supplement to the other training performed.

Numerous examples of circuits and ways of conducting them have been given. Although you can try some or all of these yourself, remember to make your own circuits specific to your needs. Pick the exercises that will help you reach your goals and train your areas of weakness. Use your imagination and see what you can come up with.

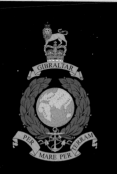

# CHAPTER 15
# IMPROVISATION EXAMPLES

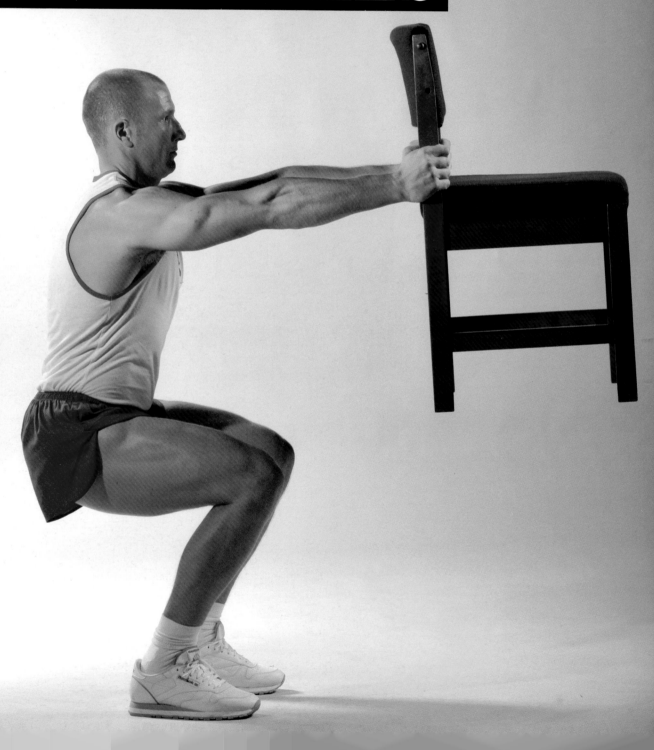

**S**ir Francis Bacon said 'knowledge is power', and in the case of improvisation I think this is true. It is so easy to improvise a physical training session with only a little knowledge. Physical training can be done anywhere, any time. From your sitting room to sitting in traffic in your car, physical training is available to you – you just have to use your knowledge. To use another quote, 'Trust yourself. You know more than you think you do.' (Benjamin Spock.) Whether you have dipped in and out of a gym over the years or you have read this book and nothing else, you will know more than you think. With a little knowledge of what the body does and the way it does it, you can train anywhere in the world with anything or nothing at your disposal.

I knew from an early age that I wanted to be fit and strong. Strangely I now realise that I started improvising even back then. I would wedge my toes under the sofa and perform sit-ups while watching TV, I would pick up the wooden footstool and perform what I now know are front and lateral raises, and then, of course, there were press-ups and pull-ups on a bar I bought and fitted in the kitchen doorway. If I could improvise in childhood without any real understanding of anatomy or physiology, then you, with the knowledge that you now have, will definitely be able to come up with something, no matter where you are.

### A chair or bed

A chair or stool adds a whole range of exercises that can be done alongside those mentioned above, even if you cannot leave the

## No kit

Let's just imagine you are in a prison cell and you have no kit at all. What could you do? Press-ups and all their variants are open to you. The different circuits for press-ups (down and ups, gainers, overload endurance etc) are all available, the plank and all its variations, all the various abs exercises, not to mention squats and lunges. Then think of all the CV/all-over body exercises: the burpee and all its variants, squat jumps, star jumps, ski jumps etc. With a little more space, plyometric exercises could be achieved, although some could be done on the spot. If you think about it, that list is pretty extensive. A simple circuit session could easily be put together which could be done as a one-off, or if staying in a hotel on business for a week or two could be done every day for the duration.

room. Press-ups with feet raised, dips with feet rested, box (or chair) jumps, step-ups, step-overs or plank exercises with the feet raised. Then there are all the exercises using the weight of the chair: squats holding it out in front with arms straight (effects the shoulders and core), using it as a light weight for biceps curls, one-arm lateral raise, front raise. With a little knowledge and a little imagination, a physical training period is very easily improvised.

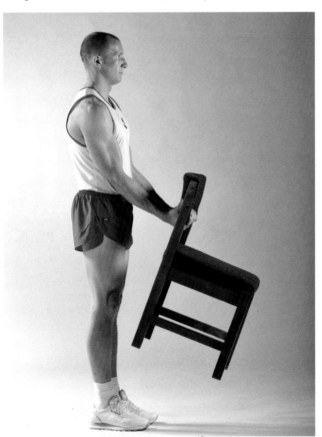
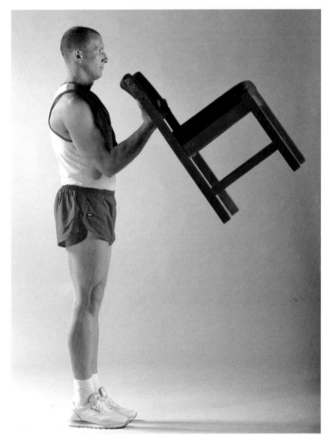

### A bag

A simple bag, no matter where you are, can provide an endless stream of improvised exercises. Fill the bag with anything you can use to make it heavy: sand, bags of flour or sugar, clothing, books, or stones wrapped in a towel.

Once you have a bag full of weight use it as such. You can perform all the various weighted legs exercises with it on your back: step-ups, squats, lunges etc. By holding it in the hands you can perform biceps curls, triceps extension, shoulder press (all two-arm or one-arm). Lie on your back and bench press the bag, again two-arm or one-arm. Stay on your back and hold the bag across your chest and perform sit-ups. Basically look at the list of exercises in Chapter 13 and work out how you could do them by improvising with whatever you have, in this case a weighted bag.

If you are away abroad for a while with no weights or kit, collect some juice or milk cartons, fill them up, and off you go. All the various exercises from Chapter 13 using dumbbells could be done with one carton in each hand. If you can find a bar, attach one carton to each end (or two bags full of sand instead) and all the barbell exercises can be performed as well. Actually, due to the crude nature of the weights used more muscles are often exercised than usual, specifically the core! Buckets full of water or earth are a good alternative to milk cartons (however, if using two it is more difficult to get the weight equal than with cartons). Once again, only your imagination need hold you back.

### Where you live

When I was a teenager I had some playing fields nearby, and I would use the pitch and its facilities. I would run what I now know to be Fartlek-style around the outside of all the pitches. In the corners of the playing fields I would do press-ups and sit-ups, at the goal posts I would perform pull-ups and at the spectators' benches I would perform step-ups or basic feet rested dips. At other times I would go to a disused children's playground and use the monkey bars for pull-ups and put my feet on the swings and perform press-ups.

If you open your eyes and look around it is simple to improvise sessions even in the environments in which we live. They often provide us with so much in terms of facilities to maintain and improve our fitness levels. Furthermore, if you move to or are visiting a new area, by going out and looking for places to train you are exploring and getting to know the place as well. Wherever I have stayed for more than a week I have sourced somewhere decent to go and train: in Barcelona I found an athletics track with a few 'trim trail' exercises around it, in Los Angeles I stumbled across the rings, pull-up bars and dip bars near Santa Monica pier (no, not Muscle Beach!), and in other areas I have searched for scaffolding to perform pull-ups. The moral here is, get out and explore, but don't forget your imagination – improvise, adapt and overcome.

In general, when training the upper body having a pull-up

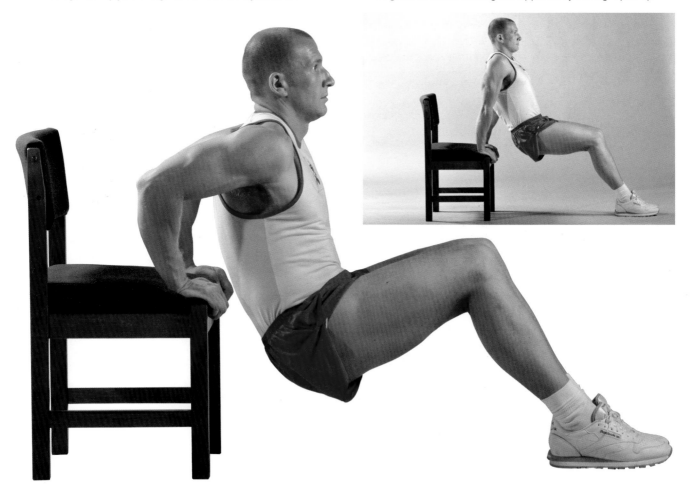

bar is best. So what could be used if a pull-up bar is unavailable? Tree branches, the backs of large road signs, (strong) signs above shops, ledges over stairwells, door heads and porches. But be careful, when selecting areas to use, to ensure that they are safe and that you will not get into trouble. Scaffolding is a personal favourite of mine – a decent bit of scaffolding provides you with all the pull-up bars you will need. If you are away from home for a week, and all you have is some scaffolding nearby, then a week of body-weight exercises and pull-up progression is by no means a wasted week. Again, open your eyes and look at the environment you are in, and make the most of what is around you.

### Kit at home

Once your physical training becomes as habitual as it is for most Royal Marines you will want to have a certain amount of kit at home. Then you can at least improvise some small circuits, either in the sitting room, garage, back garden or even the local park. I would say a pull-up bar is a must, and a fitball is really useful, not only for training the core, abs and lower back, but also for using as a makeshift bench or seat for upper body exercises. A skipping rope is a great piece of kit that can be taken anywhere, and a couple of small dumbbells or kettlebells will allow you to perform basic curls, extensions, raises, rows and presses. A pair of boxing gloves and a punchbag is excellent if you have space in the garage. A set of press-up stands, ankle weights, a rollout wheel and some elastic resistance tubing or cables will also be of considerable use.

### ■ Staying away from home

Get out and explore! The best way to do this is to go for a run in a different direction every time. Get to know the surrounding area, get to know the different ways in and out of where you are staying. Get to know the areas to avoid, spot new supermarkets or restaurants, and, of course, perform a good fitness session. In the hotel room or wherever you are staying, use the stairs for steps-ups, incline press-ups, box jumps etc, or to run up and down (with due consideration for other people). If you are staying in a rural area try to find a log. This can be used as a crude weight for all sorts of exercises – shoulder press, bench press, squats etc. If you tie a rope to it, it can be dragged, or if the rope is fashioned right, handles can be made and it can be curled.

I always try to take a set of elastic tubing with me for specific exercise purposes when I go away. This is made by one of the top sports kit manufacturers in the world, and the three different-coloured and differently shaped elastics allow pretty much all the normal directional cable/resistance exercises you would do in a gym to be done virtually anywhere. As they are just elastic they are also very light and take up hardly any space – very worthwhile for the fitness enthusiast who spends a lot of time on the road.

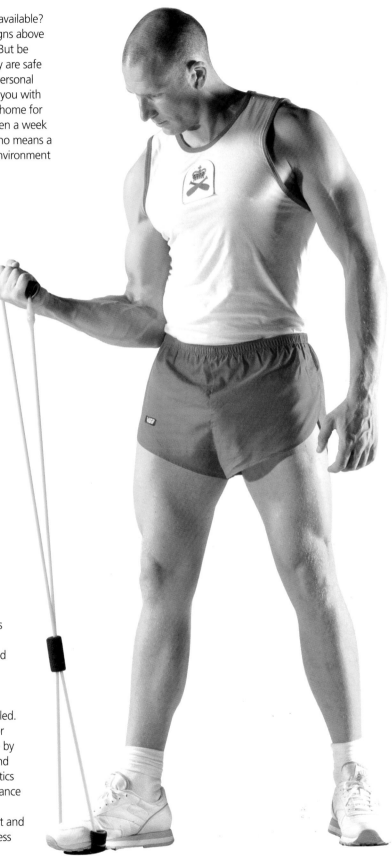

## Just walk

As should by now be clear, part of fitness training is just getting the heart rate up and keeping it there for a set amount of time. So whether at home or away, if some countryside, moorland or mountains are close by, use them. Instead of going for a run, put a rucksack on your back and yomp across varied, off-road terrain. It is worth planning a good route, and most of the time it is also worth having a map of the area and a compass (as long as you know how to use it), just in case. A day's yomping at a steady pace with weight on your back is an excellent form of continuous low intensity training.

Make sure you have well-fitting, made-for-purpose boots that are appropriate for the terrain. Plenty of water should also be taken, and if possible try to carry 10kg or more on your back. If you have only a few hours, try to jog on the downhill sections as well some of the flat (like Recruits do on the 30-Miler). Work hard on the uphill sections and try not to stop or give up.

Always ensure you leave details with someone of where you are going and approximately what time you will be back, so that if you get hurt or lose consciousness for any reason, someone will eventually realise and get help. Where possible, take a mobile phone and some snacks with you as well.

## Running

It is easy to exercise the legs using the local environment, either by running, sprinting, walking or yomping. If you want to push the session a little, look for specific features that will add difficulty: hills, sets of steps, off-road elements etc. Furthermore, look for areas where you can sprint along a road from one end to the other, using cracks in the road, lamp posts and trees to gauge distances.

Hill sprints or hill intervals can be performed on each hill you come to on a run – sprint up it, then jog down, sprint back up, jog down again, and repeat for a set amount at every hill (four to ten hill sprints should be attempted, depending on fitness and available time).

## Cycling, paddling, swimming and climbing

Depending on where you are all of these may be available. If you are at home, it is likely you have a bike or can borrow one. Cycling is an excellent form of CV training as it is non-impact and often gives the joints, bones and connective tissue a break from the impact of running. If you are away or on holiday, look around the tourist areas – generally there is somewhere you can hire a bike and perform your session that way. A bike session can incorporate any of the other CV session elements: intervals, hill sprints, low intensity etc.

Paddling, be it kayaking or canoeing, is obviously only available near a river, canal or the coast. However, in these areas it should again be possible to hire the kit for a half or full day to go out and test the upper body and CV system. Ensure you wear a life jacket and are sensible. It is often better to exercise in a pair or group, but is still an excellent and different session to try.

Swimming is generally available in most places (Third World excepted), even if you are not near the coast. Whether it is a local council pool, a hotel pool or the pool associated with a gym, it is usually possible to find somewhere to swim. As long as you pack a pair of trunks and some goggles swimming is an excellent strength and CV session, which, like cycling, is again non-impact so good for the body. Any of the various types of CV sessions can be performed for swimming. Additionally, by the coast these sessions can be done in the sea. However, a word of warning: stick to the designated swimming areas and be aware that all beaches have their own set of hazards, such as currents, tides and hidden dangers. Where possible ask a lifeguard or local what these are. Let someone know you are going for a swim and when you will be back. When I am swimming in the sea alone (at home or abroad) I often ask the lifeguards if I can leave my bag or clothes next to them or their vehicle. In that way they are more inclined to watch you and notice if you get into any trouble. No matter how good a swimmer you are, currents can catch you out.

Climbing is usually reserved for the crags on mountains and cliffs or for indoor climbing walls. If any of these exist near you then superb, you have another excellent training tool to use. Climbing provides so many elements of fitness rolled into one – skill, strength, muscular endurance, stamina and flexibility to name but a few, often outside of your comfort zone! If you have an interested friend then learn how to climb safely from a local instructor and go and try it. If you are training on your own, then bouldering (just traversing left or right and solving little problems no more than one to two metres off the ground) could be for you.

If you live in the city like me, you can still get out and boulder – old city walls and some buildings offer just as many problems and areas to test your strength. Just remember, as with Parkour (explained opposite), to start slow and stay low, and be careful as regards what is legal and illegal.

Here is a quick example programme that could be done in any hotel room or university dorm:

| Exercise | Explanation | Reps/Time |
|---|---|---|
| Chair dips | Dips with hands on chair, feet on floor | 10–20 |
| Chair curl | Using the chair as a weight perform biceps curl | 10–15 |
| Sit-ups (fixed) | Put feet under bed and perform sit-up | 10–30 |
| Squat/ Squat jumps | Perform regular squats with or without rucksack on or squat jumps | 10–20 |
| Leg raises | Lie on floor and raise straight legs up to 90° | 10–20 |
| Lunges/ Lunge jumps | Perform regular lunges with or without rucksack on or lunge jumps | 10–20 each leg |
| Press-ups | Regular press-ups or incline press-ups with feet raised | 10–30 |
| Bent over chair/bag row | Using a chair or a rucksack (with weight in it) perform bent over row | 10–20 |
| Plank | Perform the regular plank exercise | 30sec–2 mins |
| Step-up | Using chair, bed or a step perform step ups | 10–20 each leg |
| Chair lateral raise | Hold chair in one hand and raise to the side, keep core tight do not lean to 1 side | 10 each arm |
| Chair front raise | Hold chair in 1/both hands and riase to front of body | 10 each/10 - 20 both hands |
| Russian twists | Perform regular Russian twist using a bag or chair as the weight | 10–15 |
| Side plank | Regular side plank | 30sec–1min each side |
| Plyometric chair/bed jumps | Ensure ceiling is high enough and chair/ bed is sturdy enough. Stand in front of either, jump up, step down and repeat | 10–15 |

## Running exercise session

A combination of running, sprints and other exercises can produce an excellent improvised session. To do this, go out for a run, but incorporate sprints and interval training into the run, either planned or as you feel like it (but ensure you work hard). As you run, look around for obstacles or challenges – for example, when you see a park bench perform step-ups, bench jumps, incline press-ups or dips. When you see nice patches of grass perform an abs exercise. When you see some scaffolding or a tree branch big enough perform some pull-ups. You can even take this a step further and, say, whenever you see a dog, perform 20 press-ups (depending on where you are) – this could soon add up! Again, your imagination is the key. If you find a suitable area, incorporate plyometrics. Just keep a look out for anything you can use, and try it.

## Parkour and Freerunning

Carrying on from the above are Parkour and Freerunning. These two slightly different activities basically take a running exercise session and turn it into an activity or sport. I was lucky enough to be taught and coached Parkour by Urban Freeflow, the world's premier Parkour/Freerun organisation, courtesy of the Royal Marines. Parkour takes all the elements of tackling Assault Courses and combines them with gymnastics, plyometrics, co-ordination and balance to allow participants to use the world around them to train and work out. Thus sessions consist of balancing on natural features such as walls, bars and fences, jumping from wall to wall and from wall to bars, performing pull-ups on ledges, muscle-ups on bars, climbing walls, scaling scaffolding and so on. Basically, Parkour sees exercisers taking on all the physical challenges that the world around us presents, but that the average member of the public never even notices. If you decide to give this a go, just remember to start slow and stay low.

Parkour is the true essence of improvisation for physical fitness. Just going out for one, two or three hours in trainers, tracksuit bottoms and a T-shirt, with a bottle of water and a mobile phone and just running, exploring, jumping, climbing or vaulting over everything that comes your way.

## Conclusion

Improvising, adapting and overcoming the restraints of time and resources facing you in order to train are very much in line with what being a Commando is all about. In a sense we need to improvise every time we have a busy day and come home tired and not feeling like training. Use everything at your disposal, but remember above all that your most important tool is your brain – be it your imagination that enables you to come up with sessions, or your strength of mind that ensures you train, despite the difficulties of doing so.

# RECRUITMENT

The Royal Marine Commandos is relatively unique in terms of recruitment, as it attracts recruits from all parts of the globe and from all walks of life. It is not uncommon to have a Recruit Troop containing men from Scotland, Wales, Cornwall, London, Manchester, Newcastle (and everywhere in between), South Africa, New Zealand, the Caribbean or any number of Commonwealth countries. Additionally the men will have a wide variety of backgrounds, from those with no qualifications to speak of to those with PhDs. Age and experience can range from 16–32, and includes many who have served in various armies from around the world, such as the Foreign Legion, the Australian Army, the Irish Army, and even members of the British Army. It is this wide range of characters and backgrounds that gives the Royal Marines both its personality and, despite its small numbers, the huge standing it enjoys within the UK forces.

## Recruiting by fitness

The Royal Marines has a culture of selecting in rather than selecting out. But In fact it does have a number of tests with set standards. If a potential Recruit passes those standards he will be on a list to start training. If he fails them he will be given a time frame in which to train before he is due to return. In truth, there are very few people who have the commitment to come and attempt the PRMC (Potential Royal Marines Course) who do not already have what it takes physically to be a Royal Marine Commando (medical problems aside); it is usually their strength of mind that lets them down. It must be reiterated that the PRMC and POC (Potential Officers Course) are, as their names signify, 'Potential' courses – in other words we are looking for potential, we do not want the finished product. A fresh canvas that has shown potential is easy to train, easy to instruct and, generally speaking, produces great results. In many cases, highly tuned athletes are too polished already and frequently sustain injuries as a result of the arduous nature of training.

As you might imagine, there is a very wide range of physical abilities amongst young men who aspire to become Royal Marine Commandos, but this is not an issue. As already stated, it is just potential we are looking for, and in many cases if somebody struggles physically, they often excel in other areas – people always have hidden talents they do not even know about. A recruit who has never touched a firearm before training may well be an excellent shot and end up as a Royal Marine sniper later in his career.

Having said all that, the majority of men who approach the Royal Marines have played a specific sport to a high level – we just seem to attract those types of men. Those who have not played a specific sport at a high level will often be a real jack of all trades at a variety of sports; the key is that they are still very active and fit individuals.

To prepare themselves physically for their PRMC many potential Recruits may have spent some money joining a high-profile city gym; others may have trained on their own in their bedroom, garage or local playing fields, going for runs and performing press-ups and pull-ups wherever they can. It does not matter how they have made the effort to get fit enough to pass the PRMC, just that they have. Although we will be interested in their background once they are in training, at the PRMC we do not need to know how they trained sufficiently to pass; we just want to see them pass. However, the use of performance-enhancing drugs such as steroids is definitely unnecessary and not condoned. Furthermore, all Recruits and Royal Marines are randomly drug tested to ensure that they are not tempted by such methods.

There are pros and cons to training both in a city gym and out in the open fields. We will look at both and compare them later in this book. However, in the meantime, relating the issue specifically to the selection of RM Recruits, it must be said that either can lead to a pass and that is all that matters. The tests on the PRMC or POC do not involve any fancy gym equipment that will make it necessary to join a gym in order to practice. All that is required on the PRMC is a best effort over 3 miles, a best effort on press-ups, a best effort on pull-ups, and a best effort on sit-ups, all of which can be trained for at home or in the local park. Don't get me wrong, there are a lot of good reasons to join a local gym, but it is not a necessity. For example, if you are really struggling with pull-ups, most gyms have machines that allow you to do a pull-up but offer support under the knees to make it easier, which can be increased or decreased as needed. These machines are great, but there are also ways of doing this yourself (using physio therabands), which I explained in Chapter 12.

To give a personal example, I used both a city gym and no gym at all to prepare for life in the Royal Marines. I trained for my POC as a 19-year-old student during my first year at university in London, and except for the odd long run on Hampstead Heath at the weekends I used the university gym for all my training. I did this as it was over the road from where my lectures took place, and allowed me to train between lectures. As well as concentrating on press-ups, pull-ups and sit-ups (I tested myself on these once a week) I also used weights to improve my strength and muscular endurance, treadmills to ensure I was hitting the exact number of miles per hour that I wanted to, and rowing machines to push my cardiovascular stamina to a credible level. It was certainly not the case that I would have failed my POC without the use of a gym, but it certainly didn't hinder me.

Prior to joining training, having just finished university as a 21-year-old 'student', I decided to travel a little bit, but also trained to ensure that my fitness had not dropped significantly in the two or so years

since my POC. Obviously I could not join a gym while travelling, but I also decided not to waste my money when I was at home. My training consisted of long runs with a rucksack containing plastic milk cartons full of water, press-ups every night, sit-ups every night and pull-ups wherever I could (scaffolding was always a favourite). I also concentrated on interval sessions around football pitches and circuits, using benches and climbing frames in parks. Again, I do not believe I needed a gym; I was certainly not unfit when I joined the Royal Marines, and my motivation was such that I did not need a nice warm gym. One observation I would make, however, is that with no training partner a gym is often the more appealing of the two – other people will be there, and even if you do not talk to them their presence still provides some form of motivation. An empty playing field can be a lonely place when you have to sprint around it ten times!

## Reasons for joining

The reasons young men choose to join the Royal Marines are so varied it would be impossible to list them all in this book. However, there are some commonalities we tend to encounter. Additionally, it is often the case that you can look at a Recruit or a trained Royal Marine and tell why they chose to join the Corps.

For many, like me, it was the physical challenge. Having heard that the Royal Marines offer the hardest initial infantry training course in the world, I knew that if I was going to join the forces, it had to be the Royal Marines. The challenge of whether or not I could complete the training and wear the green beret was a huge draw for me and, unsurprisingly, for many of those alongside me. The Corps is full of physically fit men, and for as long as it is it will continue to be one of the fittest and strongest military forces in the world.

Many young men that join have some link to the Royal Marines already. As has already been stated, the Royal Marines family is far-reaching, and there is also a strong draw for family members. I know many Royal Marines whose fathers were also Royal Marines, or who have brothers in the Royal Marines, and even guys whose sons are in the Royal Marines.

For some, joining the Royal Marines was a way of escaping another life. Please do not see this in the same way as the Foreign Legion worked some 20 or 30 years ago, and think that we have a Corps full of criminals – this is certainly not the case. What I mean is that many young men who perhaps did not achieve the success they would have liked at school, or became stuck in a dead-end job for a minimum wage, have transformed their lives by joining the Corps. The draw of being able to change your future is a big one, and if a change of life is what is wanted then the Royal Marines and all that it offers is a good choice.

Young people have always been attracted to

excitement and adventure, and joining the Royal Marines will certainly provide that. Whether in Recruit training, working in a Commando Unit, on exercise in Norway, Belize or the USA, or on Operations around the globe, life in the Royal Marines provides all the excitement and adventure that anyone could want. These days we see a lot more young men, especially university graduates, joining the Royal Marines for their minimum four years simply with the idea of having some fun and adventure, and a bit of life experience before they settle down to a job and a family. Yes, there is adventure to be had travelling, working or studying abroad, but there is some adventure that only service in the armed forces can provide.

Although these days it is relatively inexpensive to purchase a round-the-world plane ticket and backpack for one or two years, many young men still join the forces to see the world. As one of the most active forces in the British military, the Royal Marines will certainly allow young men to do that. Added to which, there are certain places that the Royal Marines will take you that not even the most experienced backpacker would be able to reach. I myself have been lucky enough to visit Canada, the United States (Washington, Virginia Beach, Norfolk, California, Las Vegas), Northern Ireland, Afghanistan, South Korea, Egypt, Malaysia, Germany and Cyprus to name but a few. A friend of mine has, in the last month alone, been to Egypt, Malaysia, the South of France and Florida. Other friends who have served on board ship have been on such amazing trips, visiting such an astonishing list of ports across the globe, that even I was jealous. The Royal Marines really does offer some amazing chances to travel if you have the audacity and inclination to look for them.

Some young men join the Royal Marines for the friends and comrades they will make, while others who might join for other reasons entirely also soon realise what an amazing bonus comradeship is to life in the Corps. Whether it is friends who you have been through training with, or friends you have worked with in specific places for long periods of time, some lifelong and really strong friendships are made while serving in the Royal Marines. Indeed, for many who leave the Royal Marines their friends are the single greatest thing they miss about the Corps. One of the best things about such friendships is the common bond and understanding you share. If you do not talk to a friend in the Corps for a couple of years, he will not hold it against you, and as soon as you meet up again the jokes and dits start up and it is just like old times.

Due to its small size, the Royal Marines family is small enough that near enough everyone knows everyone, or knows everyone through someone else, which means that even once you've left, wherever you are in the world somewhere there will be a 'Bootneck' ready to help you out.

### The process

The first step in the process is go to the website (www.royalnavy.mod.uk) to find out more information then contact an advisor on the recruiting telephone number who checks eligibility. Once that initial step has been taken the process is relatively straightforward. As long as the individual passes the initial basic medical assessment, interview and other criteria tests at the careers office, he will find himself at the Commando Training Centre on a PRMC or POC lasting three to four days. His potential is already being tested, as if he pulls out at this early point it proves that his strength of mind did not have the potential to go the distance.

On the PRMC and POC – providing he has prepared physically – it is just a case of doing whatever he is asked to do, whenever he is asked to do it, to the very best of his ability. At some points on the course all that this will require is for him to provide information on a deluge of forms and in medicals. In short, a positive mindset will most likely be the difference between passing and failing the course.

### Training for a PRMC or POC

There are specific areas of physical and mental training that should be focused on:

#### ■ Cardiovascular endurance

Aim to do steady runs of three miles or more wearing good training shoes. Incorporate the odd sprint/interval session and incorporate hills into some runs where you can. Run at least two, and at most five times per week, and aim to achieve at least two runs per week of over four miles.

#### ■ Muscular strength and endurance

Aim for 5–8 pull-ups, 50–80 sit-ups and 40–50 press-ups. The majority of training should be done using your own body weight rather than weights. However, the odd session a week involving weights will not do any harm.

#### ■ Using the mind to push the body

Wherever possible train with a friend or training partner. You will find you push each other to achieve more by natural competition. Even now, I find when training with a fellow Commando that I work harder than on my own, even though I can push myself very hard when training individually. It is important to learn as soon as possible that you can always train harder even when you feel like stopping.

Be careful not to overtrain. It does more harm than good, and it is only potential that you need to prove on these courses, not that you are a finished product.

### Strength of mind

The most recent Royal Marines advertising campaign has the slogan 'It's a state of mind', which is absolutely true. People have always said to me, 'You have to really want to be a Royal Marine; it is not something you fall into.' Every Royal Marine Commando has had to put himself through real hardship to earn his green beret and the right to do his job. This is such a great working environment that very rarely do Royal Marines backstab, steal, or act in a selfish way. We all have a great deal of respect for each other.

On the PRMC and POC, strength of mind is vital. After the importance of physical preparation, the rest is all down to mental strength. In fact, the mind can be the strength when the body wants to give in physically. It has to be remembered that trained Commandos are just humans in a military organisation; they too have been that man on a PRMC or POC. Additionally you must remember, if you are finding it hard, that the culture and style of instruction is very different from those of school, college or family life – and in the opinion of most Royal Marines it is also far better once you get used to it. Royal Marine training is nothing to be anxious about. All of the instructors on the training teams *want* you to succeed.

### Success at PRMC or POC

Success at POC is slightly different to success at PRMC. For the Young Officers, there is now only one intake a year (in September), and there are only between 50 and 60 places, depending on the needs of the Corps at the time. However, success at POC does not mean an automatic entry into the next batch. Following a successful POC all applicants must attend the AIB (Admiralty Interview Board). This is a set of tests and interviews, taken by all officer applicants to the Navy to see if they have the necessary skills required of officers. As with the POC, at the end of the three-day AIB the attendee is told if he is successful or unsuccessful. If successful, again this does not guarantee a place in YO training. If you imagine that 200 young men were successful at POC and AIB, but only 56 places exist, then only the top 56 would be able to join the Royal Marines YO batch for that year. Basically the top 56, using combined scores from POC and AIB, would be loaded on to the course.

For PRMC candidates, all the scores for fitness tests, interviews and medicals are added together, and at the end of the course all candidates are told if they have passed or failed. If they have failed, they will be given an indication of why, and how to better themselves. They will also be given a time frame in which to do so prior to coming back; for example, some people may be told 12 months, others six, and for some minor failures only three months.

A similar system may be in place for those that pass, depending on the need for numbers. Let me explain. All successful candidates will be given a level of pass, ie high pass, low pass or pass. This will then relate to how long it will be before they will join a Recruit Troop. At times when Recruiting figures are low, a successful candidate with any form of pass could find himself in a Troop within four weeks. At other times when Recruiting figures are up, it may only be the strong passes that are loaded inside three months, and the weaker passes may have to wait 6–12 months. There have also been occasions – although not since the late '80s and early '90s – where numbers were so good that only those with a strong (or 'superior', as it is called) pass got into a Troop, and we could pick and choose exactly who we wanted.

The Recruitment figures are always changing, and so is the manning state of the Royal Marines, so the best approach is to train as hard as you can, prepare as best you can, and do your very best at the PRMC. If you do all that, you will be successful.

## Working heart rate calculations

### Estimated working heart rate equation

Our maximum heart rate decreases with age; consequently we need the following crude but usable equation to estimate our maximum, and therefore working, heart rates. The equation provides our EMHR (estimated maximum heart rate), and this can then be multiplied by the required percentage to estimate the WHR (working heart rate). NB: This method is not individualistic and is therefore not very accurate.

Males    220 minus age (in years) x % = WHR
Females  226 minus age (in years) x % = WHR

### Karvonen working heart rate equation

This is an alternative calculation that should be far more accurate. To use it, a measured maximal heart rate (MMHR) is first required, which can be obtained from an exercise stress test. To perform this test, after warming up thoroughly a best effort one-mile run is performed. However, the last half to quarter of a mile should be to absolutely maximum effort. The time and heart rate should be noted during the last ten seconds and at the finish.

This test can be performed on a bike or in the pool, either a five-minute best effort cycle, all out over the last 30 seconds, or a best effort 400m swim, of which the last 150m is performed as fast as possible.

Next, the measured resting heart rate (MRHR) is obtained. Immediately on waking from a good nights' sleep, the pulse should be taken. This should be done on three consecutive mornings and an average taken. Some people find that a full bladder leads to a higher heart rate, so it may be necessary to empty the bladder and then return to bed for a few minutes before taking the pulse.

Next it is necessary to determine your heart rate reserve (HRR). To find this, it is necessary to subtract the measured resting heart rate from the measured maximum heart rate, ie MMHR minus MRHR = HRR. However, it is also possible to find your HRR by taking the measured resting heart rate from the estimated maximum heart rate, ie EMHR minus MRHR = HRR.

Once the HRR has been calculated it is possible to work out some very accurate working heart rates. To do this, multiply the heart rate reserve by the percentage wanted and then add the measured resting heart rate. This will give the working heart rate, ie (HRR x %) plus MRHR = WHR. For example, a 40-year-old male starts an endurance programme, working at 60% MHR:

EMHR     220 minus 40 = 180bpm
MRHR     = 70bpm
HRR      180 minus 70 = 110bpm
WHR      110 x 60% = 66 plus 70 = 136bpm

Where possible, use this equation to get the accuracy you need for your training. Remember, attention to detail, effort and dedication will help your goals become a reality.

## Examples of plyometric training

The most important part of any plyometric session is the warm-up. Following this, it is best to start slow and build up. This will allow your muscles to adjust, avoid injuries (such as jumper's knee/patella tendinitis), and make your gains progressive and therefore longer lasting. At first pick three or maybe four different plyometric exercises and do three sets of six repetitions of each. Next increase this to three sets of eight repetitions, and then three sets of ten repetitions. Then up the repetitions to twelve, or add another set of ten, or add another exercise. If you are looking at improving a specific aspect, say your vertical jump height, measure it prior to starting your plyometric training programme. Then after a set time – say six or eight weeks – do the same vertical jump again. You should see an improvement.

### Jump to higher level
- Find a higher level or a sturdy box about 1ft to 3ft high.
- Stand in front of the box or higher level and jump up two-footed.
- Land softly on two feet.
- Step back down (do not jump) and repeat.

### Lateral jump to higher level
- Same as above but start next to box/higher level facing either left or right side on to it (not facing it). Jump up and to the side and land on box.
- Step down and repeat.

- Ensure you train both sides equally.

### Multiple two-footed low hurdle jumps/bounds
- Set out some low hurdles, cones, or even six to eight markers (jumpers or whatever) in a row, with about a foot between each.
- Jump two-footed between each from one end to the other.
- Repeat.

### One-legged same leg bounds
- As above but one-footed.

### One-legged alternate leg bounds
- As above, but switch legs between each hurdle. So take off right-footed, land left-footed, take off left-footed, land right-footed, etc.

### Lateral two-footed hurdle bounds
- As above, but stand two-footed side-on and bound sideways on both feet.
- Repeat.
- Try not to pause between hurdles.

### Two-footed bounds up slope
- Same as two-footed low hurdle bounds, but this time performed up a relatively steep slope.
- Start on slight slope and increase angle over time.

### Multiple two-footed high hurdle jumps/bounds
- Set out six to eight hurdles, boxes or something else about one to two feet high. Place them about a foot apart.
- Start two-footed at one end and jump two-footed over each.
  NB: If you need to pause between each hurdle until you are competent then do so.
- Repeat.

### Drop/depth jumping
- Stand on either a sturdy box or a higher level.
- Start off at 1ft height and increase over time.
- Drop (don't jump) off the box or higher ground. Absorb the impact but jump up in the air as soon as you hit the ground.
- Land safely back on the ground.
- Step back up on to the box and repeat.

### Drop jumping over a hurdle
- As above, but instead of dropping off and jumping up into the air, drop off and jump

over a hurdle or a second box.

## Two-footed long jumps

- Also called a precision jump.
- Start on a marked spot and try to jump as far horizontally as possible, but under control.
- Mark your landing point.
- Repeat and try to beat or at least match your first jump.

## One-footed hop long jump

- As above, but one-footed take-off, two-footed landing.
- Repeat.

## Two-footed on the spot tuck jumps

- Stand upright on an open piece of ground.
- Jump straight up into the air, as high as possible, bringing your knees up to your chest.
- Land on the balls of the feet and repeat immediately.
- Try to reduce ground contact time by landing softly on your feet and springing back into the air straight away.

## One-footed on the spot tuck jumps

- As above, but on one foot. Make sure you exercise both legs.

## One-footed lateral jumps

- As above, but instead of jumping straight up jump from side to side, from your start point to one side, then back to your start point.
- Exercise both legs equally.

## Lunge jumps

- Start in an open piece of ground. Stand with one leg around 2ft further back than the other, standing on the ball of the hind foot.
- Keep your head up and back straight.
- Lunge into the exercise, by bending at the right hip and knee until your thigh is parallel to the floor, and then immediately explode vertically up in the air.
- Switch feet in the air so that the back foot lands forward and front foot lands backward in a mirror image of the start position. Land softly.
- Repeat equally for both sides.

## Lateral push-ups

- Start side-on to a box or higher platform with your nearer foot on top of the box and your further foot on the floor.
- Use the foot on the box to drive up and jump vertically as high as possible.
- Land on the opposite side of the box, with the other foot on top of it and the foot previously on the box now on the floor.
- Repeat to come back to your original position.
- Exercise both sides equally.

## Two-footed jumps up steps

- Find a set of steps.
- Start at the bottom, feet together.
- Jump up the steps, keeping your feet together.
- When you reach the top, turn round, run to the bottom and repeat.

## Multiple jumps after run in

- Sprint from one marked point to another marked point between 3m and 10m away.
- When you hit the second point, take off two-footed to jump vertically and horizontally.
- Perform three jumps like this, taking care to land safely each time.
- Stop, walk back and repeat.

## Zigzag bounds

- Find a convenient straight line (such as the white lines in a car park or at the side of playing field).
- Start on one side at one end with your feet together.
- Bound forward at an angle to cross over to the opposite side of the line.
- Land and immediately bound forward again, crossing back to the original side of the line.
- Repeat all the way along the length of the line.
- Turn around and repeat back to your starting point.

## Training Programmes

### General Training Prg 1

| Day | Session |
| --- | --- |
| Monday | All over body strength (weights) sessions |
| Tuesday | Continuous CV session |
| Wednesday | Rest day |
| Thursday | All over body strength (weights) session |
| Friday | Interval session |
| Saturday | Rest day |
| Sunday | Flexibility (stretching session) |

### General Training Prg 2

| Day | Session |
| --- | --- |
| Monday | All over body strength (weights) session |
| Tuesday | Rest day |
| Wednesday | Continuous CV Hard |
| Thursday | Rest day |
| Friday | All over body strength (weights) session |
| Saturday | Rest day |
| Sunday | Continuous CV Easy |

### Strength Specific Prg 1

| Day | Session |
| --- | --- |
| Monday | Chest and Triceps |
| Tuesday | Rest/CV light |
| Wednesday | Shoulders and Legs |
| Thursday | Rest/CV light |
| Friday | Back and Biceps |
| Saturday | Continuous CV and Abs |
| Sunday | Rest |

### Strength Specific Prg 2

| Day | Session |
| --- | --- |
| Monday | Chest, Back, Shoulders |
| Tuesday | Legs, Biceps, Triceps |
| Wednesday | Rest/CV light |
| Thursday | Chest, Back, Shoulders |
| Friday | Legs, Biceps, Triceps |
| Saturday | Continuous CV and Abs |
| Sunday | Rest |

In the exercises chapter there are many variations of exercises for the same body part. It is not necessary to perform every single exercise when training an area. Pick two or three exercises per bodypart, use these for 4–12 weeks for your programme, then put a new programme together and change some/all of your chosen exercises.

### Long Distance Running Specific Prg

| Day | Session |
| --- | --- |
| Monday | Short moderate Intensity |
| Tuesday | Rest/Flexibility |
| Wednesday | Intervals High Intensity |
| Thursday | Rest/Strength training |
| Friday | Short high intensity |
| Saturday | Rest |
| Sunday | Long continuous low intensity |

### Sport Specific Prg

| Day | Session |
| --- | --- |
| Monday | Technique/Skill training |
| Tuesday | Plyometric/Strength training |
| Wednesday | Rest |
| Thursday | Technique/Skill training |
| Friday | Rest |
| Saturday | Match/Competition |
| Sunday | Rest/Flexibility/Light CV |

These are just examples. Many programmes could include morning sessions and lunchtime/ evening sessions. Strength or CV training could be substituted for circuit training depending on the aim of the individual and the type of circuit on offer. Again, it is important you put together a programme that will suit you and your gains, just as each Royal Marine will do until a PTI has to get him ready for a specific role or Operation.

# APPENDIX 3
# GLOSSARY

| | |
|---|---|
| AIB | Admiralty Interview Board. |
| AMF | Advanced Military Fitness. |
| ATP | adenosine tri-phosphate. |
| Bergen | standard Royal Marines/British Military rucksack. |
| BFT | Basic Fitness Test. |
| bpm | beats per minute. |
| BPT | Battle Physical Training. |
| BST | Battle Swim Test. |
| CDT | compulsory drug testing. |
| CQC | Close Quarter Combat. |
| CS95 | Combat Soldier 95, UK forces camouflage uniform. |
| CTCRM | Commando Training Centre Royal Marines. |
| CV | cardiovascular. |
| DEs | daily exercises. |
| Dit | Royal Marines argot for a story. |

| | |
|---|---|
| DOMS | delayed onset muscle soreness. |
| FITT | mnemonic for training overload principles: frequency, intensity, time, type. |
| 5BX | 'five basic exercises'. |
| HRM | heart rate monitor. |
| IMF | Initial Military Fitness. |
| IMFC | Initial Military Fitness Circuit. |
| IMFS | Initial Military Fitness Strength. |
| Kipping | gyrating the body. |
| MHR | maximum heart rate. |
| ML | Mountain Leader. |
| 1RM | one repetition maximum. |
| POC | Potential Officers Course. |
| PRMC | Potential Royal Marines Course. |
| PT | Physical Training. |
| PTI | Physical Training Instructor. |
| Regain | technique for righting yourself while crossing a horizontal rope. |

| | |
|---|---|
| Rep | repetition. |
| RM | Royal Marines. |
| RMFA | Royal Marines Fitness Assessment. |
| SAID | 'specific adaptations to imposed demands'. |
| SBS | Special Boat Service. |
| Set | a number of exercises performed one after another. |
| SMART | mnemonic for setting training goals: specific, measurable, achievable, realistic, timed. |
| SPORT | mnemonic for designing a training programme: specificity, progression, overload, reversibility, tedium. |
| VO2 max | volume of oxygen used during maximal exercise. |
| YO | Young Officer. |
| Yomping | walking carrying full kit on the back. |

# APPENDIX 4
# THE AUTHOR

Sean Lerwill was born in South-East England, but moved with his mother to the South-West at an early age, where he was raised and educated. He attended Wellington School, Somerset, where he succeeded in both academic subjects and sports. He represented the county at a number of sports and was a school captain and house captain in his final year. He was awarded an army scholarship prior to his 16th birthday to support him in his A-level studies at Wellington.

Sean is a graduate of King's College London, with a BSc (Hons) in molecular genetics. While studying at university he attended and passed his POC and AIB to join the Royal Marines. His success at both meant he was awarded a Bursary, which not only secured a place for him in Royal Marines Young Officer training, but also helped with meeting the cost of his university education.

After joining the Royal Marines Sean served in various Royal Marines Units around the country, as well as taking part in numerous exercises and Operations across the globe. He specialised in the Physical Training Branch of the Royal Marines at the earliest opportunity, and after joining the PT Branch gained numerous qualifications in the fitness, teaching and coaching industries, including a post-graduate Certificate of Education from the University of Plymouth.

Having left the Royal Marines in Autumn 2009, Sean now co-owns a physical training company with another Ex-Royal Marines PTI.

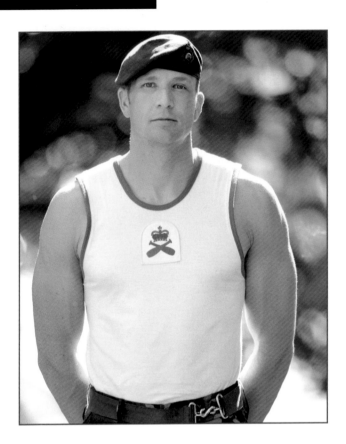

## Author's Acknowledgements

I would like to thank everyone involved in helping me to make this book a reality, in particular: Dave 'Tweety' Silvester, Phil 'Simo' Simister, Rob 'Beau' Beauchamp, Paul Curry and Andy Garland. I would also like to thank, 'Delicious' Dave Hartley, Paul 'Nobby' Clarke, Mark 'Reidy' Reid, Warren 'Essence' Keays-Smith, Justin 'Kirbs' Kirby and Tony Hands, without who I would know next to nothing. Thanks go in addition to Jonathan Falconer and Louise McIntyre for putting the pieces together, and to a truly 'Bootneck' Navy Commando, Andy Cheal, for spotting my mistakes. Thanks to my mother Gill for giving me the opportunities to be where I am today to write this book, and last but by no means least thanks to Nicola, not just for putting up with me in general but for all your help and input. I couldn't have done it without you. Above all I would like to thank all Royal Marine Commandos for giving me something to write about.

# INDEX